THE MIGRAINE REVOLUTION:

"WE CAN END THE TYRANNY!"

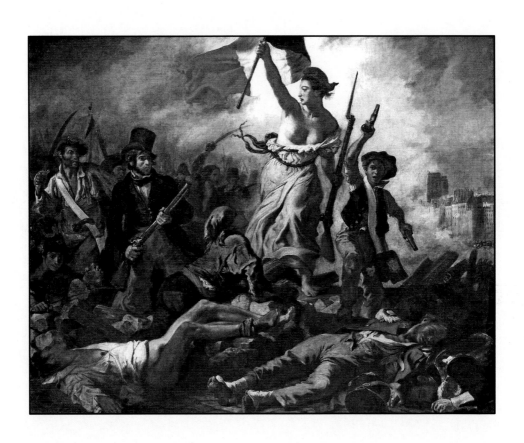

Martin Brink

THE MIGRAINE REVOLUTION:

"WE CAN END THE TYRANNY!"

Scientific Guide to Effective Treatment
and Permanent Headache Relief

**(WHAT THE CURRENT REGIME DOES
NOT WANT YOUR BRAIN TO KNOW)**

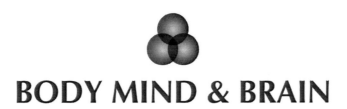

BODY MIND & BRAIN

Copyright © 2012 by Martin Brink

All rights reserved. No portion of this book may be reproduced — mechanically, electronically or by any other means including photocopying, reciting off by heart, singing, whistling or miming — without written permission of the publisher.

First Edition 2012

ISBN-10: 0-9873471-2-8 (Monochrome Edition)

ISBN-13: 978-0-9873471-2-1 (Monochrome Edition)

Publisher:

BODY MIND & BRAIN
69 Cheltenham Drive
Robina, QLD 4226
Queensland / Australia
Phone: +61 7 5593 3955
Fax: +61 7 5593 1928
e-mail: info@BodyMindAndBrain.com.au
website: www.BodyMindAndBrain.com.au

Please visit the book's website:
www.TheMigraineRevolution.com

Legal Disclaimer:

This book is intended as an informational guide. It is sold with the understanding that neither author nor publisher nor any other person involved are hereby rendering medical, health or any other kind of personal professional service to the individual reader. It is the reader's own responsibility to consult with competent health care professionals or doctors, whenever so indicated. The author, the editor, the graphic artist, the publisher, the printing service, the bookseller, the blokes involved in dispatch and shipping, the postman or delivery guy or anybody else cannot be held resposible for any liability, loss or risk, personal or otherwise, which is incurred as a consequence, directly or indirectly, of the use of any of the contents of this book. In other words: If you follow the book's advice and all goes well, it's your own fault!

Dedication

This book is dedicated to all those fed up migraine sufferers who have been waiting for this book; to the despairing ones who will feel encouraged to take their destiny into their own hands; and to the determined ones who can recognize this as their opportunity to finally end their migraine tyranny.

In order to make future editions even more better, I'm asking for your kind help. Please fill out the Reader's Feedback form on the book's website www.TheMigraineRevolution.com. Also, join TheMigraineRevolution yahoo group to share your experiences and benefit from the support of a rebellious community.

Acknowledgements

I'd like to take this opportunity to express my gratitude to all who've contributed to this book in one way or another. Names that spring to mind are (in alphabetical order):

- Ann Marie Brown, Mental Health Counsellor and Neurotherapist
- Dr. Gil Winkelman (ND, MA) Naturopathic Doctor, Neurotherapist, Counsellor
- Dr. Jeffrey Carmen (PhD) Psychologist, Inventor and Biofeedback Therapist
- Dr. Lucas Korbeda (MD, PhD) Neurologist and Assistant Professor of Neurology
- Dr. Richard Soutar (PhD) Psychologist and Neurotherapist
- Dr. Sharrie Hanley (ND) Naturopathic Doctor and Neurotherapist
- Dr. Siegfried Othmer (PhD) Physicist and Chief Scientist EEG Institute
- Susan Othmer (BA) Neurobiologist and Clinical Director EEG Institute

This book wouldn't have been possible without the work of countless researchers in the fields of medicine, pharmacology, genetics, physiology, psychology and neuroscience; and it wouldn't be the same without the many marvellous painters whose timeless works of art I've snatched from past centuries and incorporated.

A big thanks to the German company Brain Products who donated one of their top notch EEG signal acquisition systems. I'm deeply indebted to my publisher, editor and graphic artist ☺, but my most special thanks goes to my wonderful wife, who forced me to write this book and looked after everything else: Gosh, I love you.

"But what we call our despair is often only the painful eagerness of unfed hope."

George Eliot

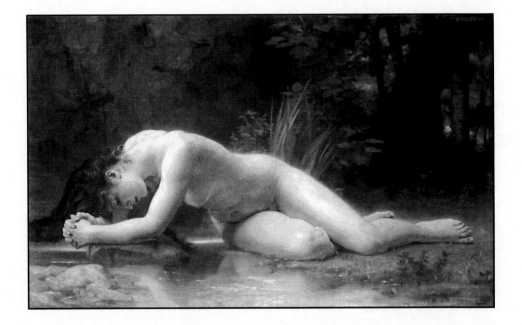

Table of Contents

Warning	This Book is Not for Everyone!	9
Foreword	Are You Ready for the Migraine Revolution?	11
Introduction	The Tyranny: Suffering from Migraine	13

Part I: The Current Regime 15

Chapter 1	The Many Faces of Migraine	17
Chapter 2	The Impact and Burden of Migraine	29
Chapter 3	Medical Treatments for Migraine Symptoms	37
Chapter 4	Avoid Life and You'll be Right	65
Chapter 5	Psycho Terror in Migraine Land	83

Part II: Preparing for Battle 119

Chapter 6	Dealing with Difficulties	121
Chapter 7	On Top of the Barricades	135
Chapter 8	Know Your Tyrant	171
Chapter 9	Thinking about Strategy	203

Part III: Weapons for the Revolution 213

Chapter 10	Choose Your Weapons!	215

Section One: Weapons for the Body 221

Chapter 11	Let's get Physical	223
Chapter 12	Passing Gas	227
Chapter 13	Making a Difference	231
Chapter 14	Thought for Food	235
Chapter 15	Doping for Migraine	243
Chapter 16	Being Watched by Angels	263

Table of Contents

Chapter 17	Balancing Your Urges	269
Chapter 18	Points of Pain	281
Chapter 19	Pricks with Benefits	285
Chapter 20	Pandora's Chest of Treasures	289

Section Two: Weapons for the Mind 297

Chapter 21	Reflecting your Thoughts	299
Chapter 22	Escaping your Traps	305
Chapter 23	Healing Shocks	309
Chapter 24	Feeling Heavy and Warm	315
Chapter 25	When the Mind Sees what the Body Does	317

Section Three: Weapons for the Brain 345

Chapter 26	Show Me Some Warmth!	363
Chapter 27	Listening Through the Wall	369
Chapter 28	Wiping Migraine Off the Map	375
Chapter 29	Recipes for the Brain	383
Chapter 30	On the Crest of Slow Waves	387
Chapter 31	Overpowering the Migraine Beast	395
Chapter 32	The Magic of a Whisper	403
Chapter 33	The Side Effects of Change	413
Chapter 34	Guide to Victory	425

Section Four: Join the Migraine Revolution! 443

Cast of Characters	448
List of Paintings	450
Picture Credits	452
Index	458

Warning

This Book is Not for Everyone!

> "There is always a well-known solution to every human problem –
> neat, plausible, and wrong."
>
> H. L. Mencken

3 steps to beat an incurable disease?

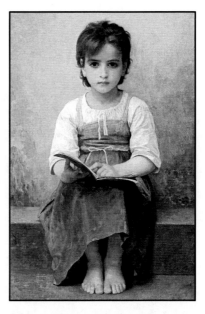

If you or a loved one suffer from severe migraine attacks and you are looking for a booklet about the "*Easy 3-Step-Breakthrough-Self-Help-Program*", which gives you a neat and plausible explanation for *headaches*, lists some catchy instructions as to which foods to avoid and promises to solve your entire *headache*-problem in one fell swoop, then this is not the right book for you. Whilst head pain is a common symptom during attacks, migraine is not "*just a headache*", at least not for us. Good news, booklets like that do exist!

Severe migraine is a serious problem that needs a savvy approach to make matters better, not worse. This is a sincere book that offers the interested reader a comprehensive, comprehensible, constructive, helpful and occasionally humorous, science-based *migraine education*. It thereby empowers the fed up sufferer with the deep understanding necessary to end the migraine tyranny.

Prerequisites are the ability to *read* and *understand* sentences with more than three words, a minimal amount of *healthy common sense* and openness to the possibility that positive statements might sometimes actually be true. The Dark Lords from the cult of hopelessness, who love dismissing anything that is different from their attitude of doom and gloom, will not enjoy this book.

If you firmly hold and cherish the unshakable conviction that **"MIGRAINE IS A GENETIC NEUROLOGICAL DISEASE THAT CAN'T BE CURED"**, then you may find this book very disconcerting and I advise against reading it.

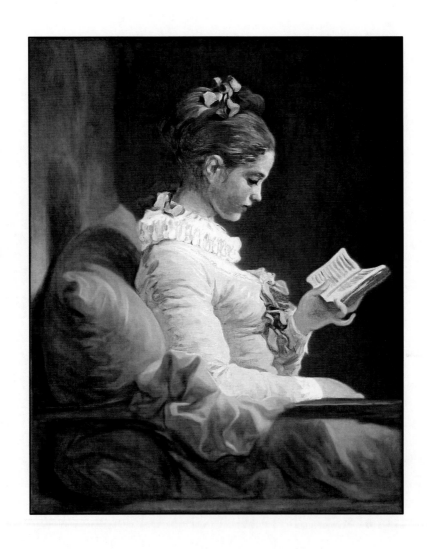

Foreword

Are You Ready for the Migraine Revolution?

> "Enlighten the people generally,
> and tyranny and oppressions of body and mind will vanish
> like evil spirits at the dawn of day."
>
> Thomas Jefferson

What's the best way to deal with a bomb in the house?

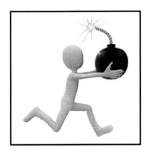

A) Get rid of the bomb!
B) Use a fire extinguisher once the bomb goes off and starts a decent fire.

If you have your answer, what would a sales rep for fire-extinguishers say?

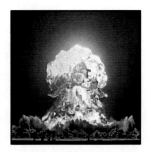

Migraine attacks are a bit like explosions in the head. So it is no surprise that the sales reps from the medical industry do their very best to make sufferers believe that 'fire-extinguishers' (= meds for the 'attack-explosion') are the best available solution.

In order to get away with this obvious nonsense, the pharma-medical propaganda-machine has caught millions of migraineurs in a trap, made of lies and misleading misinformation. For example, they speak of the attack symptom 'head pain' as "*migraines*" to imply that migraine is *just a bad headache* and you're best off with medication. Not a bad solution for very rare "*migraines*"; just like fire-extinguishers are quite okay for infrequent explosions.

Yet, three quarters of migraineurs have at least one 'explosion' per month, 15% have more than one attack per week and are helplessly caught in the propaganda-trap of the current regime:

"MIGRAINE IS AN INCURABLE GENETIC HEADACHE-DISEASE CAUSED BY SWELLING AND INFLAMMATION OF BLOOD VESSELS AROUND YOUR HEAD"

In other words: **"THERE IS NOTHING THAT YOU CAN DO ABOUT THE EXPLOSIONS IN YOUR HEAD OTHER THAN BUYING PLENTY OF FIRE-EXTINGUISHERS."**

Isn't that pretty much exactly what we would expect from the sales reps for fire-extinguishers? We'd say the same in their shoes.

As a result three quarters of migraineurs worry that they'll have to put up with "MIGRAINE DISEASE" and its consequences for the rest of their lives.[1] From a sufferer's perspective, three aspects make this grim prognosis unbearable:[2]

- *"Being besieged by the attacks"* describes the experience of vulnerability, incapacitation and loss of control of one's life as well as the embarrassment and sadness about the isolation from others.
- *"Struggling in a life characterized by uncertainty"* refers to having to live in a state of constant alertness and readiness as well as dissatisfaction with and worry about medication.
- *"Living with an invisible illness"* expresses the fear of not being believed, of not being recognized as truly suffering, of exaggerating a mere headache as well as feelings of shame and guilt.

The intention of this book is to give migraineurs and their families, but also interested doctors and therapists, a very thorough and goal-oriented *migraine education*: The complete and current, science-based knowledge to gain the deep understanding necessary to pursue answer A ("Get rid of the bomb!") enabling the reader to eventually end the migraine tyranny.

However, knowing how much hurt, disappointment and frustration most long-term migraineurs have experienced, I find it crucial to emphasize that this is *not* a catalogue of *miracle cures for everyone*. Attentive and diligent 'students' will benefit tremendously and find their way out, others will complain that three chapters into the book they still have "migraines": "IT DIDN'T DO MUCH TO ME."

I very strongly recommend reading this book from front to back and rather skim-read boring bits than jumping back and forth. Later chapters build upon the info and insights from earlier parts, not dissimilar to a *self-study course* with lessons (but more fun!).

Despite the many scientific references, the style is mostly conversational and deliberately colloquial. This book is also very *international*: written in Australia with German precision in American spelling and British-inspired, anarchic punctuation on an iMac built in China. Have fun and make the most of it!

Martin Brink, Queensland

---

[1] Harris Interactive online poll, cited in Brandes JL "The Migraine Cycle: Patient Burden of Migraine During and Between Migraine Attacks" Headache 2008;48:430-441

[2] Rutberg S et al "Migraine--more than a headache: women's experiences of living with migraine" Disabil Rehabil 2012;34(4):329-36

Introduction

The Tyranny: Suffering from Migraine

> "No greater burden can be borne by an individual than to know:
> no one cares or understands."
>
> Arthur H. Stainback

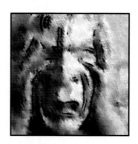

Migraine is a cruel tyrant. The people under his volatile rule periodically experience excruciating head pain (agony) in combination with dreadful nausea (misery) and extreme revulsion at the relentless persecution and invasion by the outer world in the form of glare, noise and odor (assault).[1]

It's this unique combination of agony *and* misery *and* assault that rattles the self, the core of one's being, the innermost center of spirit and soul, creating a sense of torture and defeat. And so migraineurs withdraw from life during an attack and hide in a quiet dark room, like a wounded animal in a cave.

Between the torturous episodes, patients are shaken by the latest attack and tormented by the primal fear of the next ride to hell.[2] They feel vulnerable and abandoned for not getting the protection they beg for. This lack of care makes them feel undeserving and unworthy.[3]

On top of that they struggle with shame and guilt, for being a disappointment to their children, for being a burden to their partner and for being unreliable and unproductive at work. In essence, they feel like a failed version of the person they want to be and could have been.[4]

---

[1] Rutberg S et al "Migraine – more than a headache: Women's experiences of living with migraine" Disabil Rehabil 2012;34(4):329–336
[2] Freitag FG "The cycle of migraine: patients' quality of life during and between migraine attacks" Clin Ther 2007;29(5):939-49
[3] Leiper et al. 'Experiences and perceptions of people with headache: a qualitative study' BMC Fam Pract 2006; 7:27
[4] Cottrell et al. 'Perceptions and Needs of Patients with Migraine: A Focus Study Group' J Fam Pract 2002; 51(2): 142-147

And then there is the intolerable horror of feeling not understood, of being a nuisance, a spoilsport, a party pooper, a drama queen, a nutcase with hysteria or a whining malingerer; partly unwanted and somehow outcast.[1]

But the really sour icing on this bitter cake, adding insult to injury, is the hurt and humiliation caused by words that pierce the heart like a dagger, fuel resentment and fury and add something extra to the already callous burden.

It's the merciless abuse by dismissive words like:
"You're exaggerating. It's just a headache. You'll have to live with it."

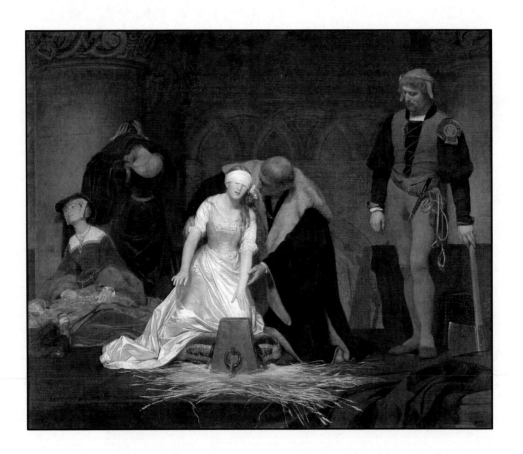

---

[1] Rutberg S et al "Migraine – more than a headache: Women's experiences of living with migraine" Disabil Rehabil 2012;34(4):329–336

Part I:

The Current Regime

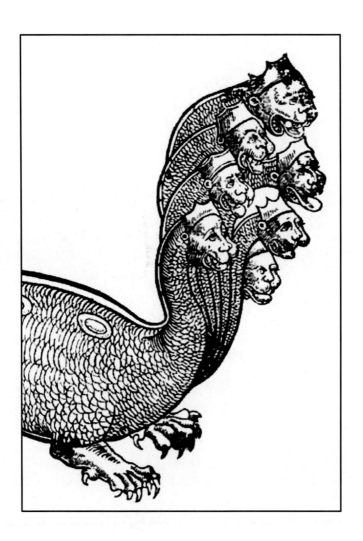

Chapter 1

The Many Faces of Migraine

"Suffering is one very long moment. We cannot divide it by seasons."
Oscar Wilde

Patients typically experience two distinct phases of migraine: the *suffering during* the attacks and the *worrying between* the attacks. Considering the unpredictable timing of the onslaughts and the varying vulnerability to normally benign components of life—like sleep, meals, weather and moderate stress—who wouldn't worry about the question: "When will the next one strike?"

Nevertheless, clinical descriptions of migraine typically refer to *the attack only*, which can be divided into four phases, similar to those of epileptic seizures. As is the case in epilepsy, not all patients experience a *complete attack* with all four phases (or five, if you count the unease of the interval).

The premonitory phase or prodrome

About 60% of migraineurs display some of the suspicious clues of an oncoming attack:

- Changes in *mood*: irritability, depression or euphoria
- *Cognitive* changes: slow thinking, difficulty concentrating
- *Speech*: reduced fluency, low motivation to talk
- Impaired *self-control*: restlessness, hyperactivity, impulsivity
- Reduced *alertness*: tiredness, fatigue, drowsiness
- Changes in *appetite*: food cravings (esp. sweets and other carbs), increased or decreased appetite
- *Water* balance: thirst and/or polyuria (= peeing a lot)
- *Digestion*: constipation or diarrhea
- Body *temperature*: feeling chilly or hot, clammy or sweaty
- Muscle *coordination*: stiffness (esp. stiff neck), clumsiness
- Aches and *pains*: neck pain, shoulder pain, back pain
- *Sensory* system: photophobia, phonophobia, osmophobia (= intolerance of light, sound or smell)

Feeling tired (72%), difficulty concentrating (51%) and stiff neck (50%) are the most common prodromal symptoms.

Most migraineurs recognize prodromal symptoms and so correctly *predict* the imminent attack. Some can even *feel* the attack coming, whereas others don't notice anything until other people tell them that they're different.

The range of strange alterations of brain function is reminiscent of a stroke or a sprawling brain tumor, presenting like a transitory selection from an encyclopedia of neurology.[1] Quite peculiar is that some symptoms can even show opposite expressions, e.g. euphoria or depression, diarrhea or constipation, unrest or fatigue. It is *characteristic* of migraine that the symptoms not only occur in puzzling diversity, but also vary greatly between patients and between individual attacks in quality, intensity and duration.

The aura phase

Only about one third of migraineurs experience an aura, typically on the last stretch before the headache phase. Of those patients some have an aura sometimes, very few have one with every attack. The symptoms tend to develop slowly over 5 to 20 minutes and last up to an hour.

- Visual aura is the most common form and consists either of *visual hallucinations* (e.g. bright dots, zigzag lines, flashes, oscillating patterns and so forth) or of *disturbances of the visual field itself* (e.g. blurred or tunnel vision, blind spots, holes and the like). One or both sides may be affected.
- Somatosensory aura refers to the perception of *tingling* or *numbness*, typically beginning in one hand or in the face.
- Motor aura means *weakness* or *paralysis* of muscles.
- Olfactory aura is the term for the illusion of *smelling* scents and odors that aren't actually there.
- Auditory aura is *hallucinations* of various *sounds* or noise.
- Speech can be affected big time and that includes difficulty *finding* and *saying* words as well as language *comprehension*.

More common in children than in adults is the *Alice-in-Wonderland* syndrome, which describes curious distortions of one's own body image, sense of space and time, and of all other sensory channels (= senses: vision, hearing …).

---
[1] Sacks OW "Migraine" First Vintage Books Edition 1999 New York, page xvii

The headache phase

The gradual onset of the headache marks the beginning of the most dreaded part of an attack for most sufferers.

- 85% get hammered by a throbbing head pain of moderate to very severe intensity which usually gets worse with movement and activity, in 60% it's the typical unilateral (one-sided) pain, 25% have it on both sides of the head (bilateral), untypical, yet common
- 80% can't stand bright light (photophobia)
- 70-90% feel extra-miserable due to nausea
- 30% enjoy the ambiguous pleasure of vomiting, some have diarrhea

Other common symptoms are dizziness, phonophobia (= noise intolerance), osmophobia (= odor intolerance), stuffed or runny nose, teary eyes, allodynia (= even light touch is painful), chills and hot flashes, dehydration or fluid retention, mental confusion and any form of emotional turmoil up to panic attacks.

Another symptom is very common, but rarely mentioned as such: the *social withdrawal* and wish to be alone, which is partly understandable, given the presenting symptoms, but still not fully explained. One could still wish for silent company in the quiet, dark room; but migraineurs typically seek solitude.

The headache phase lasts from a few hours up to three days. After that it's called *status migrainosus* (= migraine state) and warrants hospital admission.

Interestingly, headache does *not* occur in 15% of attacks. So, considering the numbers, you could also call it the *nausea phase*.

The postdrome

Most migraineurs experience a decent 'hangover' after the headache is gone and this may last for days.

- Energy: feeling tired, washed-out and lethargic
- Mood: depression, irritability
- Cognition: impaired concentration and comprehension
- Pain: scalp tenderness, feeling sore

There are suspicions that these so-called postdromal symptoms are not true attack symptoms, but indeed a hangover and mainly caused by migraine medication.

Interesting to note that, once nausea and headache are gone, some migraineurs feel ...

- refreshed, renewed, alert, even euphoric. This condition of miraculous recovery may well be the natural state after or even the purpose of a migraine attack.[1]

The interictal phase

'Ictus' is the medical term for attack and is used for epileptic seizures and migraine attacks; so the 'interictal phase' or 'interictum' is simply the period *between* attacks.

Many people — including many doctors — erroneously believe that once the headache is gone, migraineurs are symptom-free. Unfortunately that is not the case. The majority of patients feel that they don't even recover from the attacks completely.[2]

Migraineurs usually experience more symptoms and greater emotional distress than non-migraineurs, as well as disturbed contentment, vitality and sleep in the interictal phase.[3]

One major factor of emotional distress for many is the worry about the next attack, which is an expression of the understandable *conscious fear* and apprehension.[4] Besides, it is reasonable to assume that every patient with recurrent nasty symptoms is also under *unconscious* distress due to the uncertainty of the next flare-up.[5]

Surprisingly many migraineurs negate vehemently being even the slightest bit emotionally distressed, which is in stark and obvious contrast to the emotional charge with which this denial is normally expressed:[6] **"I'M NOT DISTRESSED AT ALL!"**

This contradiction indicates that many migraineurs are deeply concerned that, if they admitted their emotional tension, they might get classified as a 'psychological' case with all its awkward implications. It is appalling that many people — including doctors — still equate 'psychological' with 'not real' or 'fake' or even 'nuts'.

---

[1] Sacks OW "Migraine" First Vintage Books Edition 1999 New York, page 8 and page 202
[2] Buse DC "Assessing and Managing All Aspects of Migraine: Migraine Attacks, Migraine-Related Functional Impairment, Common Comorbidities, and Quality of Life" Mayo Clin Proc 2009;84(5):422-435
[3] Dahlöf CG et al. "Migraine patients experience poorer subjective well-being/quality of life even between attacks" Cephalalgia 1995;15:31-36
[4] "New survey reveals worrying between attacks can extend suffering for migraineurs" (press release) Titusville, NJ: Ortho-McNeill; June 8, 2006
[5] Brosschot JF "Daily worry is related to low heart rate variability during waking and the subsequent nocturnal sleep period" Int J Psychophysiol. 2007;63(1):39-47
[6] Cottrell et al. 'Perceptions and Needs of Patients with Migraine: A Focus Study Group' J Fam Pract 2002; 51(2): 142-147

Migraine and comorbidities

'Morbus' is the Latin word for ailment; 'co' means with, so a 'co-morbidity' is an *ailment that comes with*. There are quite a few ailments that tend to come with migraine, meaning that they occur *more frequently in migraineurs than in non-migraineurs*. That implies that migraine and the comorbidity are somehow related through a variety of possible mechanisms.[1]

One of those mechanisms is, that migraine can lead to the comorbid condition, as is the case for these:

| Tension-type Headache[2] | Medication Overuse Headache | Chronic Migraine |

Tension-type headache and migraine officially are separate diagnostic categories, but in reality rather form a continuous spectrum of symptoms including head pain.[3]

Another explanation why a condition is comorbid with migraine is, that both are 'brain-instabilities':[4]

Epilepsy[4]

Based on the similarity of electrical events in the brain, migraine attacks are also considered as 'non-epileptic seizures' and some forms of migraine have epilepsy-like characteristics.[5]

Epilepsy and migraine are often connected with too much 'excitement' in certain layers of brain cells.[6] And when the brain is too excited, the mind also gets revved up and we experience …

| Distress[7] | Insomnia[7, 8] |

---

[1] Scher AI et al "Comorbidity of migraine" Curr Opin Neurol 2005;18:305–310
[2] Russel MB "Genetics of tension-type headaches" J Headache Pain 2007; 8(2): 71–76
[3] Cady RK "The Convergence Hypothesis" Heache 2007;47 Suppl 1:544-551
[4] Bigal ME et al "Epilepsy and migraine" Epilepsy Behav. 2003;4 Suppl 2:S13-24.
[5] Carreño M "Recognition of Nonepileptic Events: Migraine" Semin Neurol. 2008;28(3):297-304
[6] Lipton RB et al. "Comorbidity of migraine: the connection between migraine and epilepsy" Neurology. 1994;44(10 Suppl 7):S28-32
[7] Sevillano-García MD et al "Comorbidity in the migraine: depression, anxiety, stress and insomnia" Rev Neurol. 2007;45(7):400-5
[8] Vgontzas A et al "Are sleep difficulties associated with migraine attributable to anxiety and depression?" Headache 2008;48(10):1451-9

Another mechanism linking migraine to a whole group of mood disorders is a common 'weakness' in a chief brain area, the prefrontal cortex (PFC), which I'll discuss later in this book. With a 'weak' PFC migraineurs have a higher statistical 'risk' (= chance) than non-migraineurs to also suffer from a mood disorder:

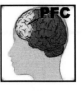

Major Depression: 3-fold risk[1]	Bipolar Disorder: 5-fold risk[2]	Panic Disorder: 4-fold risk[3]
General Anxiety Disorder: 5-fold risk[4]	Agoraphobia: 2.4-fold risk[5]	Social Phobia: 3.4-fold risk[5]

'Agora' is the Greek word for marketplace and agoraphobics were thought to be afraid of open spaces. Now we know that many patients with anxiety disorders avoid certain locations, where they fear they will have anxious or panicky feelings and this behavior of *experiential avoidance* is called agoraphobia.[6]

Now you might think: "Okay, I have migraine, but I don't have depression or panic disorder. So these statistical risks have nothing to do with me." That is a clever thought, but unfortunately what hasn't happened yet, can still happen:

new onset of depression 5.8-fold risk[7]	new onset of panic disorder 3.5-fold risk[8]

Migraineurs are not only at a higher statistical risk of *having* depression or panic disorder; they are also at a higher risk of *developing* depression or panic disorder during the course of their migraine odyssey.

---

[1] Breslau N et al "Migraine and major depression: a longitudinal study" Headache. 1994;34(7):387-93.
[2] Breslau N et al "Migraine, psychiatric disorders, and suicide attempts: an epidemiologic study of young adults" Psychiatry Res. 1991;37(1):11-23
[3] Breslau N et al "Headache types and panic disorder: directionality and specificity" Neurology. 2001;56(3):350-4
[4] McWilliams et al "Depression and anxiety associated with three pain conditions: results from a nationally representative sample" Pain 2004;111(1-2):77-83
[5] Merikangas KR "Migraine and psychopathology. Results of the Zurich cohort study of young adults" *Arch. Gen. Psychiatry* 1990;47: 849–853
[6] Wittchen HU et al "Agoraphobia and panic. Prospective-longitudinal relations suggest a rethinking of diagnostic concepts" Psychother Psychosom. 2008;77(3):147-57
[7] Breslau N et al "Comorbidity of migraine and depression: investigating potential etiology and prognosis" Neurology 2003;60(8):1308-12
[8] Breslau N et al "Headache types and panic disorder: directionality and specificity" Neurology 2001;56(3):350-4

Especially migraine and depression have a close relationship, each disorder increasing the likelihood of developing the other one. And if you think "Of course you get depressed with frequent headaches", think again: Patients with tension-type headaches do *not* have the same risk of developing depression as migraineurs.[1] This confirms that one of the underlying mechanisms of migraine is also involved in depression: a functional deficit in the prefrontal cortex (PFC), a crucial brain area behind the forehead. Who would have thought.

In the horrible state of major depression one might wish to "end it all", and in the absence of promising alternatives and driven by feelings of *hopelessness*, two sad steps can become tempting: contemplating suicide and actually doing it. Especially migraineurs with aura carry a higher risk of taking those two sad steps:

contemplating suicide 4.3-fold risk[2]	suicide attempt 3-fold risk[2]

Please note that these numbers are adjusted for depression, substance abuse and other psychiatric disorders that could explain the wish to die; this is the (statistical) effect of migraine only.

Sure, it is unpleasant to write and read about suicide, but we can't close our eyes to the fact that 23% of migraine kids with aura (13-15 years young) consider taking their own life.[3]

These shocking and awful figures should be sufficient evidence that the current treatment regime for migraine is completely unacceptable; it's simply not good enough; it's time for a migraine revolution.

Another option for adult migraineurs is to wait and see what destiny has in store. These are the odds:[4]

Migraine without aura Heart attack: 1.9-fold risk	Migraine with aura Heart attack: 2.9-fold risk

The medical term for heart attack is 'myocardial infarction': heart muscle cells die due to blocked coronary blood flow.

---

[1] Breslau N et al "Comorbidity of migraine and depression: investigating potential etiology and prognosis" Neurology 2003;60(8):1308-12
[2] Breslau N et al "Migraine, psychiatric disorders, and suicide attempts: an epidemiologic study of young adults" Psychiatry Res. 1991;37(1):11-23
[3] Wang SJ et al "Migraine and suicidal ideation in adolescents aged 13 to 15 years" Neurology. 2009;72(13):1146-52
[4] Bigal ME et al "Migraine and cardiovascular disease: a population-based study" Neurology. 2010;74(8):628-35

The well-known risk factors for cardiovascular diseases are also worse in migraineurs:[1]

Diabetes: 1.4-fold risk

High blood pressure: 1.4-fold risk

High cholesterol: 1.4-fold risk

Following the logic of cardiovascular risk factors, further trouble with perfusion has to be expected. What about the blood flow to the legs?

Claudication: 2.7-fold risk[1]

Claudication (= Latin for limping) is a disease of the peripheral arteries, a narrowing of the blood vessels, thereby restricting blood flow. Migraineurs have a 2.7 times higher risk *after* adjusting for other vascular factors. That's not good.

The brain also needs blood flow and, as expected, that is affected by migraine as well. Here are the numbers for migraineurs with aura:[2]

Stroke symptoms: 5.5-fold risk

TIA symptoms: 4.3-fold risk

verified stroke: 2.8-fold risk

TIA stands for 'transient ischemic attack', which is a temporary lack of oxygen in the brain; a precursor to a proper stroke.

Even without an ischemic stroke, migraine causes various forms of brain damage. Numerous studies in recent years have consistently found:

damage in the Gray Matter[3] (brain cell bodies)

damage in the White Matter[4] (cell connections)

damage and iron contamination in the brain stem[5, 6]

---

[1] Bigal ME et al "Migraine and cardiovascular disease: a population-based study" Neurology 2010;74(8):628-35
[2] Stang PE et al "Headache, cerebrovascular symptoms, and stroke: the Artherosclerosis Risk in Communities Study" Neurology 2005;64(9):1573-7
[3] Valfré W "Voxel-based morphometry reveals grey matter abnormalities in migraine" Headache 2008;48(1):109-17
[4] Swartz RH "Migraine is associated with magnetic resonance imaging white matter abnormalities: a meta-analysis" Arch Neurol 2004;61(9):1366-8
[5] Kruit MC "Migraine is associated with an increased risk of deep white matter lesions, subclinical posterior circulation infarcts and brain iron accumulation: the population-based MRI CAMERA study" Cephalalgia 2010;30(2):129-36
[6] Tepper SJ et al "Iron deposition in pain-regulatory nuclei in episodic migraine and chronic daily headache by MRI" Headache 2012;52(2):236-43

This damage is visible in brain scans with different technologies and it gets worse with increasing migraine frequency and duration.[1] That urgently indicates that the migraine actually *causes* the abnormalities that were found. Researchers now highlight this long-term damage and call migraine a *"progressive brain disease"*.[1]

One would think: "That should be it, enough comorbidities and additional damage." But wait, there is more. All these conditions are also more frequent in migraineurs:

- ADHD[2]
- Asthma[4]
- Back pain, chronic[6]
- Bronchitis, chronic[8]
- Cervical artery dissection[10]
- Cognitive impairments[12]
- Enuresis (=bed-wetting, in children)[15]
- Fibromyalgia[17]
- Hostility[18]
- Irritable bowel syndrome[20]
- Lupus erythematosus[22]

- Anger[3]
- Atrial septal aneurysm[5]
- Balance disorders[7]
- Celiac disease[9]
- Chronic fatigue syndrome[11]
- Endometriosis[13] / Menorrhagia[14]
- Excema (in children)[16]
- Hay fever[8]
- Impaired working memory[19]
- Kidney stone[21]
- Meniere's disease[23]

---

[1] Schmitz N et al "Attack frequency and disease duration as indicators for brain damage in migraine" Headache 2008;48(7):1044-55
[2] Fasmer OB et al "Comorbidity of Migraine With ADHD" J Atten Disord 2012;16(4):339-45
[3] Perozzo P et al "Anger and emotional distress in patients with migraine and tension-type headache" Headache Pain 2005;6(5):392-9
[4] Davey G et al "Association between migraine and asthma: matched case-control study" Br J Gen Pract 2002;52(482):723-7
[5] Carerj S et al "Prevalence of atrial septal aneurysm in patients with migraine: an echocardiographic study" Headache 2003;43(7):725-8
[6] Von Korff M et al "Chronic spinal pain and physical-mental comorbidity in the United States: results from the national comorbidity survey replication" Pain 2005;113(3):331-9
[7] Balaban CD "Neurologic bases for comorbidity of balance disorders, anxiety disorders and migraine: neurotherapeutic implications" Expert Rev Neurother 2011;11(3):379-94
[8] Aamodt AH et al "Is headache related to asthma, hay fever, and chronic bronchitis? The Head-HUNT Study" Headache 2007;47(2):204-12
[9] Gabrielli M et al "Association between migraine and Celiac disease: results from a preliminary case-control and therapeutic study" Am J Gastroenterol 2003;98(3):625-9
[10] Rist PM et al "Migraine, migraine aura, and cervical artery dissection: A systematic review and meta-analysis" Cephalalgia. 2011;31(8):886-96
[11] Peres MF et al "Fatigue in chronic migraine patients" Cephalalgia 2002;22(9):720-4
[12] Waldie KE "Migraine and cognitive function: a life-course study" Neurology 2002;59(6):904-8
[13] Tietjen GE et al "Endometriosis is associated with prevalence of comorbid conditions in migraine" Headache 2007;47(7):1069-78
[14] Tietjen GE et al "Migraine is associated with menorrhagia and endometriosis" Headache 2006;46(3):422-8
[15] Carotenuto M et al "Migraine and enuresis in children: An unusual correlation?" Med Hypotheses 2010;75(1):120-2
[16] Mortimer MJ et al " The prevalence of headache and migraine in atopic children: an epidemiological study in general practice" Headache 1993;33(8):427-31
[17] Peres MF "Fibromyalgia is common in patients with transformed migraine" Neurology 2001;57(7):1326-8
[18] Bag B et al "Examination of anxiety, hostility and psychiatric disorders in patients with migraine and tension-type headache" Int J Clin Pract 2005;59(5):515-21
[19] Kalaydjian A et al "How migraines impact cognitive function: findings from the Baltimore ECA" Neurology 2007;68(17):1417-24
[20] Cole JA et al "Migraine, fibromyalgia, and depression among people with IBS: a prevalence study" BMC Gastroenterol 2006;6:26
[21] Le H et al "Co-morbidity of migraine with somatic disease in a large population-based study" Cephalalgia 2011;31(1):43-64
[22] Appenzeller et al "Clinical implications of migraine in systemic lupus erythematosus: relation to cumulative organ damage" Cephalalgia. 2004;24(12):1024-30
[23] Cha YH et al Migraine Associated Vertigo" J Clin Neurol 2007; 3(3): 121–126

We are not done yet. Here are a few more conditions that are comorbid or otherwise associated with migraine:

- Morbus Raynaud[1]
- Narcolepsy[3]
- Obesity[5]
- Oppositional defiant disorder[7]
- Psoriasis[10]
- Rheumatoid arthritis[12]
- Scleroderma[12]
- Tinnitus[14]
- Tremor, essential[16]
- Multiple sclerosis[2]
- Neck pain, chronic[4]
- Obsessive compulsive symptoms[6]
- PTSD[8] / Persistent nightmares[9]
- Restless leg syndrome[11]
- Rhinitis (in children)[13]
- Sjögren's syndrome[12]
- Tourette's syndrome[15]
- Vertigo[17]

This concludes the disconcerting overview of the co-morbidities of migraine. You can skip to the next chapter now, unless you are female and/or would like to have children. If that is the case, you might find the following interesting or concerning:

- Women with migraine experience more **severe nausea and vomiting** during pregnancy than pregnant non-migraineurs[18] and have a higher risk of:
- **short sleep** duration (1.6 x risk; if also overweight: 2.4 x)[19]
- excessive **sleepiness** (1.4 x risk; if also overweight: 2.3 x)[19]
- experiencing vital **exhaustion** (2 x risk; if also overweight: 2.8 x)[19]
- feeling more **distressed** (1.6 x risk; if also overweight: 2.6 x)[19]

---

[1] Bartelink ML et al "Raynaud's phenomenon: subjective influence of female sex hormones" Int Angiol 1992;11(4):309-15
[2] Kister I et al "Migraine is comorbid with multiple sclerosis and associated with a more symptomatic MS course" J Headache Pain 2010;11(5):417-25
[3] Dahmen N et al "Increased frequency of migraine in narcoleptic patients: a confirmatory study" Cephalalgia 2003;23(1):14-9
[4] Hagen K et al "The co-occurrence of headache and musculoskeletal symptoms amongst 51 050 adults in Norway" Eur J Neurol 2002;9(5):527-33
[5] Peterlin BL et al "Obesity and migraine: the effect of age, gender and adipose tissue distribution" Headache 2010;50(1):52-62
[6] Perozzo P et al "Anger and emotional distress in patients with migraine and tension-type headache" Headache Pain 2005;6(5):392-9
[7] Pakalnis A "Comorbidity of psychiatric and behavioral disorders in pediatric migraine" Headache 2005;45(5):590-6
[8] Peterlin BL et al "PTSD, combat injury, and headache in Veterans Returning from Iraq/Afghanistan" Headache 2009;49(9):1267-76
[9] Lateef TM et al "Physical Comorbidity of Migraine and Other Headaches in US Adolescents" J Pediatr 2012;161(2):308-13
[10] Le H et al "Co-morbidity of migraine with somatic disease in a large population-based study" Cephalalgia 2011;31(1):43-64
[11] Rhode AM et al "Comorbidity of migraine and restless legs syndrome--a case-control study" Cephalalgia 2007;27(11):1255-60
[12] Pal B et al "A study of headaches and migraine in Sjögren's syndrome and other rheumatic disorders" Ann Rheum Dis 1989;48(4):312-6
[13] Mortimer MJ et al " The prevalence of headache and migraine in atopic children: an epidemiological study in general practice" Headache 1993;33(8):427-31
[14] Dash AK et al "Migraine and audiovestibular dysfunction: is there a correlation? Am J Otolaryngol 2008;29(5):295-9
[15] Kwak C et al "Migraine headache in patients with Tourette syndrome" Arch Neurol 2003;60(11):1595-8
[16] Silberstein SD " Shared mechanisms and comorbidities in neurologic and psychiatric disorders" Headache 2001;41 Suppl 1:S11-7
[17] Lempert T et al "Vertigo as a symptom of migraine" Ann N Y Acad Sci 2009;1164;242-51
[18] Bánhidy F et al "Pregnancy complications and delivery outcomes in pregnant women with severe migraine" Eur J Obstet Gynecol Reprod Biol 2007;134(2):157-63
[19] Williams MA et al "Sleep duration, vital exhaustion and perceived stress among pregnant migraineurs and non-migraineurs" BMC Pregnancy Childbirth. 2010;10:72

Pre-eclampsia is a pregnancy-induced high blood pressure condition with very serious risks for mother and fetus; eclampsia leads to convulsions and coma and has a high mortality rate.

Pregnant women with migraine are more likely than those without migraine …

- … to develop pre-eclampsia (2.3[1]- to 3.5[2]-fold risk)
- … to suffer a heart attack (2.1-fold risk)[1] or stroke (15-fold risk!)[1]

In other words, migraine is not good for pregnant women. But it is also pretty bad for the offspring. The risks are:

- placental abruption = tearing of the placenta (2.1-fold risk)[3]
- pre-term delivery = premature birth (3.5-fold risk)[4]
- poor intra-uterine growth = low birth weight (2[5] to 3-fold[6] risk)

Moreover, if the woman has severe migraine attacks during the first trimester, there is an increased risk of the child being born with a limb deficiency.[7] And even when all goes well: Children of migraineurs are twice as likely to have asthma.[8]

A promising solution for all these issues is marrying a male migraineur; they have up to twice the risk of *erectile dysfunction*![9]

Summary

▶ Many different *symptoms* can occur during a migraine attack; nausea, head and neck pain are the most common.

▶ Migraine has a bewildering number of *comorbidities*, covering all biological functions of the human body; problems with mood regulation (anxiety, depression) are the most prevalent.

▶ Migraine poses a threat to *mother and child*. Consider getting rid of it before becoming pregnant. Do your child that favor, please.

▶ **It is unacceptable to call an attack "*a migraine*" and thereby to imply that "*migraines*" are just bad headaches**. Analogue to *epilepsy*, *migraine* is the name of the condition, an episode is called *attack*. You wouldn't say "I had **an epilepsy** last night", would you?

---

[1] Bushnell CD et al "Migraines during pregnancy linked to stroke and vascular diseases: US population based case-control study" BMJ 2009;338:b664
[2] Sanchez SE et al "Headaches and migraines are associated with an increased risk of preeclampsia in Peruvian women" Am J Hypertens 2008;21(3):360-4
[3] Sanchez SE et al "Risk of placental abruption in relation to migraines and headaches" BMC Womens Health 2010;10:30
[4] Blair EM et al "Migraine and preterm birth" J Perinatol 2011;31(6):434-9
[5] Facchinetti F et al "Migraine is a risk factor for hypertensive disorders in pregnancy: a prospective cohort study" Cephalalgia 2009;29(3):286-92
[6] Olesen C et al "Pregnancy outcome following prescription for sumatriptan" Headache 2000;40(1):20-24
[7] Bánhidy F et al "Maternal severe migraine and risk of congenital limb deficiencies" Birth Defects Res A Clin Mol Teratol 2006;76(8):592-601
[8] Chen TC et al "Asthma and eczema in children born to women with migraine" Arch Neurol 1990;47(11):1227-30
[9] Huang CY et al "Migraine and erectile dysfunction: evidence from a population-based case-control study" Cephalalgia 2012;32(5):366-72

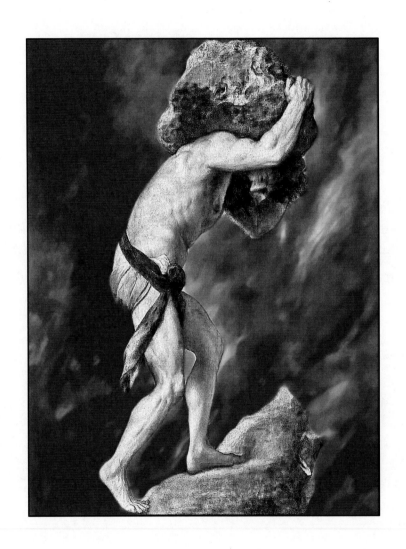

Chapter 2

The Impact and Burden of Migraine

> "I do not pray for a lighter load, but for a stronger back."
>
> Phillips Brooks

According to the official classification criteria set forth by the International Headache Society (IHS), 14.7% of the US-population[1] are affected by *strict* episodic migraine. Another 14.5% don't quite fulfill the 'strict' criteria and are declared to have *probable* migraine.[1] Including the 2% that have earned the title *transformed/chronic* migraine,[2] almost *one third* suffer more or less from migraine.

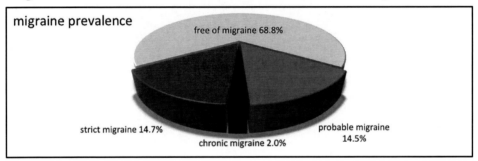

Migraine and gender

It is no secret that women are more prone to having migraine than men. The ratio is roughly 3:1 for strict migraine and 2:1 for probable migraine, both ratios in favor of women.[1]

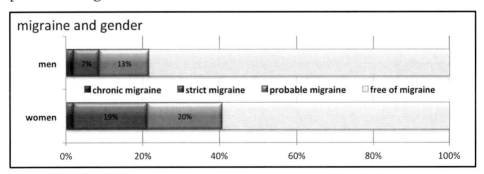

Women are more affected than men; does this mean that men have a genetic advantage at avoiding migraine triggers? Weird.

---

[1] Patel NV et al. "Prevalence and impact of migraine and probable migraine in a health plan" Neurology 2004;63:1432-1438
[2] Scher AI et al. "Factors associated with onset and remission of chronic daily headache in a population-based study" Pain 2003;106:81-89

Migraine and disability

The World Health Organization has classified migraine attacks as amongst the most disabling illnesses, comparable to dementia, quadriplegia and active psychosis.[1] Almost all patients are functionally impaired during an attack,[2] more than half are too disabled to go on with their daily business; they need bed rest.[3]

Apart from the severity of the symptoms, it's the *frequency* of attacks that determines the disabling impact of migraine on someone's life.

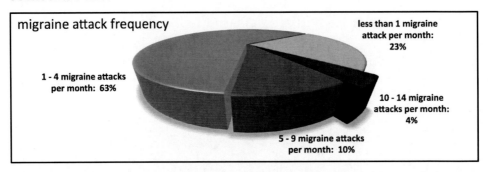

Three quarters of the migraineurs have at least one attack per month. Although in most cases an attack only lasts for a day, around 37% lose *five or more days* to migraine every month.[4]

Migraine and health-related quality of life

In medical research *quality of life* is understood as physical, mental and social well-being. Migraine has a substantial impact, which intensifies with the frequency of attacks. In comparison to the population average, migraineurs are significantly worse off.[5]

Migraineurs on average ...	feel less vivacious and energetic	have more bodily pain	are more nervous, sad and unhappy
are limited due to emotional stress	are limited due to physical problems	are restricted in social activities	feel overall less healthy

---

[1] Menken M et al. "The global burden of disease study: implications for Neurology" Arch Neurol 2000;57:418-420
[2] Lipton RB et al. "Migraine prevalence, disease burden and the need for preventive therapy" Neurology 2007;68:343-349
[3] Brandes JL "Global trends in migraine care: results from the MAZE survey" CNS Drugs 2002;16(suppl 1):13-18
[4] Lipton RB and Bigal ME "The social impact and burden of headache" in Headache – Handbook of Clinical Neurology Vol. 97 3rd series 2011 Nappi/Moskowitz Editors, Elsevier B.V.
[5] Terwindt GM et al. "The impact of migraine on quality of life in the general population." Neurology 2000; 55:624-629

Once episodic migraine has transformed into *chronic migraine* (= more than 15 headache days/month) the health-related quality of life goes pretty much down the drain. The following graph shows the results of a study group with chronic migraine, who reported an average of 23.6 headache days per month and an average pain rating of 6.4 out of maximal 10 points: Three out of four in this group were classified as *severely disabled*.[1] For comparison you see the U.S. average, which by itself is not overly impressive (if I may say so):

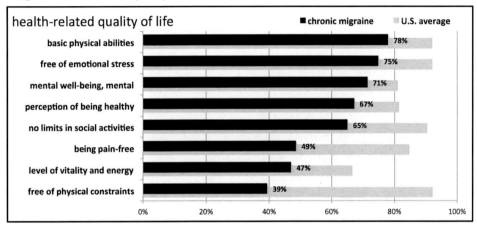

Migraine is rarely fatal, yet these results show that severe episodic migraine can develop into a *'quality-of-life-threatening'* disorder. In that sense the chronic migraineurs in the study were only 47% 'alive' (= level of vitality); you could say *'half-dead'*.

Migraine and the partner

The next group of people suffering from someone's migraine are the partners (boyfriend, girlfriend, husband, wife). A British survey found that 44% of them *worry* about their migrainous loved ones but also hold *negative feelings* towards them. Every fifth partner didn't have much understanding, but only 3% *admitted* being annoyed.[2]

A different study revealed that partners of migraineurs were significantly more *dissatisfied* with the conditions at *their own* workplace, as well as with *their own* work performance.[3]

---

[1] Lipton RB and Bigal ME "The social impact and burden of headache" in Headache – Handbook of Clinical Neurology Vol. 97 3rd series 2011 Nappi/Moskowitz Editors, Elsevier B.V.
[2] Dowson A et al. "The UK migraine patient survey: Quality of life and treatment" Curr Med Res Opin. 1999;15:241-253
[3] Lipton RB et al: "The family impact of migraine: population-based studies in the USA and UK" Cephalalgia 2003;23: 429-440

Close to one third of partners — migraine-free themselves — also felt that *arguments* were more common because of the migraine. Up to 60% reported *other negative effects* on the relationship.

In the same study half of the interviewed migraineurs confirmed more *arguments* with their partner; 36% believed they would be better company, if they didn't have migraine.

Too often the relationship suffers from the migraine too:[1]

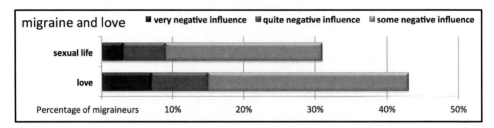

Migraine, family and leisure time

Two thirds of patients concede that their migraine has a negative effect on their family:[1] 90% have to postpone or delegate household chores during an attack.[2] Depending on circumstances, this may or may not be a problem for other family members.

In particular it's the indirect impact of the migraine on their *children* that causes patients regrets, resentment and guilt.[3] In surveys many migraineurs acknowledge that they are...

- ... less available for their children
- ... less understanding as parents
- ... less capable of supporting their offspring (e.g. homework)
- ... more likely to argue with their kids[4].

In other words, in the eyes of migraineurs, it's not so much the '*caring for*' but the '*being with*' the children that is compromised.

Also, migraineurs sometimes *miss out* on family time, social events and leisure activities. Many of them stop making plans for fear of short-notice cancellation due to an attack.[5] So the mere *unpredictability* of a migraine attack has an effect all of its own.

---

[1] Linde M et al. "Attitudes and burden of disease among self-considered migraineurs: a nation-wide population based survey in Sweden" Cephalalgia 2004;24(6):455-465

[2] Edmeads J et al. "Imapact of migraine and tesnion-type headache on life-style, consulting behavior and medication use: a Canadian poulation survey" Can J Neurol Sc 1993;20:131-137

[3] Cottrell et al. "Perceptions and Needs of Patients with Migraine: A Focus Study Group" J Fam Pract 2002; 51(2): 142-147

[4] Lipton RB et al: "The family impact of migraine: population-based studies in the USA and UK" Cephalalgia 2003;23: 429-440

[5] Brandes JL "The Migraine Cycle: Patient Burden of Migraine During and Between Migraine Attacks" Headache 2008;48:430-441

Some migraineurs are afraid of *travelling*, because they are concerned about jet-lag, weather and foreign food as additional triggers for an attack. This has the sad potential to hold the entire family back from exploring new parts of the world.

An extra source of tension, especially within the family, is the perceived lack of *empathy*, the feeling of not being fully understood or even of being *dismissed*, which many migraineurs report.[1] Dismissed? Would anybody 'dismiss' panic attacks or epilepsy?

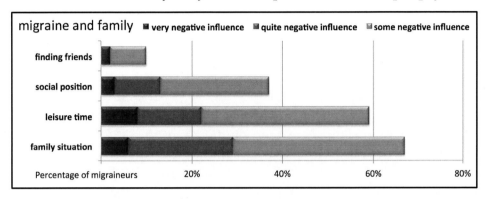

The burden of migraine on the entire family can only partly be expressed with *statistics*: How do you quantify the missed opportunities, the compromises and disappointments? Who wants to count the days without laughter in the house, but with *silent tears* instead? (Okay, that was a bit corny, but you get the idea.)

Migraine and money

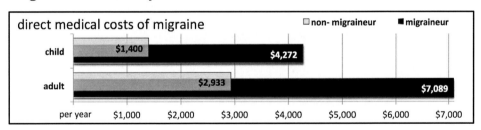

Migraine also has financial consequences for the family. The average medical expenses for an adult migraineur are almost 2½ times as high as for non-migraineurs and three times as high, if it's a child.[2] Of that money about 30% is spent on medication.[3] Note: That is based on figures from 1999, before triptan medication!

---

[1] Cottrell et al. "Perceptions and Needs of Patients with Migraine: A Focus Study Group" J Fam Pract 2002; 51(2): 142-147
[2] Pesa J et al. "The medical costs of migraine and comorbid anxiety and depression" Headache 2004;44:562-570
[3] Hu XH et al. "Burden of migraine in the United States: disability and economic costs" Arch Intern Med 1999;159:813-818

Migraine and work

Nobody can really work during a full-blown migraine attack and so 76% report a negative influence of their migraine on work *attendance*.[1] This negative influence can be quantified and studies find averages of 4 to 12 lost work days per migraineur each year.[2]

"Headache", including "migraine", is the most common cause of *lost productive time*, leading other pain conditions like arthritis or back pain.[3] One study calculated the cost of migraine to U.S. employers between $5.6 billion and $17.2 billion per year.[4] That was for 1992 and does not include productivity lost by *family members* to migraine care. In stark contrast to these facts, only 27% of patients believe that their migraine has a negative influence on their professional career.

A different study found that migraineurs lost on average only 2.2 work days per year to migraine attacks, but another 9 days for other reasons.[5] It was found that migraineurs miss more work days than average employees, not so much because of migraine attacks, but because of *other medical conditions*. In fact, they *avoided* taking sick leave on days with headache. This behavior—called *presenteeism*[6] – appears to be *more 'brave' than helpful*: It is an extra torture for the patient, the productivity is still reduced, colleagues get annoyed and it *doesn't solve the problem*. It seems as if migraineurs are either trying to *ignore it away* or they don't know what else to do.

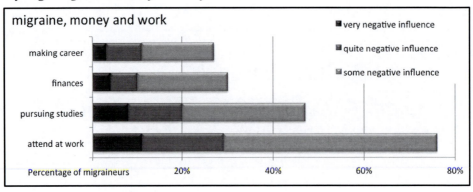

[1] Linde M et al. "Attitudes and burden of disease among self-considered migraineurs: a nation-wide population based survey in Sweden" Cephalalgia 2004;24(6):455-465
[2] Lipton RB and Bigal ME "The social impact and burden of headache" in Headache – Handbook of Clinical Neurology Vol. 97 3rd series 2011 Nappi/Moskowitz Editors, Elsevier B.V.
[3] Steward WF "Lost Productive Time and Cost Due to Common Pain Conditions in the US Workforce" JAMA 2003;290(18):2443-2454
[4] Osterhaus J et al. "Health care resources and lost labor costs of migraine headaches in the United States" Pharmaeconomics 1992;2:67-76
[5] Michel P et al. "Incremental absenteism due to headaches in migraine" Cephalalgia 1999;19:503-510
[6] Dahlöf CG "Impact of the Headache on the Individual and Family" in Olesen et al.: The Headaches, 3rd Edition 2006 LWW

Migraine and society

Migraine has an enormous impact on society. An analysis of data from 1989 and 1990 revealed that migraineurs had …

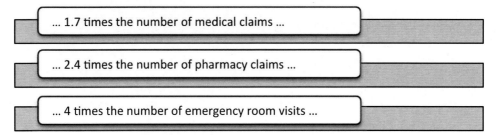

… in comparison to the population average.[1] Estimates based on figures from 1994 came to $1 billion in direct costs for the *United States*.[2] The same authors gave a conservative estimate for the indirect costs (loss of productivity) of $13.3 billion, mostly due to presenteeism, not to absenteeism (= sick-leave).

The healthcare costs of migraine in the *UK* are estimated at £150 million per year, including the cost of prescription drugs, as well as visits to general practitioners. Adding the loss of productivity and the costs of disability the author reaches an estimate of £3.42 billion per year[3] (≈ $5.5 billion US).

For *Australia* the total costs were estimated between $300 million and $720 million per year in 1990 already.[4]

Summary

- about *30%* of the population has strict or probable migraine
- *women* are 2-3 times more affected than men
- migraine can cause considerable *disability*
- migraine is a '*quality-of-life-threatening*' condition
- the *partners* suffer with, and so do the *children*
- the burden on the *family* can be heavy
- the *average* sufferer spent about $4000/year on *migraine* (in 2004 already)
- migraine also has an impact at the *workplace*
- the burden on *society* is enormous

---

[1] Berg J "Societal Burden of Headache" in Olesen et al.: The Headaches, 3rd Edition 2006 Lippincott Williams & Wilkins
[2] Hu XH et al. "Burden of migraine in the United States: disability and economic costs" Arch Intern Med 1999;159:813-818
[3] Headache UK "The economic cost of migraine and headache" based on a presentation by Dr. Tim Steiner, Imperial College, London to the All-Party Parliamentary Group on Primary Headache Disorders 19 November 2008, Westminster
[4] Parry TG. The prevalence and costs of migraine in Australia. Centre for Applied and Economic Research working paper. Sydney: CAER, University of New South Wales, 1990-1991, www.headacheaustralia.org.au

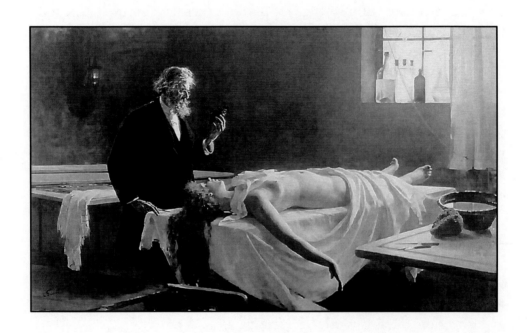

Chapter 3

Medical Treatments for Migraine Symptoms

"Formerly, when religion was strong and science weak, men mistook magic for medicine; now, when science is strong and religion weak, men mistake medicine for magic."

Thomas Szasz

Coffee or tea to wake up in the morning, a beer after work to wind down. We commonly use substances to regulate our state of mind. The inattentive student takes Ritalin® and the anxious and depressed rely on psychopharmaca. We take tablets when our blood pressure is too high or when our libido is too low. Whatever plagues us, chances are, there is at least one 'helpful' drug available. When we're not well, we're trained to assume a 'medical' problem and we've become used to the fact that medical treatment mostly means *medication only*. That's convenient and saves time. Awesome!

For some health problems conventional medicine has come up with excellent pharmaceutical solutions: Anesthesia, antibiotics and vaccines are just three of the many milestones in the history of pharma-medicine. Alas, the pharmaceutical treatment of migraine does not belong to that proud list. Strictly speaking, there is *no pharma-medical treatment* for migraine: No drug can stop the attacks once and for all.

Medication which can help with attack symptoms is highly appreciated—thank you—but migraineurs deserve much better. They deserve not only reliable and complete relief from the suffering during an attack, but especially, effective therapies to fully finish off the migraine-tyrant in their brains. Patients with migraine not only have a right to these therapies, but they are entitled to be educated about them and encouraged to take full advantage of what is possible today: to end the migraine tyranny.

Unfortunately, it's neither patients' rights nor migraineurs' well-being which makes the world go round. Conventional medicine—once on the patient's side—has transformed into a drug delivery network for the pharma industry. In this system, doctors are just as lost and helpless as their patients and so they comply with the industry's instructions: MEDICATION ONLY, is that clear?

Sure, the pharma companies don't send out thugs, they send invitations to free lectures and workshops, to 'educate' doctors about developments in their respective field, drug developments of course. Would anyone expect a pharma company to finance a workshop that spreads a message like this one?

> "Our drug is quite okay to suppress the symptoms of a migraine attack, but we recommend that all doctors and patients familiarize themselves with the established behavioral and the emerging neuroscientific therapies which actually open up the opportunity to end the migraine tyranny. That is something our drug simply can't do. We are strongly committed to your patients, our customers, and we'd like to invite you to discuss the amazing advancements in non-drug therapies for migraine during this complimentary five-star South Sea cruise to Bora Bora."

Pharma companies are committed to their shareholders and their task is to make as much money as possible by promoting and selling their products. That's the way it is. It is pointless to criticize them for their excellent marketing or for taking advantage of their influence on doctors. In their shoes, we would do the same.

What has to be criticized here is not the treasured migraine medication, which often is the only help that migraineurs dare to hope for. It is the current regime's policy to keep migraineurs in this holding pattern of *total reliance on drugs only* which is to be condemned. Cynically, it's the doctors themselves who are the first to point their fingers at the "irresponsible" patients, when the *dependence on drugs* has developed into *drug dependence*.

I find this behavior of *blaming the victim* not as atrocious as it probably appears to patients. It rather indicates that doctors still feel a little bit guilty, when they recognize what they've done in their role as drug servants. Shall we criticize doctors then, for not following their Hippocratic Oath (you know: "for the benefit of the sick", "never do harm", "responsibility"; all that sort of antique stuff, mate)?

"He that is among you without sin, let him cast the first stone" is still a valid line. Isn't it us, the patients, who only want the quick fix from the doctor, the convenient and time-saving patch-up? Isn't it our responsibility to take better care of ourselves in sickness and in health? Isn't it us who decide which road to travel? Isn't it us who choose liposuction over food reduction and drugging over jogging? Isn't it us who choose cosmetic surgery over sanity and spirituality, medication over meditation? It is us. It's our choice.

Medical Treatments for Migraine Symptoms

It is just a headache!

In the first two chapters of this book we've learnt that migraine produces a wide variety of symptoms in body, mind and brain. We've looked at the puzzling number of comorbidities, at migraine as a *complex and progressive brain disorder* and at the impact on the lives of the sufferers and their families.

In contrast, according to the IHS classification (IHS = International Headache Society), migraine is a *primary headache disorder*,[1] which only means that the head pain has been promoted from 'symptom' to 'disorder', for lack of a better explanation. It is not uncommon in medicine to call a group of unexplained symptoms a 'syndrome' or 'idiopathic' or 'essential' or 'primary'. That way, docs don't have to admit "We don't really know". Would that be so bad?

The first line of treatment: self-medication

Since migraine is officially declared to be a primary headache and because it is widely known that there is no diagnostic test that would influence treatment choices anyway, it's not surprising that many migraineurs can't be bothered consulting a doctor:[2]

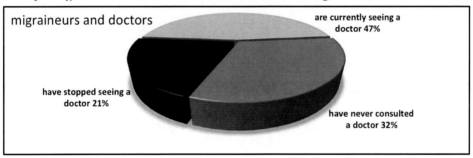

According to studies, about half of the non-consulters think it's not worth the effort because ...

- "... doctors can't help me" or
- "... doctors aren't interested in migraine treatment."[2]

One could think that the majority of these doc-avoiders are patients with mild symptoms, but we know that two thirds of the non-consulters actually have *severe* or *very severe* complaints.[3]

---

[1] http://ihs-classification.org/en/02_klassifikation/02_teil1/
[2] Lipton BR et al. "Acute Migraine Therapy: Do Doctors Understand What Patients With Migraine Want From Therapy?" Headache 1999;39(suppl 2):S20-26
[3] Lipton RB et al. " Medical consultation for migraine: results from the American Migraine Study" Headache 1998;38(2):87-96

A wide selection of OTC medication is freely available (OTC = over-the-counter = prescription-free). Patients who self-medicate, should know what to watch out for and when to see a physician. According to experts' recommendations[1] a doctor visit is indicated when headaches ...

- ... occur on more than 10 days per month
- ... are accompanied by additional symptoms such as motor weakness, sensory, visual or balance disturbances, double vision or vertigo
- ... are accompanied by mental or cognitive changes such as disturbances of short-term memory or of orientation to time, place and person
- ... manifest for the first time beyond age 40
- ... are unusual in intensity, duration and/or localization
- ... first appear during or after physical exercise and/or are very severe and radiate out from the neck
- ... are accompanied by high fever
- ... appear after a head injury
- ... increase in frequency, intensity and duration despite treatment
- ... occur together with epileptic seizures and disturbances of consciousness
- ... no longer respond to previously effective medication.

Recommendations about specific drugs and dosages for self-medication can be found (in English!) on the website of the *German migraine and headache society* (DMKG): "www.dmkg.de/therapie-empfehlungen" under "Migräne" (= migraine, duh).

After reviewing a few, I've chosen the German guidelines as the main reference for this chapter, because they actually represent the evidence-based advice of several reputable Swiss, Austrian and German societies. Also, these guidelines seem less obsequious to the pharma industry and even advise about self-medication.

And still, one adjustment must be made: One of the listed products contains *caffeine*. Caffeine has *no place* in migraine medication, because caffeine is associated with medication-overuse-headache[2] and chronification,[3] which is a major concern of mine.

---

[1] Haag G et al "Self-medication of migraine and tension-type headache: summary of the evidence-based recommendations of the Deutsche Migräne und Kopfschmerzgesellschaft (DMKG), the Deutsche Gesellschaft für Neurologie (DGN), the Österreichische Kopfschmerzgesellschaft (ÖKSG) and the Schweizerische Kopfwehgesellschaft (SKG)" J Headache Pain 2011;12:201-217, available in English on the website of the German migraine and headache society: www.dmkg.de/therapie-empfehlungen

[2] Meng ID "Pathophysiology of medication overuse headache: insights and hypotheses from preclinical studies" Cephalalgia 2011;31(7):851-60

[3] Aguggia M et al "Pathophysiology of migraine chronification" Neurol Sci 2010;31 Suppl 1:S15-7

Self-diagnosis of migraine

This leaves us with the question of self-diagnosis: Is it really migraine or could it be a different form of headache? The symptoms of a *typical* migraine attack (see chapter 1) are very different from a *typical* tension-type headache:

typical features	migraine	tension-type headache
prodrome and/or aura	possible	never
head pain intensity	moderate to severe	mild to moderate
head pain location	left or right or front	all-over or both temples
pain characteristic	deep throbbing, pulsating	dull, pressure-like
nausea	very common	uncommon
sensitivity to light, sound	typical	untypical
runny or stuffy nose	typical	not related
physical activity, sport	typically impossible	often helpful

Yet, migraineurs can also have tension-type headaches and some migraine attacks can be mild and untypical. The distinction between the two types can occasionally be quite difficult. This is not critical, since the recommendations for self-medication are pretty much the same. There is one exception: Immigran Recovery®, an OTC Triptan drug, available in the UK, is for migraine only.

It can be a smart move for migraineurs who don't want to see a doctor to at least consult with a qualified pharmacist and not to buy *unfamiliar* medication at the supermarket or petrol station.

The distinction between migraine and so-called *sinus headaches* is easy. Unless there is a proven sinus infection, e.g. as a consequence of a nasty cold, it is most likely a migraine:[1] Nasal symptoms and a 'feeling of sinus headache' is typical for migraine.

The risk to mistake a *cluster headache* for a migraine attack is rather low. Cluster headaches feel like a hot knife in one eye, are of unparalleled pain intensity and last between 15 minutes and three hours. The unlucky sufferers are typically *agitated* and walk around, literally banging their head against the wall. This is very different to a migraine attack, where you don't want to move.

---

[1] Foroughipour M et al "Causes of headache in patients with a primary diagnosis of sinus headache" Eur Arch Otorhinolaryngol 2011;268(11):1593-6

The second line of treatment: seeing the family doctor

Patients who want medical care and advice typically see their family doctor or GP (general practitioner). GPs receive little formal education regarding migraine.[1] Consequently, many family doctors rate their own knowledge about migraine treatment as average or below.[2] This lack of depth of knowledge is no surprise, given the complexity of migraine on the one hand and the breadth of ailments that GPs have to deal with on the other hand.

Unless they specialize in migraine and develop their own opinions and expertise, general practitioners can only follow the official treatment guidelines or risk getting in trouble for not adhering to the so-called standards of care.

Those treatment guidelines are typically put together by recognized migraine and headache doctors. They come together in societies and associations and develop recommendations based on their interpretation of selected evidence, mainly drug studies.

Let's be realistic: Doctors are trained in *pharmacological* medicine and are familiar with countless medications for numerous conditions. Prominent expert doctors frequently conduct clinical drug trials for pharmaceutical companies. It would be silly to expect of these experts to maintain a balanced view between the meds which they've helped to register[3] and non-drug therapies.

Naturally, so-called 'treatment' guidelines for migraine are therefore predominantly *medication guidelines*.[4] Only the patients are unaware of the strong influence of pharma companies on their doctor's prescriptions and recommendations and instead expect their doctor to be an objective expert with comprehensive advice.[5]

This inherent and strong bias towards *drugs only*[6] must suit the GPs reasonably well, since *consultation time* is far too limited[7] to fully engage with the entire spectrum of a patient's sorrows (symptoms, disability, comorbidities, impact and burden, ...).

---

[1] Shapero G "Improved migraine management in primary care: results of a patient treatment experience study using zolmatriptan orally disintegrating tablet" Int J Clin Pract 2006;60(12):1530-1535
[2] Kern R "There is a Strong Unmet Need for Improved Headache Education among Primary Care Physicians: Results from a Primary Care Needs Assessment" Headache Care 2004(2)1: 47-50
[3] Lexchin J et al "Pharmaceutical industry sponsorship and research outcome and quality: systematic review" BMJ. 2003;326(7400):1167-70
[4] Smulders YM "The influence of the pharmaceutical industry on treatment guidelines" Ned Tijdschr Geneeskd. 2007;151(44):2429-31
[5] Tattersall et al "Patients expect transparency in doctors' relationships with the pharmaceutical industry" Med J Aust. 2009;190(2):65-8
[6] Lexchin J "Interactions between physicians and the pharmaceutical industry: what does the literature say?" CMAJ. 1993;149(10):1401-7
[7] Britt H et al "Time for care – Length of general practice consultations in Australia" Aust Fam Phys 2002;31(9):876-880

Medical Treatments for Migraine Symptoms

Therefore GPs tend to ask closed-ended (= yes/no) questions[1] about the attack symptoms; a prescription for an abortive drug is written quickly. Usually there is no time for anything else.

In contrast, many migraine patients are concerned about medication risks and side effects and want to discuss treatment alternatives. [2] They have *many questions* and expect qualified answers and compassionate support.[3] Unfortunately, all too often these understandable needs remain unmet.[4]

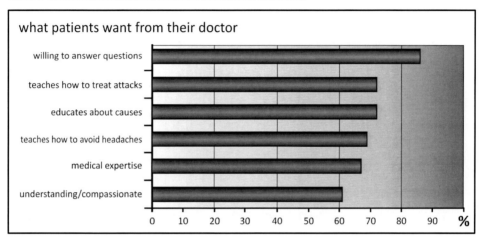

This illustrates that their encounter is pre-programmed for a bit of annoyance on the side of the doctor and a decent degree of disappointment on the side of the migraine patient.

It speaks volumes for the outstanding quality of some doctors that, given this blatant mismatch, surprisingly many patients (28%) are even *"very satisfied"* with their treatment[5] (or just polite in polls.)

Migraineurs shouldn't expect too much from their family doctor. On average it can be considered a success when a GP finds the right headache/migraine diagnosis, is familiar with current guidelines and willing to write the prescriptions necessary to try one after the other, until one drug or a drug combination is found that has a reasonable ratio between effectiveness and side effects.

---

[1] Lipton RB et al "In-office discussions of migraine: results from the American Migraine Communication Study" J Gen Intern Med 2008;23(8):1145-51
[2] Cottrell CK et al "Perceptions and Needs of Patients With Migraine: A Focus Group Study" J Fam Pract 2002;51(2):142-7
[3] Lipton BR et al. "Acute Migraine Therapy: Do Doctors Understand What Patients With Migraine Want From Therapy?" Headache 1999;39(suppl 2):S20-26
[4] Belam et al "A qualitative study of migraine involving patient researchers" Br J Gen Pract 2005;55(511): 87–93
[5] Lipton BR et al. "Acute Migraine Therapy: Do Doctors Understand What Patients With Migraine Want From Therapy?" Headache 1999;39(suppl 2):S20-26

The expectation that every family doctor should be a migraine expert, offer thorough patient education about the latest neuro-scientific findings, as well as compassionate psychotherapeutic support in a collaborative partnership and guidance to effective non-drug therapies, is understandable but unrealistic.

The directive "in migraine treatment, medication has to be combined with non-drug therapies" is part of several official guidelines, but in reality doctors are simply not that interested in other therapies.

A miracle treatment?

The goal of pharma-medicine under the current regime is the attack abortion, e.g. with triptans — hailed by some as *"a major breakthrough"* or even as *"miracle treatment"*.[1] The marketing slogan "Triptans are highly effective, reducing the symptoms or aborting the attack within 30 to 90 minutes in 70-80% of patients"[2] even snuck into Wikipedia.

Nevertheless, reality looks slightly different:[3]

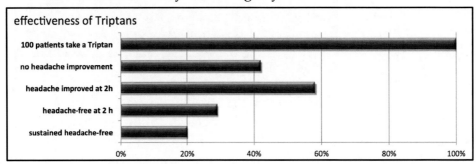

A comparative study shows: Of 100 patients taking a triptan[4] only 20% become and remain headache-free. In up to 57% the headache improves at first, but comes back later[5], asking for more.

And for 30%[6] to 40%[7] of patients a triptan doesn't cut it at all. Nevertheless, for a minority of patients, triptans seem to work like a charm, so that only the price hurts ($20-43 per single dose)[8], which indeed is *a major breakthrough* — for the pharma industry.[9]

---

[1] Bernstein C "The Migraine Brain" Free Press 2009; 160
[2] http://en.wikipedia.org/wiki/Triptan
[3] adapted from Goadsby P et al. "Migraine – current understanding and treatment" N Engl J Med. 2002;346(4):257-70
[4] e.g. Imitrex®, Imigran®, Cinie®, Illument®, Migriptan®, Maxalt®, Amerge®, Naramig®, Zomig®, Relpax®, Axert® etc.
[5] Aurora SK et al. "Headache Recurrence and Treatment" Curr Treat Options Neurol 2002;4(5):335-342
[6] Dodick DW "Triptan nonresponder studies: implications for clinical practice" Headache 2005;45(2):156-62
[7] Goadsby P et al. "Migraine – current understanding and treatment" N Engl J Med. 2002;346(4):257-70
[8] http://www.consumerreports.org/health/best-buy-drugs/triptan.htm
[9] Map Pharmaceuticals Inc 10-K 2008 on www.wikinvest.com/stock/Map_Pharmaceuticals_Inc_(MAPP)/Migraine_Market

Medical Treatments for Migraine Symptoms

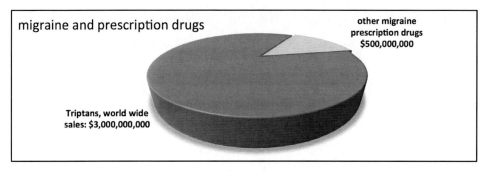

Triptans earn 86% of the $3.5 billion in the market of migraine prescription drugs for the pharma companies. In several countries some triptans are now available OTC without a prescription. Like every other medication, they are neither indicated nor effective for every patient and, like every other medication, come with certain side effects. Sadly, there is no miracle here.

In general the advice is to take triptans at the earliest warning signs of an attack at a high enough dose, but to avoid doing this too often, since medication-overuse leads to chronic headache.[1] Migraineurs with frequent attacks are thus left in an impossible bind and deeply frustrated. Many end up complementing triptans or other prescription drugs with OTC medication to get relief:[2]

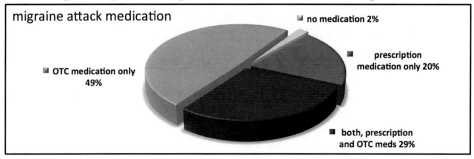

Only 2% manage their migraine attacks without medication. Perhaps that is the group of pregnant women or young children, where doctors suddenly discover non-drug therapies. Or is that the group of patients, who have become chronic due to medication overuse and now have to ride it out without drugs? Who knows? The best solution is not to have migraine attacks in the first place, but there are no drugs for that, so doctors have nothing to offer.

---

[1] Aurora SK et al "Headache Recurrence and Treatment" Curr Treat Options Neurol 2002;4(5):335-342
[2] Diamond S et al "Patterns of diagnosis and acute and preventive treatment for migraine in the United States: results from the American Migraine Prevalence and Prevention study" Headache 2007;47(3):355-63

Principle problems with puppies and potions

Imagine you've just picked up your brand-new puppy dog. The entire family is excited and so is the little pooch. After a bit of running, barking, licking and playing, the cute canine kid squats down on that amazing Oriental rug of yours and...ooops... pees. The wee-wee creek streams into a petite piss pond; the sodden Syrian silk suddenly starts smelling.

What do you do? Even if you have no idea how to handle this, there is one thing that you *do* know, which you should *not* do, and that is *rewarding* the puppy for the piddle puddle, right? So you can't give it attentive affection after the 'accident' and certainly no 'tinkle treat'. And you know that without being a dog trainer: Reward leads to the repetition of the rewarded behavior (= operant conditioning). Can you see a connection to migraine attacks?

Apparently, 38% of acute migraine medication prescribed by Australian GPs are *short-acting* opioids like codeine, hydrocodone or pethidine (Demerol®). **"Opioids and tranquilizers"** (e.g. barbiturates) **"should not be used in the treatment of migraine attacks"** say the German guidelines.[1] A review states: **"Opioids and butalbital"** (Butalbital = barbiturate tranquilizer) **"should be avoided in acute migraine treatment."**[2]

The problem with some substances is, that they are involved in the *reward system* of the brain.[3] And like the brain of the peeing puppy would learn from a 'tinkle treat' to go to the bathroom on the carpet again, so can the migraine brain learn from being rewarded with opioid medication to produce a migraine attack again. This explains why opioids (and barbiturates too) are associated with migraine chronification.[4,5] Please, don't take them!

In addition, opioid medication is of limited effectiveness in migraine,[6] makes people sick and vomit and is a fair bit addictive; opioids lead to constipation and slight euphoria[7] (= 'reward')[8].

The scheduled and constant use of *long-acting* opioid meds in the treatment of chronic pain is an entirely different kettle of fish.

---

[1] Evers S et al "Akuttherapie und Prophylaxe der Migräne" Nervenheilkunde 2008;27:933-949
[2] Tepper SJ "Acute treatment of migraine" Neurol Clin. 2009;27(2):417-27
[3] Le Merrer J "Reward processing by the opioid system in the brain" Physiol Rev 2009;89(4):1379-412
[4] Bigal ME et al "Overuse of acute migraine medications and migraine chronification" Curr Pain Headache Rep 2009;13(4):301-7
[5] De Felice M et al "Opiate-induced persistent pronociceptive trigeminal neural adaptations" Cephalalgia 2009;29(12):1277-84
[6] Tepper SJ "Opioids should not be used in migraine" Headache 2012;52 Suppl 1:30-4
[7] Doyle D "Oxford Textbook of Palliative Medicine" 3rd ed. Oxford University Press 2004
[8] Stein DJ et al "Opioids: from physical pain to the pain of social isolation" CNS Spectr 2007;12(9):669-70, 672-4

Abortive medication

Triptans and ergotamines—both used for attack abortion—can also lead to an *increase* in migraine attack rate, especially when used frequently. [1,2,3,4,5,6] Apparently triptans increase the sensitivity, reactivity and the vulnerability to migraine 'triggers', e.g. stress.[7,8] Although it is quite tricky to *prove* that the development of chronic migraine was *caused* by triptans, a significant connection was found in women with more than ten days of headache per month.[9] That alone should serve as a *severe warning*. Guidelines typically allow triptans on up to three consecutive days and ten days per month.

Analgesic medication

The other group of meds used during the attack are analgesics (= pain killers). 'NSAIDs' is not an immune deficiency disorder amongst national socialists; it stands for non-steroidal anti-inflammatory drugs. Aspirin, ibuprofen and naproxen are NSAIDs.

NSAIDs don't have any narcotic or 'reward' effect. The star amongst them is Aspirin (acetylsalicylic acid), which not only can be *as* effective as a triptan,[10] but also seems to be comparably *protective* against the feared chronification process.[9]

NSAIDs are not Smarties (or m&m's) either. In medication-overuse headache (MOH), NSAIDs *sensitize* those areas of the brain that receive data about what the body feels ("somatosensory"), which could add to any already existing 'sensitivity'/reactivity.[11]

Paracetamol, also known as acetaminophen, is another first line analgesic that might help during the headache phase of the attack. Paracetamol with aspirin can be an effective combination.[12]

---

[1] Kaube H et al "Sumatriptan misuse in daily chronic headache" BMJ 1994;308:1573
[2] Evers S et al "Sumatriptan and ergotamine overuse and drug-induced headache: a clinicoepidemiologic study" Clin Neuropharmcol 1999;22:201-206
[3] Limmroth V et al "Headache after frequent use of new serotonin aganists zolmitriptan and naratriptan" Lancet 1999;353:378
[4] Gaist D "Use and overuse of sumatriptan. Pharmacoepidemiological studies based on prescription register and interview data" Cephalalgia. 1999;19(8):735-61
[5] Katsarave Z et al "Drug-induced headache (DIH) following the use of different triptans" Cephalalgia 2000;20:293
[6] Lucas C et al "Use and misuse of triptans in France: data from the GRIM2000 population survey" Cephalalgia 2004;24(3):197-205
[7] De Felice M et al "Triptan-induced latent sensitization: a possible basis for medication overuse headache" Ann Neurol 2010;67(3):325-37
[8] De Felice M wt al "Triptan-induced enhancement of neuronal nitric oxide synthase in trigeminal ganglion dural afferents underlies increased responsiveness to potential migraine triggers" Brain 2010;133(Pt 8):2475-88
[9] Bigal ME et al "Overuse of acute migraine medications and migraine chronification" Curr Pain Headache Rep 2009;13(4):301-7
[10] Diener HC "Placebo-controlled comparison of effervescent acetylsalicylic acid, sumatriptan and ibuprofen in the treatment of migraine attacks" Cephalalgia 2004;24:947-954
[11] Coppola G et al "Abnormal cortical responses to somatosensory stimulation in medication-overuse headache" BMC Neurol 2010;10:126
[12] Diener H et al "The fixed combination of acetysalicylic acid, paracetamol and caffeine is more effective than single substances ... for the treatment of headache: a multi-centre, randomized, double-blind, placebo-controlled parallel group study" Cephalalgia 2005;25:776-787

All in all, some migraineurs do okay or even well on drugs. Some others are almost in love with their meds. But many others are not satisfied and there are good reasons for that:[1]

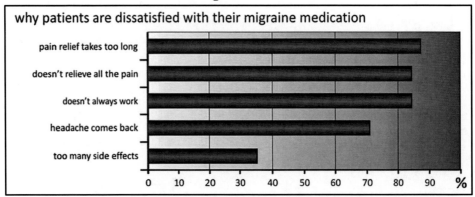

Abortive and analgesic medication may be a sufficient solution for those migraineurs with *occasional* attacks only and no other problems. If these lucky people (1) respond well to their favorite meds, (2) only need one dose to abort the attack and (3) don't see an increase in migraine frequency or severity, then I am not going to twist their arm in order to persuade them that they urgently need a migraine revolution; because they probably don't.

However, it is my impression that the good effect of triptans in a minority of patients and especially the *marketing* hype around them has clouded some doctors' judgment a fair bit, made them complacent, relying completely on medication only. And so they seem less interested than ever to motivate their patients to seek other solutions, *at least* in addition to the medication.

Even the official German 'medical' treatment guidelines for *doctors*, put together by pharma-friendly neurologists—not by bearded biodynamic energy healers—state clearly that either the medication should be *combined* with *behavioral* therapies or non-drug and *behavioral* therapies *alone* are recommended for migraine.[2]

Meds for the crippling attack symptoms are necessary, but rebound headaches and medication-overuse headaches are serious problems, so frequent attacks require a different drug strategy.

---

[1] Lipton BR et al. "Acute Migraine Therapy: Do Doctors Understand What Patients With Migraine Want From Therapy?" Headache 1999;39(suppl 2):S20-26

[2] Evers S et al "Akuttherapie und Prophylaxe der Migräne" Leitlinie der Deutschen Migräne- und Kopfschmerzgesellschaft und der Deutschen Gesellschaft für Neurologie, Nervenheilkunde 2008;27:933-949

Medical Treatments for Migraine Symptoms

Preventive medication for migraine prophylaxis

Preventive medication is usually recommended[1] when...

- ... there are more than 2 migraine attacks per month or
- ... migraine attacks last longer than 72 hours or
- ... the abortive medication doesn't really help or
- ... the side effects of the abortive medication can't be tolerated or
- ... there are prolonged auras or other other rare conditions.

Yet in real life that doesn't always happen: One study reports that 80% of the patients, who should have received preventive medication, did not.[2] Only 20% get what they need? Given the hype around triptans and the focus on attack symptoms instead of on patients' needs, it wouldn't surprise me, if it were indeed true.

On the other hand, preventive medication isn't always the hammer either. It is already considered a success, when the number of attacks is reduced by 50%.

As a rule of thumb it can be said that the more effective drugs are the ones that produce more side effects; for instance the anti-epileptic drug Valproate (e.g. Depakote®) can cause weight gain, tremor, nausea, liver problems and hair loss,[3] to name just a few. Several classes of drugs are used for migraine prevention:[1]

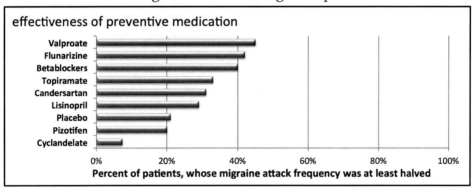

Please note that a reduction in the frequency of migraine attack by 50% is considered a success for preventive medication; an end to the tyranny should *not* be expected.

---

[1] Evers S et al "Acute therapy and prophylaxis of migraine: Guidelines of the German Migraine and Headache Society and of the German Neurological Society" Nervenheilkunde 2008;27:933-949

[2] Lipton RB et al "In-office Discussions of Migraine: Results from the American Migraine Communication Study" J Gen Intern Med 2008;23(8):1145-51

[3] Fumal A et al "Current migraine management – patient acceptability and future approaches" Neuropsychatr Dis Treat 2008;4(6):1043-57

Not that a 50% reduction is shabby, but there are still too many attacks left, which interfere with love, life and laughter. The only solution is not have migraine attacks at all; then the question "Which drug is next?" is obsolete and *smiling* replaces suffering.

The third line of medical treatment: seeing a neurologist

Intriguingly, many neurologists are migraineurs themselves[1] and apparently are quite interested in migraine treatment. Yet, neurologists also say that they find migraine a *challenging* condition to manage for the following reasons:[2]

- 60%: "complicated by comorbid mood disorders"
- 49%: "treatment is time consuming"
- 47%: "medical nomadism" (= seeing multiple doctors)
- 46%: "unrealistic patient expectations"

Migraineurs shouldn't hesitate to ask their GP for a referral to a neurologist who specializes in headache medicine. Rare and complicated forms of migraine, e.g. with frightening symptoms like partial paralysis, belong firmly in the domain of neurology.[3]

But if it's 'normal' migraine—with or without aura—and a decent amount of head pain that has become a real problem, what would the neurologist do?

A study[4] in 2004 assessed attitudes, knowledge and practice patterns of two groups of US neurologists relative to the guidelines set forth by the US Headache Consortium. The allegedly 'positive' findings were (in simplified form):

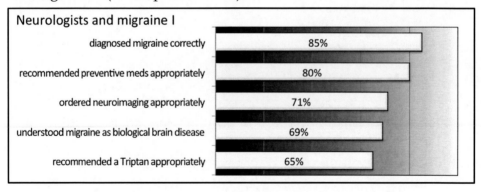

---

[1] Evans RW et al "The prevalence of migraine in neurologists" Neurology 2003;61(9):1271-2
[2] Donnet A et al "Migraine and migraines of specialists: perceptions and management" Headache. 2010;50(7):1115-25
[3] Goadsby P "The vascular theory of migraine – a great story wrecked by the facts" Brain 2009;132:6-7
[4] Lipton RB et al "Migraine practice patterns among neurologists" Neurology. 2004;62(11):1926-31

Medical Treatments for Migraine Symptoms

It is interesting that only 69% of the neurologists saw migraine as a "disease of the brain with a well-established neuro-biological basis". I would love to hear whether the other 31% have a different idea or if they just didn't understand the question.

And although the results were quite positive (as judged by the 'independent' investigator, a neurologist who frequently works for pharma companies) there were also negative findings:

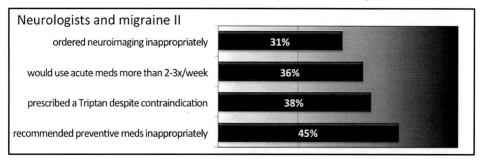

The results of this study illustrate my points:

- Neurologists too are supposed to follow *medication* guidelines
- they occasionally order expensive and useless brain scans
- too many disregard the grave danger of medication overuse
- the triptan madness too often defeats caution and knowledge
- drug-free therapies that can finish off migraine were not even mentioned.

"Why do I need a neurologist, when they can't cure migraine either?" Well, they might be able to help you with *symptom* control and — due to more training and specialization — perhaps better than GPs, who, on average, select the meds from a limited range[1] or too often prescribe the wrong kind of medication.[1]

One study from Norway[2] and one from Singapore[3] show that neurologists can generally achieve better treatment results than average family doctors, when they're *specialized* in headache medicine. It can be a good idea to do some research in order to find a neurologist who is not only qualified, but also *interested* in migraine treatment. That is not always the case; allegedly, some find treating migraine *frustrating* and blame the patients for that.[4]

---

[1] Stark et al "Management of migraine in Australian general practice" Med J Aust 2007;187(3):142-6
[2] Salvesen R et al "Aspects of referral care for headache associated with improvement" Headache. 2003 ;43(7):779-83
[3] Soon YY et al "Assessment of migraineurs referred to a specialist headache clinic in Singapore: diagnosis, treatment strategies, outcomes, knowledge of migraine treatments and satisfaction" Cephalalgia. 2005;25(12):1122-32
[4] Buchholz D "Heal your headache: The 1-2-3 Program for Taking Charge of Your Pain" Workman Publishing 2002; xix

The frustration that some neurologists ostensibly experience is easily understood. Family doctors have no reason to refer 'easy' patients on to neurologists. Referrals are typically given to 'difficult' cases with more frequent and more severe symptoms and more frequent and more severe comorbid disorders. Guess what almost all of them get more of from the experts? Here is the answer (according to a Canadian study[1]):

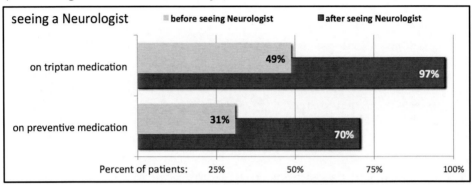

The medication treatment of severe migraine is a constant *trade-off* between symptom relief on one hand and side effects and overuse on the other hand. In this Canadian study every fifth patient was classified as a "medication overuser", 42% of those were overusing opioids, 22% were overusing triptans.[1]

Every year 2.5% of the patients with episodic migraine develop 'chronic' or 'transformed' migraine;[2] in the majority of cases due to medication overuse (but who is the *real* overuser?)

Does 'medication overuse' sound like 'drug addiction' to you? Not true. Migraineurs don't overuse medication for kicks, but because their symptoms have become too bad to endure without chemical help. In that sense they have become *dependent* upon medication, but that doesn't turn them into drug addicts. The addictive effect of *recommended* meds is negligible, yet the potential for *dependence* and *chronification* is huge and crippling.

The punch line is: Migraine medication is like a *crutch*; it helps you limp, but hinders you walking. Migraine meds relieve the pain of living with the tyrant, but they *don't end* the tyranny.

---

[1] Jelinski SE "Clinical features and pharmacological treatment of migraine patients referred to headache specialists in Canada" Cephalalgia 2006;26(5):578-88

[2] Bigal ME et al. "Acute migraine medications and evolution from episodic to chronic migraine: a longitudinal population-based study" Headache 2008;48(8):1157-68

Don't take migraine to heart!

If you have your heart in the right place, it likely has ...[1]

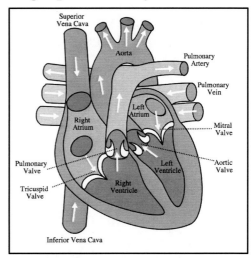

➡ ... a *right atrium* (= Latin for entrance hall), the chamber where the deoxygenated blood from the body gets collected and at the right moment pushed into ...

➡ ... the *right ventricle* (from Latin 'venter' = belly), the muscle chamber that pumps the blood into the vessels of the lungs. There the red blood cells take up oxygen and the reoxygenated blood streams back to the heart into ...

➡ ... the *left atrium* (another entrance hall) where it gets collected again and at the right moment shoved into the fourth chamber, ...

➡ ... the *left ventricle*, the muscle pump that drives our 5-7 liters of blood through the entire body, 70 beats per minute, 24/7.

During their stay in their mother's womb, babies can't breathe for they're submerged in amniotic fluid. They get their oxygenated blood via the umbilical cord from their mom. Since they don't breathe anyway, there is no need to pump blood through the lungs.

A door ('shunt') in the wall ('septum') between the left and right atrium of the baby's heart allows the blood to flow from the right atrium directly to the left atrium, *bypassing* the lungs.

Once born, babies slam that door shut with their legendary first breath and blood gushes into the lungs. Not in all cases is the door perfectly sealed and the leak that's sometimes left is called a *'patent foramen ovale'* (PFO).[2]

The rate of PFO in the general population is difficult to determine, because it rarely causes symptoms. Autopsy studies have found up to 25%, Echocardiography studies up to 24% PFOs in unselected people.[3] Let's say: every fourth one has a PFO.

---

[1] The schematic picture of the human heart was downloaded from Wikipedia and adapted; thanks to Eric Pierce, wapcaplet88
[2] Tobis J "Patent foramen ovale and migraine headaches: the saga continues" Catheter Cardiovasc Interv 2011;77(4):575-6
[3] Meier B "Catheter-based closure of the patent foramen oval" Circulation 2009;120(18):1837-41

Laypeople are usually told that a PFO is "a hole in the *heart*". That is misleading. A PFO may be *inside* the heart, but it is located in the inter-atrial septum (the separation between the two entrance halls) and not in the heart muscle itself. In order to be able to see a *leak* with ultrasound imaging (Echocardiography) the investigated owner of the heart needs to produce a favorable pressure difference between the two heart chambers.[1] That is done by inhaling and pressing as if you're 'delivering' something—if you know what I mean—and called a Valsalva maneuver. And then, with a bit of luck, you might see some blood dribbling into the left atrium.

When young people have a stroke and nobody knows why, it's called a 'cryptogenic' stroke;[2] that sounds more educated than 'mysterious'. Amongst those with a mysterious cryptogenic stroke, the rate of PFO is 40-50%,[3] which is twice as high as the general population. Therefore the idea was born that the PFO was the culprit of the stroke in those who had both, PFO *and* stroke—but not in those, who had a cryptogenic stroke *without* a PFO.

In order to close a PFO, cardiologists can thread a tiny hose (catheter) through a vein in the groin, up into the right atrium and through the PFO. After arrival in the left atrium, a little device that resembles a double cocktail umbrella can be fiddled through the catheter and placed on the septum, thereby closing the PFO more or less, with the explicit intention to prevent further strokes.

This is an awesome idea and highly beneficial for the stroke patient, conclude the studies done by the cardiologists.[4] In contrast, neurologists find that the data so far don't justify that at all:[5] When stroke patients take their medication, the presence of a PFO has no influence on the rate of further complications.[6]

Coincidentally, cardiologists also found that stroke patients with PFO and migraine with aura, who underwent the PFO closure procedure, magically and completely lost their migraine at spectacularly high percentages (e.g. 75%[7]).

---

[1] Sollman OI et al "The use of contrast echocardiography for the detection of cardiac shunts" Eur J Echocardiogr 2007;8(3):S2-12
[2] Sacco RL et al "Infarcts of undetermined cause: the NINCDS Stroke Data Bank" Ann Neurol. 1989;25(4):382-90
[3] Tobis MJ et al "Does patent foramen ovale promote cryptogenic stroke and migraine headache?" Tex Heart Inst J. 2005;32(3):362-5
[4] de Cillis et al "Recurrence of cryptogenic stroke or TIA in patients with patent foramen ovale successfully treated by using different kind of percutaneous occluder devices: five-year follow-up" Minerva Cardioangiol. 2010;58(4):425-31
[5] Thaler DE et al "Rethinking trial strategies for stroke and patent foramen ovale" Curr Opin Neurol. 2010;23(1):73-8
[6] Shunichi H et al "Effect of Medical Treatment in Stroke Patients with Patent Foramen Ovale" Circulation 2002;105:2625-31
[7] Tobis JM et al "Does Patent Foramen Ovale Promote Cryptogenic Stroke and Migraine Headache?" Tex Heart Inst J 2005;32(3):362-365

One study of "PFO closure for stroke patients" allegedly resulted in *complete* resolution of migraine in 56% of the migrainous part of the study group, irrespective of the completeness of PFO closure at one year.[1] In other words, it didn't matter that some still had a leaky septum. Isn't that weird?

Interestingly, PFO is more frequent in migraineurs than in non-migraineurs. Here are the results of a Turkish[2] study:

- 27 age and gender matched control subjects: 22.2% had a PFO
- 18 patients with migraine *without* aura: 47.4% had a PFO
- 10 patients with migraine *with* aura: 66.7% had a PFO

A Swiss study[3] found 47% PFO in migraineurs with aura in comparison to 17% in control subjects and the average size of the shunt was larger in the migraineurs. There was no difference in clinical presentation between the aura-migraineurs *with* PFO and the aura-migraineurs *without* PFO. Huh?

An Italian study sorted 65 aura-migraineurs into two groups: one group with *typical* aura, the other with *atypical* aura. Then the researchers looked for PFO and found:

- 46% PFO in the group with typical migraine aura
- 79% PFO in the group with atypical migraine aura

Does that mean migraine is caused by PFO? Or does PFO make migraine worse? What happens to the migraine when you close the PFO with a little cocktail umbrella like they did with the stroke patients?

A study in Boston[4] put migraine patients in three groups:

how many?	PFO?	intervention?	nick name
65	no PFO	nothing	controls
63	did have PFO	nothing	open PFO
41	did have PFO	PFO closure	closed PFO

The patients, who had their PFO closed, had an 85% reduction in migraine frequency and a 71% reduction in their use of abortive drugs. There was no significant change in the other two groups.

---

[1] Reisman M et al "Migraine headache relief after transcatheter closure of patent foramen ovale" J Am Coll Cardiol 2005;45(4):493-5
[2] Tatlidede AD et al "Prevalence of patent foramen ovale in patients with migraine" Agri. 2007;19(4):39-42
[3] Schwerzmann M et al "Prevalence and size of directly detected patent foramen ovale in migraine with aura" Neurology 2005;65(9):1415-8
[4] Kimmelstiel C et al "Is patent foramen ovale closure effective in reducing migraine symptoms?" Catheter Cardiovasc Interv 2007;69(5):740-6

This clearly proves that migraine is at least partially caused by patent foramen ovale, doesn't it? What do you think? There are strong arguments against this logically appealing conclusion:

- Migraine is way more prevalent in women, PFO is not.
- Migraine typically doesn't start at birth, PFO does.
- Migraine often stops during pregnancy, PFO doesn't.
- Migraine decreases with aging, the size of PFO increases.
- Migraine is episodic, PFO is constant.
- Migraineurs with aura don't always have an aura, how could a PFO possibly explain that variability?
- Migraine is often preceded by premonitory symptoms (prodrome), often days in advance; how can a PFO cause that?
- Trained migraineurs can recognize their premonitory symptoms and stop the progression into a full-blown migraine attack (e.g. with mental exercises). How is that possible, when a PFO causes the attack?

A PFO (patent foramen ovale) simply doesn't explain the phenomenon of migraine with or without aura. The higher rate of PFOs in migraineurs may be a co-occurrence and not at all related to a migraine-specific mechanism: Patients with cluster headaches, which is a very different disorder, also have higher rates (37%[1] - 54%[2]) of PFO and there is no discussion about the PFO being the cause of the cluster headaches.

A higher rate of PFO was also found[3] in patients with ...

- ... COPD (chronic obstructive pulmonary disease)
- ... OSA (obstructive sleep apnea) and
- ... decompression illness (in divers)
- ... but not in patients with tension-type headache.[4]

Okay, that's very interesting, but what does that mean for the connection between patent foramen ovale (PFO) and migraine with or without aura?

---

[1] Daila Volta G et al "Prevalence of patent foramen ovale in a large series of patients with migraine with aura, migraine without aura and cluster headache, and relationship with clinical phenotype" J Headache Pain. 2005;6(4):328-30
[2] Amaral V et al "Patent foramen ovale in trigeminal autonomic cephalalgias and hemicrania continua: a non-specific pathophysiological occurrence?" Arq Neuropsiquiatr 2010;68(4):627-31
[3] Johansson MC et al "The significance of patent foramen ovale: a current review of associated conditions and treatment. Int J Cardiol. 2009;134(1):17-24
[4] Moaref AR et al "Patent foramen ovale in patients with tension headache: is it as common as in migraineurs? An age- and sex-matched comparative study" J Headache Pain. 2009;10(6):431-4

A study[1] found a possible link: Finnish researchers measured the position of the pineal gland (a pea-sized brain area) in relation to the midline of the brain in migraineurs and control subjects. They found that the pineal gland is *significantly off-center* in migraine patients. That is a clue that migraine is more likely, when an embryo grows a bit *asymmetrically*, which is a known consequence of an altered serotonin signaling in the mother.[2] In simple words: If a mother has too much serotonin activity during the first trimester of the pregnancy, the likelihood increases that her offspring ends up slightly crooked; *with* an off-center pineal gland, *with* a PFO and *with* migraine. This surprising discovery needs to be verified with further studies, of course, but it points to an intriguing explanation.

Now we're only left with the question, whether it is helpful for migraineurs with a PFO to undergo a PFO closure operation. This question was the objective of the MIST trial[3] (= <u>M</u>igraine <u>I</u>ntervention with <u>S</u>tarflex <u>T</u>echnology, funded by the manufacturer of the little cocktail umbrella).

In total, 136 migraine patients with aura and PFO were randomly assigned to two groups. One group had a PFO closure procedure under general anesthesia. The other group had a sham (= fake) operation, also under general anesthesia, which made them *believe* that a 'cocktail umbrella' was sealing their PFO (but it wasn't).

MIST results	real PFO closure	fake procedure
reduction of headache days per 3 months	-33%	-30%
patients w/o any migraine attacks	3 out of 74	3 out of 73

Long story short: The study was a massive disappointment for everybody involved, including the manufacturer, but especially for those cardiologists, who had suddenly discovered their interest in migraine therapy (wink, wink). They are literally heartbroken.

---

[1] Kaaro J et al "Is migraine a lateralization defect?" Neuroreport. 2008;19(13):1351-3
[2] Louik C et al "First- trimester use of selective serotonin-reuptake inhibitors and the risk of birth defects" N Engl J Med 2007; 356:2675–83
[3] Dowson A et al "Migraine Intervention With STARFlex Technology (MIST) trial: a prospective, multicenter, double-blind, sham-controlled trial to evaluate the effectiveness of patent foramen ovale closure with STARFlex septal repair implant to resolve refractory migraine headache" Circulation. 2008;117(11):1397-404

> "But what about all those studies that showed amazing migraine reduction after PFO closure operations?"

Those *stroke patients* who also have migraine and a PFO might actually benefit from PFO closure. We don't know, because the way the studies were done ("retrospective" = in hindsight) doesn't allow for that conclusion. One possible explanation is that after a stroke the frequency of migraine attacks starts to decrease anyway, with or without surgery.[1] Perhaps the PFO shrinks or even disappears like a German study found.[2]

There are many possible speculations why migraine gets better after a stroke and a PFO closure operation. During the procedure the cardiologist needs to monitor the placement of the cocktail umbrella with echocardiography. He gets the best picture when he sticks the ultrasound probe down the patient's throat ("esophagus") and so general anesthesia is required. A known side effect of general anesthesia is called 'brain fog', a kind of long-term hangover after surgery.[3] It may be that the brain fog has a calming effect on overexcited migraine brains and so reduces migraine, but that's just another speculation. Further studies will shed more light on the subject—or add to the confusion.

At this point in time there is no scientific justification for PFO closure as a treatment for migraine. That doesn't mean nobody does it 'off-label' in exchange for money, but even cardiologists state that this surgery is *not* an indicated treatment for migraine.[4]

PFO summary

> ▶ Migraineurs, especially those with aura, have a higher rate of patent foramen ovale (PFO) in the inter-atrial septum. There is no evidence that a PFO creates or aggravates migraine.
> ▶ PFO closure for stroke-patients resulted in unexplained reduction of migraine headaches in several 'hindsight' studies.
> ▶ PFO closure for migraine with or without aura is not indicated. A landmark study, the MIST trial, showed disheartening results.

---

[1] Lapergue B et al "Frequency of migraine attacks following stroke starts to decrease before PFO closure" Neurology 2006;67(6):1099-100
[2] Tanislav C et al "Decrease in shunt volume in patients with cryptogenic stroke and patent foramen ovale" BMC Neurol. 2010;10:123
[3] Orser BA "Lifting the fog around anaesthesia" Sci Am. 2007;296(6):54-61
[4] Carroll JD "Is patent foramen ovale closure indicated for migraine?: PFO closure is not indicated for migraine: 'Don't shoot first, ask questions later'" Circ Cardiovasc Interv 2009;2(5):475-81

Medical Treatments for Migraine Symptoms

What would I do? If I was a weightlifter or removalist and I noticed that the majority of my headaches or migraine attacks occurred after heavy lifting (= straining), I would consult with a trustworthy cardiologist who doesn't make money from PFO closures. If that independent cardiologist could show me, that I have a relatively large PFO and indeed a fair amount of blood leaks from my right atrium into my left atrium ("RLS" = right-left shunt), especially when I'm straining, then a diagnosis of 'PFO headache' or 'PFO migraine' becomes feasible. Under these circumstances I personally *might* consider a PFO closure for myself and I would try to find a reputable cardiology clinic for that. Personally, I'd stay away from cardiologists who advertise PFO closure as a treatment for every form of migraine or headache or bad breath without establishing that the shunt is indeed the probable culprit of the targeted symptoms. Migraine is rarely a matter of the heart.

Killing migraine with poison

When in 1822 the German doctor Justinus Kerner reported 200 cases of severe food poisoning in a medical journal, he also suggested using the sausage poison therapeutically for a movement disorder. Little did he know that 170 years later, women—and some men— would pay decent money to have their wrinkles smoothed with that very sausage poison.

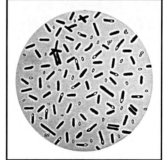

Botulism (from 'botulus', Latin for sausage) became the medical term for an infection with the bacterium *clostridium botulinum*. The symptoms are muscle weakness, paralysis and finally respiratory failure. The toxin (= poison) from the botulinum bacterium is botulinum toxin, better known under its brand name Botox®.

Botox® is not the only brand of botulinum toxin used for medical or cosmetic purposes, but the other brands (Dysport®, Myobloc®, NeuroBloc® and Xeomin®) don't play a major role in the treatment of migraine, so let's ignore them.

The weakening and paralyzing effect of Botox® on muscles is caused by interfering with the release of the neurotransmitter that is responsible for telling a muscle fiber to contract ("acetylcholine").

For many the cosmetic use of Botox® has become a regular procedure, implying it is as benign of a substance as lip-gloss or mascara. Still, botulinum toxin is a dangerous neurotoxin (nerve poison) with a frightening potency: Four kilograms (= ca. nine pounds) would suffice to kill the earth's entire human population.

The side effects are typically called 'minor' or 'transitory', but a droopy eyelid for 2-4 months is not a *minor* incidence after a temporary treatment for a few wrinkles. Other possible side effects resemble the symptoms of Botulism, like muscle weakness, difficulty speaking, breathing or swallowing.[1] Apparently, cases that required feeding by '*nasogastric tube*' (a hose through the nose into the stomach) have been rare and if the patients can't hold their heads upright anymore, they get a cervical collar.[2] Easy, ey?

The idea that the paralyzing poison will stay at the injection site, e.g. inside a muscle, is an illusion. Research shows that it migrates up the axon (the 'talking' line of a nerve cell) into the central nervous system.[3] Although that sounds frightening, it might actually be a good thing: Botulinum toxin also reduces the release of Glutamate,[4] a neurotransmitter in some 'pain' pathways,[5] and so Botox® is also used and investigated for severe pain disorders.[6,7]

There are good reasons to consider Botox® for some serious medical conditions and even as a cosmetic treatment in cases, when a few more wrinkles could mean the end of a career; but there are also good reasons not to be nonchalant about the risks: A blasé beauty brunch with bubbly and Botox® makes me uncomfortable.

The treatment of migraine with Botox® is a regular topic for the media, yet the study results can't quite keep up with the hype. In studies on patients with *episodic migraine* Botox® typically shows moderate treatment success, for instance a reduction in the rate of migraine attacks, so that it *appears* to be a viable option for treatment. So, what are you waiting for? **Call 1800-BOTOX, call now!**

---

[1] Botox® "Consumer Medicine Information" downloaded from www.allergan.com
[2] Mauskop A "Botulinum neurotoxin in the treatment of headache disorders" Handbook of Clinical Neurology Vol. 97 3rd series 2011 Nappi/Moskowitz Editors, Elsevier B.V.
[3] Antonucci F et al "Long-Distance Retrograde Effects of Botulinum Neurotoxin A" J Neurosci. 2008;28(14):3689-96
[4] Cui M et al "Subcutaneous administration of botulinum toxin A reduces formalin-induced pain" Pain 2004;107(1-2):125-33
[5] Fundytus ME "Glutamate receptors and nociception: implications for the drug treatment of pain" CNS Drugs 2001;15(1):29-58
[6] Wu H et al "A Prospective Randomized Double-Blinded Pilot Study to Examine the Effect of Botulinum Toxin Type A Injection Versus Lidocaine/Depomedrol Injection on Residual and Phantom Limb Pain: Initial Report" Clin J Pain 2012;28(2):108-12
[7] Bach-Rojecky L et al "Botulinum toxin type A reduces pain supersensitivity in experimental diabetic neuropathy: bilateral effect after unilateral injection" Eur J Pharmacol 2010;633(1-3):10-4

Unfortunately, the patients who received placebo injections, have the *same* moderate improvements *without* any Botox®; for example in this multicenter, double-blind, placebo-controlled parallel group study with multiple dosages compared to a placebo-treatment (= skillful injection of something useless):[1]

Relja et al 2007	Botox® 225U	Botox® 150U	Botox® 75U	Placebo
no of mgr. attacks before	4.3	4.7	4.7	4.4
no of mgr. attacks after	2.7	3.0	3.2	3.0
reduction of mgr. attacks	1.6	1.7	1.5	1.4

Isn't it amazing that the patients of the placebo group also had a reduction (-32%) of migraine attacks *without* any sausage poison? Some people respond really well to a bit of medicine-show. You present them with white coats and the smell of disinfectant, inject a placebo and voilà: fewer migraine attacks. In order to emphasize the 'real' effect (the drug) and reduce the 'fake' effect (without drug), you can sort those pesky "placebo-responders" out, before you inject the real Botox®. Isn't that clever?

That's what they did in a study in Seattle[2] and the result was: 50% of patients had at least 50% fewer migraine attacks in all groups; no difference between Botox® and placebo treatment other than in adverse effects (6 with Botox®, 1 with placebo). Bugger.

The punch line is that Botox® for the treatment of *episodic* migraine is off the table: Meta-analyses [3] of multiple studies conclude that it is not better than placebo, end of story.

The picture is barely different for *chronic* migraine (= more than 15 headache days per month). In 2008 the American Academy of Neurology published their findings about Botox® for *chronic* migraine:[4]

"There is presently no consistent or strong evidence to permit drawing conclusions on the efficacy of Botulinum neurotoxin in chronic daily headache (mainly transformed migraine)."

---

[1] Relja M et al "A multicentre, double-blind, randomized, placebo-controlled, parallel group study of multiple treatments of botulinum toxin type A (BoNTA) for the prophylaxis of episodic migraine headaches" Cephalalgia 2007;27(6):492-503

[2] Aurora SK "Botulinum toxin type a prophylactic treatment of episodic migraine: a randomized, double-blind, placebo-controlled exploratory study" Headache 2007;47(4):486-99

[3] Shuhendler AJ et al "Efficacy of botulinum toxin type A for the prophylaxis of episodic migraine headaches: a meta-analysis of randomized, double-blind, placebo-controlled trials" Pharmacotherapy 2009;29(7):784-91

[4] Nauman M et al "Assessment: Botulinum neurotoxin in the treatment of autonomic disorders and pain (an evidence-based review): report of the Therapeutics and Technology Assessment Subcommittee of the American Academy of Neurology" Neurology 2008;70(19):1707-14

In other words, at least six randomized, double-blind, placebo-controlled studies on botulinum toxin in the prophylactic treatment of chronic daily headache/chronic migraine could *not* show that Botox is better than placebo (= neutral substance).

Nevertheless, another big clinical trial (PREEMPT)[1] was conducted in 2009 with a slightly different methodology and finally the results were in favor of OnabotulinumtoxinA (= Botox®): At week 24 of a 56-week trial the 'verum' group (verum = real drug) showed a reduction of 8.4 headache days and — due to the large number of participants — that was *statistically* significant. So the conclusion was: "OnabotulinumtoxinA is an effective prophylactic treatment for chronic migraine." (Luckily, this time the placebo group had *only* 80% of the therapeutic effect.)

Based on the results of this *one* 'successful' study, the FDA approved Botox® in October 2010 as a treatment for chronic migraine;[2] coincidentally only one month after the producer Allergan paid a total of $600 million as a penance for illegally promoting the unapproved use of their premium product.[3] That was a good investment, since the FDA approval will increase sales of Botox® by an estimated $1 billion per year — every year.[4] Guess, who's paying?

Doctors who regularly use Botox say it is indeed beneficial for chronic refractory migraine; not so much for the frequency, but for the severity of the headaches, the intake of triptans and the number of visits to the Emergency Room.[5]

Others try to identify subgroups of patients, who benefit most from the injections and find 'pericranial tenderness' (tender neck muscles) is a sign that the patient will likely respond well.[6]

Real 'experts' suggest that Botox® should be injected into muscular trigger points for best results.[7] It's looking good for the predicted $1 billion extra for Allergan. Let's not forget, a vial with 200 IU of Botox costs more than a thousand bucks.[2]

---

[1] Dodick DW "OnabotulinumtoxinA for treatment of chronic migraine: pooled results from the double-blind, randomized, placebo-controlled phases of the PREEMPT clinical program" Headache. 2010;50(6):921-36
[2] Watkins T "FDA approves Botox as migraine preventive" CNN 2010 Oct 15
[3] Singer N "Botox Shots Approved for Migraine" The New York Times 2010 Oct 15
[4] Staton T "New migraine use for Botox could be worth $1B" FiercePharma.com 2010 Oct 18
[5] Oterino A et al "Experience with onabotulinumtoxinA (BOTOX) in chronic refractory migraine: focus on severe attacks" J Headache Pain 2011;12(2):235-8
[6] Sandrini G et al "Botulinum toxin type-A in the prophylactic treatment of medication-overuse headache: a multicenter, double-blind, randomized, placebo-controlled, parallel group study" J Headache Pain. 2011;12(4):427-33
[7] Gerwin R "Treatment of Chronic Migraine Headache with OnabotulinumtoxinA" Curr Pain Headache Rep 2011;15(5):336-8

I fully agree that every effective therapy option for treatment-resistant chronic migraine with or without medication overuse is welcome. Botox® is an option for those who (1) have a positive attitude towards injections into face and neck, (2) who 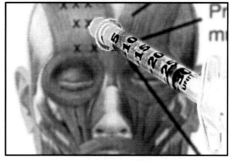 insist on *passive* treatments to evoke a slightly enhanced placebo effect and (3) are happy to fork out big bucks for it.

On the other hand, there are less expensive and more established treatments for painfully tender neck muscles and *myofascial trigger points*; and if you insist on having injections, then Lidocaine is just as good[1] for trigger point injections as botulinum toxin, considerably cheaper and doesn't cause paralysis.

And if the true intention is to efficiently *help* patients, have a look at the Akershus study from Norway:[2]

Chronic migraine and headache patients with medication overuse received *one short and brief explanation* about the possible role of medication overuse in headache chronification. One and a half years later they were followed up:

- 76% no longer had medication overuse
- medication days were reduced from 22 to 6 per month
- 42% no longer had chronic headache
- headache symptoms went down by 24%

Sometimes less is more.

Why do medical treatments not cure migraine?

When 100 patients with the same bacterial infection get the right antibiotic drug, you would expect success rates close to 100%. Of course, some patients forget to take their pill and some have diarrhea; but other than that, it should work for all of them.

If it doesn't work, you know that it's *not the right treatment* for that particular bug (= germ, bacterium).

---

[1] Kamanli A et al "Comparison of lidocaine injection, botulinum toxin injection, and dry needling to trigger points in myofascial pain syndrome" Rheumatol Int 2005;25(8):604-11

[2] Grande RB et al "Reduction in medication-overuse headache after short information. The Akershus study of chronic headache" Eur J Neurol. 2011;18(1):129-37

So, what does it tell you, when many medical migraine treatments struggle to beat placebo in their respective trials? It means that it's *not the right weapon* against that particular 'bug' in the migraine brain. Sure, in the case of migraine, 'bug' doesn't mean 'bacterium', but it refers to the faulty mechanism in the brain, similar to the expression 'computer bug' or 'software bug'. If you want to get rid of migraine, you have to find the migraine 'bugs', but at this point in time there is neither a *medical* diagnostic test nor a *pharmacological* treatment for migraine 'bugs', sorry.

That doesn't mean that medical treatments aren't helpful for countless migraineurs to alleviate the symptoms of an attack. Quite the opposite, many migraineurs with mild and infrequent episodes do well enough on occasional medication that they don't need anything else. Only if you don't belong to that lucky group, then it gets tricky. One of the tricky traps is the *unique* quality of migraine brains to produce new headaches from analgesic medication (= pain killers). Patients with other medical conditions, who need to take analgesics, *do not develop rebound headaches or medication-overuse headaches* from that; only migraineurs do.[1] It is, as if the migraine brain was protesting: "This is *not* what I need and want!"

Speaking of 'want', this is what patients want:[2]

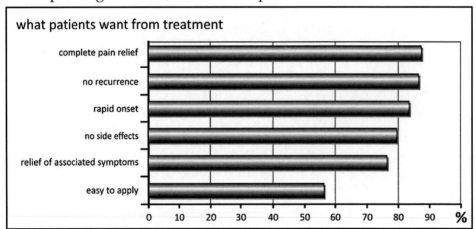

The good news is that many frustrated and discouraged migraineurs can have all that — after their migraine revolution.

---

[1] Bigal ME "The paradoxical effect of analgesics and the development of chronic migraine" Arq Neuropsiquiatr 2011;69(3):544-551
[2] Lipton BR et al. "Acute Migraine Therapy: Do Doctors Understand What Patients With Migraine Want From Therapy?" Headache 1999;39(suppl 2):S20-26

Chapter 4:
Avoid Life and You'll be Right

"One should, as a rule, respect public opinion in so far as is necessary to avoid starvation and to keep out of prison, but anything that goes beyond this is voluntary submission to an unnecessary tyranny, and is likely to interfere with happiness in all kinds of ways."

Bertrand Russell

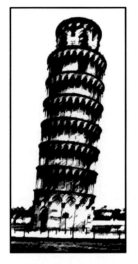

The citizens of Pisa were concerned. Their tower was leaning and every child knew, that if the lower side of the foundation continued to sink deeper into the soft ground, it was merely a matter of time until this famous bell tower, Pisa's number one tourist attraction, would fall.

The town council decided to ask for help and the most renowned architect of his time, Tomasso di Andrea da Pontedera, was hired at an exorbitant rate. Da Pontadera and his assistants spent weeks and months walking around the tower, scratching their heads. Finally, the celebrated expert, a legend in the history of architecture, asked the council to call a public meeting the next day.

Da Pontadera made his way through the crowd and walked importantly up to the stage. With poise he raised his arms and addressed the crowd in a proud voice: "*Citizens of Pisa, my name is Tomasso di Andrea da Pontadera. I am a famous architect. I have built cathedrals, bridges, town halls and bell towers all over Italy. My assistants and I have examined your tower and we've come to the finding …*" His exhilarated voice went up a notch in pitch: "*… that your tower is leaning.*" He paused to enjoy the amazed murmur of the crowd. Da Pontadera inhaled deeply and with grand gestures explicated: "*If the lower side of the foundation continues to sink deeper into the soft ground …*" He held his arms parallel as if he was holding the tower, leaned to one side, tilted the imaginary building between his arms and continued with authority: "*… it is a matter of time until this famous building, Pisa's number one tourist attraction, will fall.*" Stunned by the architect's flamboyance the crowd went silent.

The prominent architect continued in a mesmerizing voice: *"You have to avoid rain, snow, hail, strong wind and earthquakes that soften the soil even further and trigger the tower's toppling."*

The citizens of Pisa and the town council were still staring into each other's perplexed faces when Da Pontadera's horse disappeared behind the horizon. Some later said, they still had a slight ringing in their ear, like a remnant echo of the gold coins clinking in the architect's bags.

Some time thereafter the Pisa folk themselves found a solution to save the vulnerable building: They pumped concrete into the soil under the tower, increased the ground's resistance and achieved the necessary stability to withstand wind and weather.

New insights into attack prevention

Imagine that you're a doctor. You've spent a few hours on the weekend in a classroom on a course for your continued education.

Now it's Monday morning and your first patient enters the consulting room: *"Good morning, doc."* – "Good morning, Joe. What seems to be the problem?" Joe sighs and says: *"Well, doc, it started last week, when I was reading the newspaper. After a page or so I suddenly started trembling; first my hands, then my arms and after a while my whole body was trembling and shaking."*

"Wow, what a coincidence" you think to yourself "that's what the weekend workshop was about." And then you look up and tell your patient: "Joe, what you have is Morbus-Coruscus-Ataxia, a primary trembling disorder. The therapy is to avoid reading the newspaper. In fact, I've just received the updated list of trembling-triggers from the International Trembling Society. Here, avoid reading newspapers, books, brochures, letters, street-signs and everything else with letters on it, okay?" Joe is puzzled: *"But doc, this is not very practical. I'm an elementary school teacher and ..."* You interrupt: "Sorry, Joe, the waiting room is chocker's. I'll see you in two weeks and if the trembling attacks don't get better, I might have to refer you to a specialist." Joe's face lights up: *"And the specialist can help me with that darn trembling."* Now, push Joe out the door with the words: "No, he can't. But about all those things that you have to avoid?" — *"Yeah?"* — "He's got a longer list."

Tomasso di Andrea da Pontedera would be proud of you.

Learning from trembling disorder

An estimated 1% of the population have inherited the Coruscus gene, responsible for the susceptibility to trembling disorder.[1]

About one third of the carriers of the gene actually experience trembling attacks after visual stress.[2] The trembling is caused by the spreading of activity in the motor cortex (where the brain generates muscle commands) into other areas.[3] Those aberrant impulses originate in a field that drives the eye-muscles and were meant to counterbalance a slight misalignment of the axes of both eyes.[4] In combination with visual stress, like reading the small font of a newspaper, the higher pre-activation of the motor cortex and frequent corrective eye-movement impulses lead to a temporary instability and therefore to trembling attacks.[5]

After the Second World War, affected patients in Europe were instructed to avoid reading printed text like newspapers or books. A trial in France,[6] evaluating reading-avoidance versus placebo in 1972 (NOBUC), had to be stopped, because the avoidant participants had an *increase* in trembling attacks in daily life.

Shortly thereafter the Dutch eye-doctor Henk van Haaren conducted a study with an eye-exercise program that reduced trembling attacks by 93% within 4 weeks of daily eye exercises.[7] Van Haaren had recognized that—although logically appealing—the avoidance of reading was rather impractical in daily life and strict reading-avoidance led to further misalignment of the eye axes. Together with his wife Bintje, a physiotherapist, he then created the Van Haaren training, which is still the basis of every treatment program of ataxia corusci (= trembling disorder).

After her husband's death in 2004, Bintje van Haaren became President of the International Society for Foveal Alignment Training (ISFAT)[8] that educates neurologists and ophthalmologists about the Van Haaren Training for trembling disorder.

---

[1] Winterbottom FD et al "P10 CORU-48 gene promoter polymorphism in morbus coruscus" Am J Ophtalm Gen 2001;17(8):1294-9
[2] Turner H et al "Prevalence of primary trembling disorders" in Movement Disorders – Handbook of Clinical Neurology Vol. 241 3rd series 2011 Penzel/Dvorak Editors, Elsevier B.V.
[3] Li-Tao W et al "Motor Cortex Hyperexcitability in Adolescents with Coruscus Ataxia – An fMRI study" J Neurol Imag 2008;81(4):112-7
[4] Cordes M "Foveal misalignmnet and axial digressions in idiopathic trembling disorders" Brit J Ophtalm 1983;99(5):345-56
[5] Eschenbach G et al "Magnetoencephalographic findings in patients with trembling ataxia" J Kinet Disor 1994;16(10):243-8
[6] De Ballandard GB "A multi-center, double-blinded, randomized, cross-over study on treatment of ataxia corusci by reading-avoidance – the NOBUC study" Int J Atax Ther 1972;21(3) Suppl 2:16-19
[7] Van Haaren HG "The Utrecht Fovea Alignment Program – Tremble Cure With Eye Exercises?" Ophtalm Cour 1974;45(7):86-88
[8] see www.isfat.com/about_us.htm

Avoidance as therapeutic strategy?

Migraineurs with aura are in a similar position to patients with trembling disorder: Visual stress, e.g. long hours in front of a computer, can trigger a migraine attack, allegedly due to an instability of the visual cortex[1] (= the brain area where signals from the eyes get processed to create our experience of vision).

Unfortunately, Dr. van Haaren didn't invent a training program for migraineurs with aura, but at least his work reminds us that avoiding newspapers or computer monitors to prevent attacks—although logically appealing—*doesn't solve the problem* of the underlying vulnerability, rather makes it worse.[2]

Many migraineurs, with and without aura, seem to know their 'triggers'. After hours or even days with debilitating headaches they often identify in hindsight what caused the last attack, so that they can avoid repeating the horrible experience.

Theoretically, that should lead to a migraine-free life, once all migraine triggers are identified and strictly avoided. Alas, in practice that seems to hold true for very few only. Characteristic for migraine, there are always some who respond well, even to the otherwise deeply frustrating idea of 'trigger' avoidance.

Life 'triggers' migraine attacks

In studies and books these factors are frequently mentioned as potential 'triggers' of a migraine attack:

- mental/emotional distress, but also relaxation after distress
- skipped meals, but also certain foods or drinks
- lack of sleep, but also too much sleep
- menstruation, but also pregnancy or the pill, even menopause
- sensory input: bright lights, noise, odors
- alcohol, especially red wine
- weather or weather change, travel, sex, exercise ...

When forced to condense this list into one word, you would want to choose the word 'Life' for that, given that sleep, nutrition, stress and reproduction are represented.

---

[1] Chronicle EP et al "Thresholds for detection of a target against a background grating suggest visual dysfunction in migraine with aura but not migraine without aura" Cephalalgia 1995;15(2):117-22

[2] Martin PR "How do trigger factors acquire the capacity to precipitate headaches?" Behav Res Ther 2001;39(5):545-54

It doesn't require a genius like Henk van Haaren to recognize that the avoidance of life is neither viable, nor desirable, nor a successful solution to the problem of migraine attacks.

Nevertheless, migraineurs are bombarded with the advice to identify and avoid migraine 'triggers', not only by over 7.6 million websites,[1] but also by the American Headache Society,[2] the British Association for the Study of Headache,[3] Headache Australia[4] and countless books on migraine, written by medical headache experts.[5]

In contrast to Crystal Healing, the practice of medicine should not be based on intuition, superstition or personal beliefs, but on solid scientific evidence; hence the term 'evidence-based' medicine. Current treatment guidelines, issued by respectable and (certainly) independent medical organizations, are expected to be the result of the competent appraisal of the existing scientific evidence.[6] If a topic hasn't been studied enough to allow conclusions, sincere guidelines should say so. The American Headache Society declares on its website that the available treatment guidelines for migraine are indeed evidence-based,[7] yet highly qualified critics state that there is *no scientific evidence* for the concept of trigger avoidance.[8]

If it were true, that the 'trigger-avoidance advice' is lacking any substance, that could mean that migraineurs have been deceived by an elaborate bluff disguising a useless, hollow warning, like the citizens of Pisa: *Avoid the weather of life* or you will fall!

I couldn't find *any* scientific studies about the efficacy of trigger-avoidance as migraine attack prevention. That could have helped us to take a side in this dispute, but now we're left with common sense to investigate this crucial topic. The identification of 'triggers', especially 'food triggers', with the help of headache diaries, elimination diets and strict avoidance, can place quite a burden on migraineurs. Most of all, it creates additional fear, which is a powerful migraine trigger by itself.[6]

---

[1] search result of www.google.com.au to "avoid migraine triggers" on 26th of July 2011
[2] American Headache Society website: "http://www.achenet.org/tools/TriggerAvoidanceInformation.asp"
[3] British Association for The Study of Headache: "http://217.174.249.183/upload/NS_BASH/2010_BASH_Guidelines.pdf"
[4] Headache Australia website: "http://headacheaustralia.org.au/headache-management"
[5] Buchholz D "Heal your headache: The 1-2-3 Program for Taking Charge of Your Pain" Workman Publishing 2002
[6] Committee on Standards for Developing Trustworthy Clinical Practice Guidelines, Institute of Medicine "Clinical Practice Guidelines We Can trust" Graham R et al (Editors), The National Academies Press 2003 Washington
[7] American Headache Society "http://www.achenet.org/about/index.asp"
[8] Martin P et al "Behavioral management of headache triggers: Avoidance of triggers is an inadequate strategy" Clin Psychol Rev 2009;29(6):483-95

How to avoid life?

The (unproven) assumption is, that you *can* avoid 'trigger' factors and thereby reduce the overall number of migraine attacks. That is logically appealing, but how does it work in reality?

Stress/tension is mentioned in all the recent studies[1,2,3,4,5,6] and about 80% of migraineurs report that it is a 'trigger' for their migraine attacks. People typically experience stress, when they believe that they might not be able to cope with a given situation well enough to avoid negative consequences.[7] For instance, being attacked by a chihuahua—although annoying—is less threatening and stressful than being attacked by an adult tiger, because we can control the tiny dog, but we can't control the tiger. It's the lack of control that creates the stress.

Stressful events in real life are illness or death of a family member, separation or divorce, unemployment, financial pressure or inter-personal conflicts, all of which are rather difficult to avoid. The instruction to avoid the unavoidable, to escape the inescapable, and to control the uncontrollable isn't really helpful, is it?

Relaxation after stress is frequently mentioned as a migraine 'trigger', so the advice would be to maintain the stress and avoid migraine attacks due to relaxation. It doesn't make sense, does it?

Menstruation is another trigger factor, reported by 50% of surveyed migraineurs. Let's assume that one quarter of the migraineurs in all those studies were men, who rarely menstruate, and conclude that roughly two thirds of the women are affected by menstruation as a migraine 'trigger'. The thrilling question is: How does one avoid menstruation? I can think of one answer only and I wonder whether the official treatment guidelines indeed intend to recommend *continuous pregnancy* as migraine prevention.

Avoiding ***lack of sleep*** is good advice for migraine prevention, it seems. However, insomnia is a frequent comorbidity of migraine and insomniacs would love to avoid 'not sleeping', if they could.

---

[1] Spierings L et al "Precipitating and aggravating factors of migraine versus tension-type headache" Headache. 2001;41(6):554-8
[2] Ierusalimschy R et al "Precipitating factors of migraine attacks in patients with migraine without aura" Arq Neuropsiquiatr. 2002;60(3-A):609-13
[3] Deniz O et al "Precipitating factors of migraine attacks in patients with migraine with and without aura" The Pain Clinic, 2004;16:451–456
[4] Karli N et al "Comparison of pre-headache phases and trigger factors of migraine and episodic tension-type headache: Do they share similar clinical pathophysiology?" Cephalalgia. 2005;25(6):444-51
[5] Kelman L "The triggers or precipitants of the acute migraine attack" Cephalalgia. 2007;27(5):394-402
[6] Wöber C et al "Prospective analysis of factors related to migraine attacks: the PAMINA study" Cephalalgia 2007;27(4):304-14
[7] Kohlhaas JM et al "Stress revisited: a critical evaluation of the stress concept" Neurosci Biobehav Rev 2011;35(5):1291-301

The encouragement to get regular sleep[1] is however highly appreciated. I imagine a student in her premenstrual week, forced to pull an all-nighter in order to learn for an exam, who might follow this advice, go to bed early and fail the exam, only to have her migraine attack the next day anyway. Still, regular sleep is beneficial, not only for migraineurs. In addition, sleep is also known to abate migraine attacks;[2] thumbs up for sleep. On the other hand, sleep was also found to precipitate migraine attacks[2] and the question arises, whether reduced sleep quality is *a 'trigger'* or *a symptom* of migraine.[3] To be on the safe side, migraineurs should avoid sleep as well as bad sleep and sleep deprivation.

Certain *weather situations* and *weather changes* are reported by about 45% of migraineurs as an attack 'trigger' in surveys. Researchers are struggling to identify what the migraine-active ingredients of weather are. Irrespectively, in 1984 a surgeon reported his overwhelming success in treating weather-related and menstrual migraine in 42 patients with an operation, during which he crushed parts of the nasal septum (= wall) and carved out spongy bones in the nasal cavity.[4] Inexplicably, this procedure didn't enter any official treatment guidelines for migraine.

Speaking of avoidance, migraineurs should avoid moving to Alberta in Canada, since local research could show an influence of Chinook (= name of the local wind) weather conditions on the probability of migraine onset.[5] The 'Chinook-migraine-effect' was stronger for older migraineurs. So you better avoid aging!

A second Chinook-study[6] was able to identify one sub-group of patients as sensitive to Chinook-days and a second sub-group as sensitive to pre-Chinook-days. The risk of migraine attack onset was increased by an 'alarming' factor of 1.2 (= barely) and peaked on days with strong Chinook winds at 1.4 times the normal risk.

While the Canadians were focusing on windy research, German scientists investigated the effect of sferics on migraine. Sferics are electromagnetic fields in the atmosphere.

---

[1] American Headache Society website: "http://www.achenet.org/tools/TriggerAvoidanceInformation.asp"
[2] Inamorato E et al "The role of sleep in migraine attacks" Arq Neuropsiquiatr. 1993;51(4):429-32
[3] Della Marca G et al "Dysfunction of arousal systems in sleep-related migraine without aura" Cephalalgia 2006;26(7):857-64
[4] Novak VJ "Pathogenesis and surgical therapy of migraine attacks caused by weather (Foehn) and menstruation" Rhinology 1984;22(3):165-70
[5] Piorecki J et al "Effect of Chinook winds on the probability of migraine headache occurrence" Headache 1997;37(3):153-8
[6] Cooke LJ et al "Chinook winds and migraine headache" Neurology 2000;54(2):302-7

The German academics exposed 32 weather-sensitive (so they said) migraineurs to very low frequency electromagnetic fields, similar to sferics, and observed changes in brain activity, but unfortunately failed to provoke headaches or migraine attacks.[1]

A second sferics-study revealed a 'significant' correlation between natural sferics and migraine of 0.33 (= weak) between October and December, but not in July and August, when there was intense thunderstorm activity (strong sferics). In order to be safe, migraineurs should avoid sferics, thunderstorms and Germany in late autumn/fall.

Other researchers were less successful in identifying an influence of weather on migraine: No correlation was found between weather parameters and migraine-related emergency room visits in Ottawa.[2] Another study from Vienna concluded: "The influence of weather factors on migraine and headache is small and questionable."[3]

How is it possible that almost *every second* migraineur reports weather as a 'trigger' factor, but researchers can't find any evidence for that? Are weather-sensitive migraineurs liars?

A study in Berlin/Germany *could* identify a subgroup of migraineurs, who were clearly sensitive to weather changes. In those patients only, a highly significant association was found between lower temperatures and higher humidity on one side, and migraine onset and intensity on the other side. Again, that was *only* true for weather-sensitive migraineurs, 6 out of 20 in that study.[4] In order to be safe, migraineurs should avoid being weather-sensitive and trips to Berlin all year round.

Sensory stimulation (glare, noise and odors) is reported by 40-50% of migraineurs as a 'trigger'. In order to be safe, all migraineurs should avoid any sensory stimulation by living in a quiet, dark clean-room. Alternatively, surgical solutions like the removal of cranial nerves I, II and VIII should be explored. If you think "This is a bad joke", you're so right: It's cranial nerve *V* that desperate migraineurs indeed have surgically destroyed ("rhizotomy").[5]

---

[1] Schienle A et al "Electrocortical responses of headache patients to the simulation of 10 kHz sferics" Int J Neurosci 1999;97(3-4):211-24
[2] Villeneuve PJ et al "Weather and emergency room visits for migraine headaches in Ottawa, Canada" Headache. 2006;46(1):64-72
[3] Zebenholzer K et al "Migraine and weather: A prospective diary-based analysis" Cephalalgia 2011;31(4):391-400
[4] Hoffmann et al "Weather sensitivity in migraineurs" J Neurol 2011;258(4):596-602
[5] Slavin KV et al "Current algorithm for the surgical treatment of facial pain" Head Face Med 2007;3:30

So far the strategy of trigger-avoidance hasn't shown much promise, but now we're coming to a big one:

Hunger/skipped meals is, according to 60% of migraineurs, a 'trigger' factor for an attack. In addition, the occurrence of headaches after long hours of religious fasting has created expressions like "Ramadan headache" [1] and "Yom-Kippur headache"[2]. The IHS (International Headache Society) even has a classification category of its own for "Headache attributed to fasting".

Given that otherwise healthy muslims and jews suffer from headaches during fasting, it is not surprising that headache patients also get headaches during food abstinence. It would be rather surprising, if they didn't. Research confirms what we already know, hunger can cause headaches; a provocation study left no doubt.[3]

It can also be expected, that hungry headache patients experience their *typical pain pattern*, which would be bilateral, dull and pressure-like for tension-type headache patients. In contrast, migraine patients can expect their typical migraine headache, which is more often than not unilateral and throbbing. Otherwise it would be a *fasting-induced tension-type headache*[4], which patients with migraine don't want to add to their symptom list.

However, there is not a single scientific study, which proves that skipping meals triggers complete *migraine attacks*. Seriously, no researcher has ever published about a trial with migraineurs with aura, reporting how he deprived them of food and observed:

"After seven hours 36 of the 40 hungry volunteers noticed premonitory symptoms; after 12 hours, 32 ravenous individuals described their aura; by the 19th hour all of the starving 40 had horrible migraine headaches with nausea, 22 famished subjects tried vomiting but their empty bellies had nothing to give."

Not a single study proves that food deprivation actually triggers *migraine* attacks. Can you believe that?

Anyway, migraineurs don't need additional hunger headaches and so the advice to avoid fasting is completely justified.

But wait, the avoidance of fasting means eating food and as we all know, a lot of foods are known as migraine 'triggers' and need to be avoided. This is what I call a catch-22.

---

[1] Awada A et al "The first-of-Ramadan headache" Headache 1999;39(7):490-3
[2] Mosek A et al "Yom Kippur headache" Neurology 1995;45(11):1953-5
[3] Martin PR "Effects of food deprivation and a stressor on head pain" Health Psychol 1997;16(4):310-8
[4] Torelli P et al "Fasting headache: a review of the literature and new hypotheses" Headache 2009;49(5):744-52

A classic in experimental psychology

One of the many highlights of experimental psychological research was this experiment by the legendary B. F. Skinner:[1]

A very hungry pigeon is put into an isolated cage. From her cage the bird can see a little bowl with food, mounted to an arm. Being hungry, the pigeon becomes restless and moves around, flaps her wings, turns left or turns right, bounces, hops or pecks somewhere, desperate to get to the food. Suddenly the arm swings towards the cage and the food bowl ends up in a place so that the eager bird can eat a bit; but after five seconds the food-arm swings away from the cage, much to the dismay of the puzzled pigeon.

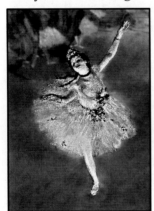

Even though the delivery is controlled by an independent timer, the reward with food leads to reinforcement of the bird's most recent behavior (= operant conditioning). In plain language: The pigeon *assumes* that her actions (e.g. turning left) *caused* the food bowl to swing towards her. Being hungry, she tries to get more food by performing the same behavior (e.g. turning left) again; and because the bird is persistent enough, after some time the next food bowl swing *confirms* the pigeon's assumption ("my left turn triggers the swing") and her persistence ("I need to turn left more often").

After a while the pigeon will have created the most bizarre dance routine as a result of multiple refinements that ultimately get rewarded by a bit of food. At least that's what the bird is convinced of and, still being hungry, it wouldn't dare to try something else.

Six out of eight pigeons in Skinner's experiment developed this kind of behavior so clearly that independent observers could agree perfectly when counting the repetitions.

The accidental co-occurrence of some random behavior with the timer-controlled reinforcement was enough to create amazing performances by the pigeons. An outside observer would think, "Bird, have you gone mad?"; but what would the pigeons say after so many *definite confirmations* of their beliefs and actions?

---

[1] Skinner BF "Superstition in the Pigeon" Journal of Experimental Psychology 1947;38:168-172

The science of 'trigger' foods

Going to bed on time and eating regularly is not too hard for migraineurs, especially given the promised reward of fewer migraine attacks. Following the advice to avoid 'trigger' foods is considerably harder. What do we do, when we want to have a good time? We invite friends for dinner, go to a nice restaurant, grab a beer or enjoy a glass of wine in front of the fireplace. We celebrate Christmas, Thanksgiving, Easter, Australia Day or Queen's birthday with a dinner, a lunch, a brunch or a barbie (= BBQ). Social gatherings are basically feedings and it's called "Gala Dinner" and hardly ever "Gala Trigger Food Avoidance Banquet".

Avoiding one or two foods is no major problem. Derek needs to lose weight and has water instead of beer, Celine has a peanut allergy and swaps her desert with Edna. In contrast, migraineurs are under constant threat, persecuted by an army of malicious foods that try to sneak onto their plates and forks, to finally wreak havoc in their vulnerable brains.

And so the headache experts warn and admonish to their heart's content: "*Stay away from trigger foods or you shall suffer!*"[1] And many migraineurs do suffer, one way or another.

Chocolate is a legendary migraine 'trigger', because it contains caffeine and phenyl-ethyl-amine. A double-blind study of chocolate versus carob (a chocolate substitute made from a different plant) found no difference.[2] The scientist concluded that chocolate doesn't trigger migraine attacks, but other experts had a different interpretation: They added carob to the list of trigger foods!

Even the most unsubstantiated warning becomes very impressive and effective, when the 'offending' ingredient is named in Latin. ***Tyramine*** or 4-Hydroxyphenylethylamine is a naturally occurring monoamine-compound derived from the amino acid tyrosine.[3] Tyramine acts as a releasing agent for catecholamines (epinephrine, norepinephrine) in the brain and therefore it is no surprise that food rich in tyramine typically 'triggers' migraine attacks. Many foods contain tyramine and they're all under suspicion, but the most famous tyramine bomb is cheese.

---

[1] Sun-Edelstein C et al "Foods and supplements in the management of migraine headaches" Clin J Pain 2009;25(5):446-52
[2] Marcus DA et al "A double-blind provocative study of chocolate as a trigger of headache" Cephalalgia 1997;17(8):855-62
[3] http://en.wikipedia.org/wiki/Tyramine

One randomized trial of 80 patients with frequent episodes showed that tyramine and a placebo induced migraine at the same rate.[1] The logical conclusion is that tyramine does *not* prompt migraine attacks, but I'm confident that some other expert will put "placebo" on a 'trigger' food list.

All biogenic amines (tyramine, phenylethylamine, histamine etc.), present in many foods, often get accused of 'triggering' attacks. Scientific evidence says that they don't,[2] but what does it matter?

Too much ***alcohol*** can cause headache in healthy people, so we can expect that in migraineurs too. On the other hand, a study found that the consumption of *beer* reduces the statistical risk of a migraine attack.[3]

The number of substances and foods that allegedly 'trigger' attacks exceeds the number of studies proving the opposite by far. It takes an educated 'expert' a few seconds only to add another food to the already long list, since scientific evidence seems not required.

There is not a single food or substance, which has scientific support to deserve the title migraine 'trigger' food, not even the legendary red wine. In a survey in London only 12% of migraineurs *reported* sensitivity to red, but not to white wine.[4]

One study investigated all the internal and external 'triggers' in 182 migraineurs in India and found the usual suspects:[5]

- Emotional stress: 70% reported stress as a 'trigger'
- Physical exhaustion: 53%
- Fasting: 46%
- Menstruation: 13%
- Weather changes: 10%
- More than one trigger: 34%

Not a single patient reported *food* or certain foods as a 'trigger' for migraine attacks. How is that possible? The concept of 'trigger' food avoidance is *unknown* in India. Nobody knows about it, nobody believes in it, nobody is scared of food. No fear equals no 'trigger'. So what should be avoided, food or fear?

---

[1] Ziegler DK "Failure of tyramine to induce migraine" Neurology 1977;27(8):725-6
[2] Jansen SC et al "Intolerance to dietary biogenic amines: a review" Ann Allergy Asthma Immunol 2003;91(3):233-40
[3] Wöber C et al "Prospective analysis of factors related to migraine attacks: the PAMINA study" Cephalalgia. 2007;27(4):304-14
[4] Peatfield RC "Relationships between food, wine, and beer-precipitated migrainous headaches" Headache 1995;35(6):355-7
[5] Yadav RK "A study of triggers of migraine in India" Pain Med 2010;11(1):44-7

The identification of 'trigger' foods

Once the idea has entered our minds that certain foods might 'trigger' migraine attacks, there is no way back anymore. After a crippling episode, Caroline naturally wants to find out, what 'triggered' the attack. By comparing her headache diary with 'trigger' food lists, she will likely find a culprit: "The orange. It was the orange, because it is the only suspect in my diary." This creates the illusion of proof, although her 'conclusion' is merely an unproven assumption.

The next time Caroline eats an orange she can't help it but be anxious and think: "I hope this orange doesn't give me the next attack." Of course, that's exactly what happens. And now it gets crazy. Caroline reports that an orange triggered her migraine attack to her internet support group and some members immediately chime in: "I've had the same experience: horrible attack after only half an orange." The next one is even more vulnerable: "My attack was triggered by an orange cookie."– "Oh, I suffered like a dog for three days after accidentally inhaling the scent of oranges." — "I WAS DREAMING I WAS WEARING AN ORANGE T-SHIRT AND WOKE UP WITH HEADACHES."

All orange-'trigger'-sufferers put oranges on their 'trigger' food list and report their orange-'trigger'-findings on websites and blogs. Additionally they inform their doctors so that physicians too can spread the warning: Oranges are a migraine 'trigger' food.

One imperious doctor even writes a book about 'trigger'-avoidance. His 'expertise' couldn't be more convincing: Avoid all triggers and you will be fine. If not, then take medication!

Desperate migraineurs now try to heal their headaches by following his authoritative advice and struggle, but their persistence is encouraged by several reports of how well this avoidance-program has allegedly worked for some.

Many diligently persevere in their avoidance of 'trigger' foods and so add more stress and fear to their already difficult lives.

Are 'trigger' foods a psychological phenomenon?

Unfortunately it's not that easy. Migraine attacks probably occur based on an irregular, yet cyclical schedule. The superstition-effect, leading to the identification of blameworthy foods, is based on the *information* and the *assumption* that food is a likely 'trigger'.

The tricky thing is that this assumption is possibly even true, but only sometimes and for a very small minority of migraineurs.

The entire concept of 'trigger'-food avoidance suffers from the idea that a food ingredient is the culprit. It makes more sense to consider the *vulnerability* to a certain substance to be the problem.

In a biochemical-pharmacological model of humans it may be inexplicable, but some people are indeed weather-'sensitive'. Why wouldn't there be people with an unusual reactivity to certain foods? There is already one disorder which is explained by a process of sensitization: multiple chemical sensitivity,[1] now called "idiopathic environmental intolerance".

Sensitization is a maladaptive learning process that leads to stronger and stronger reactions to weaker and weaker stimuli.[2] In migraineurs, sensitization *and* de-sensitization to light,[3] noise[4] and stress[5] have already been *demonstrated* by Australian researchers.

In principle, susceptible people can get sensitized to anything. Some migraineurs are not only sensitized to light, noise or stress, but also to some feared foods. Please note: The vulnerability to a migraine 'trigger' is the result of a *fear-driven learning process* ("sensitization"). The substances to which one migraineur reacts are very individual and can seem erratic from a biochemical point of view. In any case, the food to which one person may be *sensitized* has no power to 'trigger' attacks in others.

Another possible mechanism is *food allergy*. Celiac disease is an allergy to a wheat protein (gluten) and a frequent comorbidity of migraine. Neurological symptoms are common in celiac disease, with mood disorders (35%) and migraine (28%) at the top of the list.[6] Apart from these, a gluten allergy can be asymptomatic and therefore go unnoticed.[7] A gluten-free diet has been reported to improve migraine symptoms markedly in celiac migraineurs.[8]

Yet, the British Association for the Study of Headaches states in its guidelines explicitly: **"Food allergy (i.e. an immunological process) has no part in the causation of migraine."** How can they possibly know?

---

[1] Rossi J 3rd "Sensitization induced by kindling and kindling-related phenomena as a model for multiple chemical sensitivity" Toxicology 1996;111(1-3):87-100
[2] Dodick D et al "Central sensitization theory of migraine: clinical implications" Headache 2006;46 Suppl4:S182-91
[3] Martin PR "How do trigger factors acquire the capacity to precipitate headaches?" Behav Res Ther 2001;39(5):545-54
[4] Martin PR "Noise as a trigger for headaches: relationship between exposure and sensitivity" Headache 2006;46(6):962-72
[5] Martin PR et al "Stress as a trigger for headaches: relationship between exposure and sensitivity" Anxiety Stress Coping 2007;20(4):393-407
[6] Bürk K et al "Neurological symptoms in patients with biopsy proven celiac disease" Mov Disord 2009;24(16):2358-62
[7] Mazure RM et al "Early changes of body composition in asymptomatic celiac disease patients" Am J Gastroenterol. 1996;91(4):726-30
[8] Gabrielli M et al "Association between migraine and Celiac disease: results from a preliminary case-control and therapeutic study" Am J Gastroenterol 2003;98(3):625-9

The participation of an allergy-induced immune response in the migraine mechanism in some patients may well be against the financial interests of some British neurologists, but it may also be not too far-fetched:

A *desensitization* treatment for the immune system with subcutaneous (= under the skin) histamine injections was a popular migraine therapy in the 1940s and 1950s and then forgotten. Recent experimental studies showed promising preliminary results.[1,2,3]

This does not prove (beyond reasonable doubt) that the immune system *does* contribute to migraine, but it certainly does not invite absolute statements, that this can't possibly be the case.

Below the level of officially recognized allergy, gluten may well cause reactions in gluten-sensitive individuals that are similar to those seen in celiac disease.[4]

Countless other *individual intolerances* to foods, substances, chemicals or electromagnetic fields are not only conceivable, but have been observed by therapists with open eyes and minds.

The 'trigger'-food tyranny

I think it is foolish to blame particular foods for the *individual* allergies, sensitivities and intolerances of a relatively small sub-group of *sensitized and reactive* migraineurs.

I think it is misguided to compile a list of these foods and effectively hypnotize all other anxious migraineurs *without* any allergies, sensitivities or intolerances into the belief that they too are vulnerable to the malicious powers of 'trigger' foods.

I think the need to explain the occurrence of a migraine attack will inevitably lead to *superstition and more fear* in even the most un-allergic, unreactive and insensitive migraineurs and indeed make an attack more likely.

I think the current regime of 'trigger'-food avoidance is more harmful than helpful for the vast majority of migraineurs.

What do you think?

---

[1] Millán-Guerrero RO et al "Subcutaneous histamine versus sodium valproate in migraine prophylaxis: a randomized, controlled, double-blind study" Eur J Neurol 2007;14(10):1079-84

[2] Millán-Guerrero RO et al "Subcutaneous histamine versus topiramate in migraine prophylaxis: a double-blind study" Eur Neurol 2008;59(5):237-42

[3] Millán-Guerrero RO et al "Subcutaneous histamine versus botulinum toxin type A in migraine prophylaxis: a randomized, double-blind study" Eur J Neurol 2009;16(1):88-94

[4] Wills AJ et al "The neurology of gluten sensitivity: separating the wheat from the chaff" Curr Opin Neurol 2002;15(5):519-23

Are migraine attacks 'triggered' at all?

The recommendation to identify and avoid migraine triggers is based on the following *assumptions*:

1.) Migraine attacks are mainly triggered and rarely occur spontaneously or cyclically.
2.) The 'triggers' can be identified and avoided.
3.) The avoidance of migraine 'triggers' leads to fewer attacks.

The neurologist Prof. Dr. Ambar Chakravarty from the Vivekananda Institute of Medical Science elaborated in an article in the journal "Medical Hypothesis" in 2010 on his *theory* that all migraine attacks are triggered.[1] Chakravaty's *hypothesis* is not entirely new, a similar article was published by different authors in a different journal in 2005.[2] It is remarkable that the authors of both articles speak of migraine attacks as being mostly triggered as their *hypothesis* (= an interesting and unproven opinion).

In contrast to the trigger *theory*, three other prominent migraine scientists from Italy and Belgium explain the details of the migraine *cycle* as a mainly *time-based* process[3] in "Headache – Handbook of Clinical Neurology" 2011. They effectively summarize 198 studies investigating the electrophysiological behavior of migraine brains with various measurement techniques conducted over more than a decade in dozens of electrophysiological research laboratories.

German scientists from the Department of Systems Neuroscience reported in February 2011 that they could *predict* the onset of the next migraine attack, based on the activity in a certain brain area, which proves mainly *cyclical* mechanisms in migraine (timer).

Now we have no idea who is right: The authors who present an *unproven hypothesis* or the researchers who show with an *abundance of facts* — discovered in precise measurements and brain scans — that migraine is mainly a cyclical/time-based process.

Isn't it interesting, there is *no* scientific evidence *for* 'trigger' avoidance *and* lot of proof *against* it, but patients get fed the same, 'Pontadera-like' advice over and over again.

---

[1] Chakravati A "How triggers trigger acute migraine attacks: A hypothesis" Med Hypotheses 2010;74(4):750-3
[2] Burstein R et al "Unitary hypothesis for multiple triggers of the pain and strain of migraine" J Comp Neurol 2005;493(1):9-14
[3] Ambrosini A et al "Migraine – clinical neurophysiology" in Handbook of Clinical Neurology Vol. 97 3rd series 2011 Nappi/Moskowitz Editors, Elsevier B.V.

One day it will become clear that the truth lies somewhere in the middle: The migraine cycle is irregular and can be accelerated and decelerated by many factors. Sometimes migraine attacks can even be initiated, but that depends on the phase of the migraine cycle,[1] the instability of the brain and the strength of the initiating factor: Hormonal fluctuations are probably stronger than broccoli.

The danger of ignoring the cyclical nature of migraine is that understandably anxious migraineurs end up behaving like the pigeons in B. F. Skinner's experiment. They create an anxious dance around suspected 'trigger' foods, even those to which they are not allergic or sensitized, and so drive themselves deeper and deeper into the soft ground of chronification.

'Experts' who have nothing to offer but hollow warnings (like the pompous Tomasso di Andrea da Pontedera) and the advice to avoid life, are useless fear-mongers and shouldn't be listened to.

Henk van Haaren recognized decades ago that avoidance is not a therapeutic strategy. His insight made it possible that patients with trembling disorder can learn to lead a symptom-free life.

I wonder how much longer it will take until migraineurs come to the same decision and start building their own resistance against 'wind and weather' to achieve the necessary stability to cope with and enjoy life rather than avoid it.[2]

In the meantime, in order to be safe, migraineurs should eat a healthy and balanced diet and make sure they avoid everything on this list of migraine 'trigger' foods: [3,4,5,6,7,8,9,10,11,12,13,14,15,16,17,18,19,20] ➡

---

[1] Siniatchkin M et al "How the brain anticipates an attack: a study of neurophysiological periodicity in migraine" Funct Neurol 1999;14(2):69-77
[2] Martin PR "Managing headache triggers: think 'coping' not 'avoidance'" Cephalalgia 2010;30(5):634-7
[3] Buchholz D "Heal your headache: The 1-2-3 Program for Taking Charge of Your Pain" Workman Publishing 2002
[4] http://www.webmd.com/migraines-headaches/guide/triggers-specific-foods
[5] http://www.total-headache-relief.com/FoodTriggers.htm
[6] http://www.migraines.org/treatment/migraine_food_triggers.htm
[7] http://www.helpforheadaches.com/articles/migraine_food_triggers.htm
[8] http://www.chetday.com/migrainetriggers.htm
[9] http://www.nationalpainfoundation.org/articles/702/food-triggers-and-migraine
[10] http://www.beyondheadaches.com/migraine-food-triggers.html
[11] http://www.uhs.berkeley.edu/home/healthtopics/pdf/triggers.pdf
[12] http://www.bbc.co.uk/dna/h2g2/A882876
[13] http://www.thechart.blogs.cnn.com/2011/05/16/what-foods-trigger-migraines/
[14] http://altmedicine.about.com/od/popularhealthdiets/a/migrainediet.htm
[15] http://www.suite101.com/content/what-foods-can-trigger-migraines-a41662
[16] http://www.headache-adviser.com/migraine-food-triggers.html
[17] http://headache.emedtv.com/migraines/migraine-food-triggers.html
[18] http://www.netplaces.com/migraines/avoiding-triggers/food-triggers.htm
[19] http://www.bupa.com.au/health-and-wellness/hubs/health-conditions/pain/articles/doc/migraines-and-headaches
[20] http://www.help-for-migraines.com/migraine-food-triggers.html

anchovies, apple juice, aspartame, avocados, bacon, bagels fresh, banana, beans pole, board, navy, fava, lima, Italian, pinto, garbanzo, beef, beer, berries canned, bourbon, broccoli, buttermilk, carob, cauliflower, caviar, celery, champagne, cheese blue, cheese brie, cheese parmesan, cheese Romano, cheese camembert, cheese aged, cheese feta, cheese mozzarella, cheese provolone, cheese Swiss, cheesecake, chicken liver, chili peppers, chocolate light, chocolate dark, cider, clementine, cocoa, coconut, coffee, coffee cake, corned beef, cream, dates, decaffeinated coffee, decaffeinated tea, doughnuts fresh, dried fruit i.e. raisins sultanas and currents, dried meat jerky, eggplant, energy drinks, fig, fish dried, fish salted, fish smoked, fruit dried, garlic, gluten, grape juice, grapefruit, gum sugar free, ham, herring, hot dogs, ice cream, kiwifruit, lemon, lentils, lettuce, lime, liverwurst, lox, meat tenderizer, meats aged, meats cured, meats smoked, milk, miso, MSG, mushrooms, nuts, olives, onions, oranges, papaya, passion fruit, pastrami, pate, pea pods, peanut butter, peas, pepperoni, pickled food, pineapple, pizza dough, pork, potatoes, raspberries, red plums, red wine, salami, sauerkraut, sausage, seasoned salt, seeds of pumpkin, sesame and sunflower, shellfish, sherry, shrimp paste, snow peas, soft pretzels fresh, soup canned, sour cream, sourdough bread fresh, soy sauce, spinach, stock cubes, strawberry, tangerine, tea, tempeh, teriyaki sauce, tomato, vermouth, vinegar, wheat, whiskey, white wine, yeast baked bread fresh, yoghurt, zest.

Chapter 5

Psycho Terror in Migraine Land

> "When I despair, I remember that all through history
> the ways of truth and love have always won.
> There have been tyrants and murderers, and for a time they seem invincible,
> but in the end they always fall. Think of it – always."
>
> Mahatma Gandhi

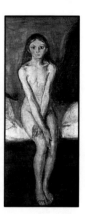

Migraine is like life; some people cope incredibly well with the difficulties they encounter. Think of a young woman—let's call her Clare—who has her first migraine attack at the end of a particularly stressful week. After a weekend of intense pain and being sick, Clare decides to limit her workload to a reasonable amount and informs her boss on Monday. She begins a regular exercise program on Tuesday and sticks with it. As a result, she never has another migraine attack ever again. This is how Clare deals with problems.

Compare that to the stories of *those* migraineurs who struggle for years and decades and can't get their migraine under control. Many of them try several doctors, countless medications and a few alternative therapies before they finally end up in a specialized headache clinic as so-called 'difficult' patients.[1]

Wouldn't it be interesting to find out what the difference is between those 'difficult' patients and Clare? Of course, Clare isn't suffering from frequent and severe migraine attacks and therefore doesn't need to see a headache specialist, but there is no question that she has the genetic 'talent' for migraine. That makes her a recovered migraineur, but not a non-migraineur.

We could say, that Clare was sickeningly *lucky*. I bet everybody has the feeling that there are some people who attract good fortune like warm cow dung attracts flies. This may even be *true*, because of an effect that we call cumulative advantage.[2]

---

[1] Loder E "The approach to the difficult patient" in Headache – Handbook of Clinical Neurology Vol. 97 3rd series 2011 Nappi/Moskowitz Editors, Elsevier B.V.

[2] O'Rand AM "The precious and the precocious: understanding cumulative disadvantage and cumulative advantage over the life course" Gerontologist 1996;36(2):230-8

The term cumulative advantage expresses that for people with more and better resources (money, knowledge, abilities, social support etc.) it is easier to be successful and even to extend their resources (more money, more knowledge, more abilities, more social support etc.) than for people with poor resources (no money, no knowledge, no abilities, no social support etc.).

Do 'difficult' migraine patients perhaps have a *cumulative disadvantage*? Are there mechanisms at play that turn migraine patients into 'difficult' ones? Let's find out!

What is a 'difficult' migraine patient?

Doctors typically find those patients 'difficult', who present with *anxiety* or *depression*.[1] A French study of over 5000 migraine patients in primary care found 67% suffered from anxiety, of which 60% also had depression. In other words, *two thirds* of migraineurs in French doctors' care were somewhat 'difficult'.

UK hospital doctors found patients 'difficult', who were *distressed, dissatisfied* and *showed up frequently*.[2] We can safely assume that the majority of migraineurs are more or less distressed and there are reasons for that: Medications for the torturous attack symptoms often don't work as well as advertised and other options are rarely offered. The fact that these patients frequently return for consultations, despite being dissatisfied, indicates that they don't see any options other than consulting an unsatisfying doctor.

UK neurologists found those patients difficult to help, whose symptoms are *not explained by organic disease*.[3] Migraine itself is not well explained by a model of 'organic disease'. Many of the comorbidities of migraine form a group of disorders with the label 'medically unexplained symptoms' or 'functional somatic syndromes': fibromyalgia, irritable bowel syndrome, chronic fatigue syndrome and idiopathic environmental intolerance etc. Just like migraine, these disorders are closely connected to anxiety and depression,[4] but can't be explained by simply *labeling* them as "psycho-somatic". There is much more to them than meets the eye.

---

[1] Hahn SR et al "The difficult patient: prevalence, psychopathology, and functional impairment" J Gen Intern Med 1996;11(1):1-8
[2] Sharpe M et al "Why do doctors find some patients difficult to help?" Q J Med 1994;87(3):187-93
[3] Carson AJ "Patients whom neurologists find difficult to help" J Neurol Neurosurg Psychiatry 2004;75(12):1776-8
[4] Henningsen P et al "Medically unexplained physical symptoms, anxiety, and depression: a meta-analytic review" Psychosom Med. 2003;65(4):528-33

Migraineurs' special sensitivity

Talking about mood disorders or migraineurs' personality traits can be dangerous in the presence of some patients who angrily insist: "MIGRAINES ARE NEUROLOGICAL, NOT PSYCHOLOGICAL."

I empathize with the apparent fear of being categorized as a 'psycho case' and I obviously support the wish to be taken seriously. It is not my intention to demolish anyone's reassuring thought model of migraine as a *'disease that spares the soul'* — unless that belief interferes with successful rehabilitation.

There comes a point in the progression of severe migraine, when it must be possible to take a factual look at the psychological *impact* of migraine, at the psychological *response* to migraine and at the psychological *profiles* and *behaviors* that help drive patients into chronification.

Denial doesn't make things go away. In very early childhood we believe that the world disappears, when we hold our hands in front of our eyes. Later we understand that things do exist, even when we choose not to look at them.

Another author asserts that "MIGRAINE IS REAL AND NOT PSYCHOLOGICAL OR EMOTIONAL ..." Is the intense emotional experience of migraine *not real*? Fake perhaps? Made up? Just a show? — He goes on by saying: "... SO NO ONE SHOULD BLAME YOU FOR YOUR HEADACHES." In contrast, I don't think that patients deserve to be *blamed*, if they find a connection between their migraine and their thoughts and emotions.

The attitudes that shine through those weird assertions seem fearful and illogical to me. We need to address these *irrational thoughts*, because they distract us from constructive questions like 'What can we learn from Clare?'

One author's defensiveness even extends to the phrase "YOUR HEADACHES ARE ALL IN YOUR HEAD", which he understands as "IT'S YOUR FAULT". Wouldn't it be an absolute blessing for migraineurs to find the 'fault' in the brain that leads to migraine, so that by correcting that very 'fault' the attacks could be stopped? What would you rather be, a 'suffering innocent victim' or an ex-migraineur with a fixed brain?

In part II of this book, we will learn that the brain doesn't really care whether we call a particular function *'neurological'* or *'psychological'*. And if the brain doesn't care, why do we bother? Let's be reasonable, rational and mature about this crucial topic.

Vicious cycles

The word 'stress' has two meanings. Often it refers to a *distressing situation*, to some form of *threat* that triggers our biological *stress response* in brain and body, which is the second meaning. In short: Distressing situations trigger a stress response.

For migraine that has massive consequences, because it can (and it does) create a vicious cycle: Stress (here: the stress response) precipitates migraine attacks and frequent severe migraine attacks inevitably create stress (here: a distressing situation). In short: Migraine causes migraine attacks.[1] That puts questions about coping with stress (here: distressing situations) and recovery from stress (here: the stress response) on the table.

In experiments, migraineurs showed a diminished capacity to recover from mental distress[2] or performance anxiety.[3] Does this mean that—on average—the migraineurs experienced the same mental challenge as more 'threatening' than did the controls, and therefore had a *stronger stress response*? This would be in harmony with findings of lower self-esteem in migraineurs,[4] which is a known consequence of chronic illness,[5] or feelings of unworthiness ("I'm not good enough"), which are associated with depression.[6]

The idea sounds plausible. However, the body's stress response is actually not stronger in migraineurs.[7] The delayed recovery after stress is not even related to shortfalls in calming the body,[8] but due to *deficits in calming the brain*.[9] This in turn is in accordance with a tendency towards anxiety.

In this context the term anxiety should not be understood as anxious feelings, but rather as a form of *brain arousal*, which can show as restlessness, nervousness, apprehension, tension, irritability, impatience, agitation, annoyance and so on. Perhaps one should rather think of 'anxiety' as 'too much energy'.

---

[1] Sauro KM et al "The stress and migraine interaction" Headache. 2009;49(9):1378-86
[2] Stronks DL et al "Personality traits and psychological reactions to mental stress of female migraine patients" Cephalalgia 1999;19(6):566-74
[3] Holm JE et al "The stress response in headache sufferers: physiological and psychological reactivity" Headache 1997;37(4):221-7
[4] Bormann M et al "Coping with stress and pain in migraine patients" Schmerz 1989;3(4):195-203
[5] Huurre TM et al "Long-term psychosocial effects of persistent chronic illness. A follow-up study of Finnish adolescents aged 16 to 32 years" Eur Child Adolesc Psychiatry 2002;11(2):85-91
[6] Shapiro MB "Self-reported feelings in clinical depression: an analysis of published data" Br J Med Psychol. 198;56 (Pt 3):211-23
[7] Shechter A et al "Migraine and autonomic nervous system function: a population-based, case-control study" Neurology 2002;58(3):422-7
[8] Benjelloun H et al "Autonomic profile of patients with migraine" Neurophysiol Clin 2005;35(4):127-34
[9] Kröner-Herwig B et al "Psychophysiological reactivity of migraine sufferers in conditions of stress and relaxation" Source J Psychosom Res 1988;32(4-5):483-92

In fact, migraineurs — on average — were found to have a low awareness of their emotional state,[1] a reduced mindfulness, which academics call *alexithymia* (= Latin for 'no words for feelings').[2,3] In plain words: Many migraineurs don't really know how they feel, because their brains are too 'revved up' for that.

Because of the higher brain arousal, alexithymia plays a role in many migraineurs' high reactivity.[4] It is involved in elevated pain sensitivity[5] and correlated to the level of unpleasantness of chronic pain.[6] In migraineurs alexithymia is associated with anxiety and depression,[7] factors that make them appear 'difficult'.

Another long-term consequence of the persistent distress of severe migraine is the development of a personality trait called 'secondary *neuroticism*'.[8] The terms 'neurotic' and 'neuroticism' sound almost 'gaga', but they merely express a stronger than average tendency to *experience negative emotions* like fear, sadness, anger, shame, guilt and so on; basically all the unpleasant emotions, that one would expect in chronic illness and pain.

This negative emotional load ("neuroticism") obviously adds to the distress and now we're facing a second and very vicious cycle: Migraineurs with 'hidden anxiety'[1] (alexithymia), who do not respond well to treatment, get distressed and get worse, and are increasingly burdened by their developing neuroticism and therefore get even '*worser*'. That is exactly what studies show.[9,10,11]

Migraine is a progressive brain disorder, affecting body and mind; whether it responds well to treatment or *does* progress into a quality-of-life-threatening condition, depends on emotions, beliefs, thoughts and behaviors.[12] That's good news: Room for change!

---

[1] Muftuoglu MN et al "Alexithymic features in migraine patients" Eur Arch Psychiatry Clin Neurosci 2004;254(3):182-6
[2] Taylor GJ "Alexithymia: concept, measurement, and implications for treatment" Am J Psychiatry 1984;141(6):725-32
[3] Baiardini I et al "Alexithymia and chronic diseases: the state of the art" G Ital Med Lav Ergon 2011;33(1Suppl A):A47-52
[4] Karlsson H et al "Cortical activation in alexithymia as a response to emotional stimuli" Br J Psychiatry 2008;192(1):32-8
[5] Nyklícek I et al "Alexithymia is associated with low tolerance to experimental painful stimulation" Pain 2000;85(3):471-5
[6] Lumley MA et al "The relationship of alexithymia to pain severity and impairment among patients with chronic myofascial pain: comparisons with self-efficacy, catastrophizing, and depression" J Psychosom Res 2002;53(3):823-30
[7] Yalug I et al "Correlations between alexithymia and pain severity, depression, and anxiety among patients with chronic and episodic migraine" Psychiatry Clin Neurosci 2010;64(3):231-8
[8] Huber D et al "Personality traits and stress sensitivity in migraine patients" Source Behav Med 2003;29(1):4-13
[9] Mongini F et al "Personality traits, depression and migraine in women: a longitudinal study" Cephalalgia. 2003 Apr;23(3):186-92
[10] Lucas C et al "The GRIM2005 study of migraine consultation in France II. Psychological factors associated with treatment response to acute headache therapy and satisfaction in migraine" Cephalalgia 2007;27(12):1398-407
[11] Radat F et al "Anxiety, stress and coping behaviours in primary care migraine patients: results of the SMILE study" Cephalalgia 2008;28(11):1115-25
[12] Passchier J et al "Evaluation of the Dutch version of the migraine quality of life instrument (MSQOL) and its application in headache coping" Cephalalgia 2001;21(8):823-9

The power of the mind

At the time when God took his holy soldering iron out of the celestial toolbox to create the circuits in Adam's and Eve's brains, the world was a different place. Dangerous predators were roaming the savannah and the human fight for survival would be an uphill-battle against faster and stronger creatures with considerably larger teeth. And so God designed the stress response, which enables us to quickly climb up a tree, whenever hungry lions can't be bothered to run after antelopes and choose to hunt humans instead.

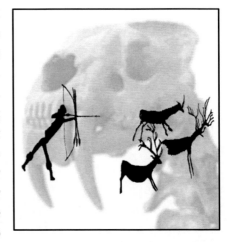

"Thou shalt not deliberate, when beasts are coming for you" God murmured and installed a control circuit that turns down the activity of our thought processor in the prefrontal cortex[1] (PFC) in favor of more primitive, yet faster actions.[2] Typically these simple behaviors are running away or climbing a tree, thereby escaping the threat, since humans are rather fragile in comparison to lions, bears or a pack of wolves. So we tend to lose our ability to think straight, when our brains are in a state of high distress and fear.

This emergency effect — simple when stressed — still shows up occasionally, for instance as stage fright (a nervous actor forgets his lines) or test anxiety (a scared student can't find the answer).

In situations that are only moderately upsetting, but not life threatening, the prefrontal cortex normally keeps its astuteness by putting a lid on stress and anxiety.[3] However, when the prefrontal cortex (PFC) is a tad 'weak-ish', as is the case in migraineurs,[4] it can't quite control distress and anxiety. The unfortunate effect is a certain loss of sharpness, logic and sound judgment.[5,6]

---

[1] Mobbs D et al "When fear is near: threat imminence elicits prefrontal- shifts in humans" Science 2007;317(5841):1079-83
[2] Murray EA et al "Interactions between orbital prefrontal cortex and amygdaly: Advanced cognition, learned responsive and instictive behaviors" Curr Opin Neurobiol 2010;20(2):212-20
[3] Marsh R et al "A developmental fMRI study of self-regulatory control" Source Hum Brain Mapp 2006;27(11):848-63
[4] Mongini F et al "Frontal lobe dysfunction in patients with chronic migraine: a clinical-neuropsychological study" Psychiatry Res 2005;133(1):101-6
[5] Camarda C et al "Interictal executive dysfunction in migraineurs without aura: relationship with duration and intensity of attacks" Cephalalgia 2007;27(10):1094-100
[6] Karceski SC "How migraines affect cognitive function" Neurology 2007;68(17):E23-4

As a consequence many migraineurs don't see when they get duped by fanciful fairy-tales and misleading myths about migraine mechanisms or offered treatments that are illogical, invasive and ineffective, such as the amputation of muscles accused of causing migraine by allegedly pinching and squeezing facial nerves.[1]

People whose judgment is not handicapped by their brain's emergency mode have a chance to spot the holes in the surgeon's fairy-tale of the pinched nerves and might ask probing questions:

"Mister Surgeon, how does the alleged nerve-pinch cause all the other symptoms of a migraine attack? Let's start with premonitory symptoms like changes in mood, thinking, speech, self-control, alertness, appetite, water balance, digestion, body temperature, coordination and sensory tolerance. After that, can you explain how the pinched nerve produces an aura with visual disturbances or visual hallucinations, somatosensory symptoms like tingling or numbness, funny smells, awkward sounds and those remarkable difficulties with speech and language comprehension? Finally, Mr. Surgeon, when I get my headaches, how can the allegedly pinched nerve cause dizziness, nausea, vomiting, diarrhea, sensitivity to glare, noise and odor, runny or stuffy nose and all the other symptoms, plus that feeling of being very very ill? How does the nerve-pinch do that? And if my face muscles are responsible for pinching those nerves, how come there is not a single grimace that causes any discomfort: smiling, frowning and so on, how can that possibly be the case, if your story were even the tiniest bit true?"

In this example, all we're doing is comparing the hypothesis ("migraine attacks are caused by pinched nerves") to the real world observations that every migraineur has made too many times.

I don't expect everybody to know that nerves get pinched all the time all over the body; that's normal for a nerve. Also, pinched nerves can't hurt, because they don't have 'pinch' receptors. When nerves get a whack, it feels 'electric' or tingly, which you know from "bumping your funny bone" (the nerve outside your elbow). Long-term compression of nerves can lead to a loss of sensation, but nerves — in spite of the frequent blame — rarely cause pain.

So-called migraine surgeons are very clever. They prey on severe and *desperate* migraineurs by announcing that surgery is an option, "when optimal medical management has failed". Then the dubious pinch muscle gets paralyzed with Botox®, supposedly in order to verify that the carving will be helpful. As we've seen in chapter three, success with Botox® is 80-100% due to the placebo effect.

---

[1] Kung TA et al "Migraine surgery: a plastic surgery solution for refractory migraine headache" Plast Reconstr Surg 2011;127(1):181-9

That means the surgeons select those patients, who have a good placebo response to Botox®, which makes it likely that they'll also have a good placebo response to the mutilation. Surgery achieves the highest placebo effects known to man and for that, migraine surgery *might even work* on carefully selected responders. It would be more humane to create impressive placebo treatments without the amputation of face muscles. But back to migraineurs:

Robbed of their astute judgment,[1] most severe migraineurs can't help but accept misleading information and adopt *unhelpful beliefs*, which promotes further aggravation. In contrast, a sharp mind in a calm brain can recognize the *cognitive distortions* in some of the messages floating through migraine land.

Disturbing thoughts

Cognitive distortions are also called *bad thinking habits* or 'errors in thinking'. They lead to additional fear, anxiety, hostility and depression[2] and become *massive* obstacles for any attempt to escape the migraine tyranny. For a suffering mind in a distressed brain, burdened by neuroticism and alexithymia, the last anchor to protect sanity is *logical thinking* to make smart decisions and to find pragmatic solutions. Bad thinking habits (cognitive distortions) can be *detrimental* in such a difficult situation. For that very reason we need to look into some of these *unhelpful* thought patterns[3] as they show up in books and on websites about migraine:

Absolutistic thinking is the term for mixing up thoughts with reality, based on the narcissistic belief "If I think so, then it is so." Since this type of overbearing thinking categorically rules out the possibility of errors and thereby insight and learning, it can't adapt to new knowledge or changing circumstances.

One migraine-book author explicitly writes about his diet program: "NO 'SCIENTIFIC DATA' TO THE CONTRARY, FROM A RANDOMIZED CONTROLLED TRIAL OR ANY OTHER SOURCE, WOULD EVER CONVINCE ME OTHERWISE." When you look at history you'll find many examples of how extreme ideologies based on rigid beliefs in overly determined persons have brought a lot of suffering to mankind.

---

[1] Calandre EP et al "Cognitive disturbances and regional cerebral blood flow abnormalities in migraine patients: their relationship with the clinical manifestations of the illness" Cephalalgia 2002;22(4):291-302
[2] Brent DA et al "Suicidality in affectively disordered adolescent inpatients" J Am Acad Child Adolesc Psychiatry 1990;29(4):586-93
[3] Doverspike WF "How Cognitive Distortions Cause Emotional Distress" Georgia Psychological Association 2011 www.gapsychology.org

Arbitrary inference is drawing a conclusion without any evidence or even *against* existing evidence, and also failing to test a thought against reality. "MIGRAINE CAN'T BE CURED." is an example of such an *unhelpful*, unsubstantiated and untrue declaration.

Catastrophizing refers to imagining the worst possible scenario and dwelling on related worries and fears without even considering the likelihood of the pictured disaster. Endless "what-if"-questions about the potential negative consequences of a decision can result in a 'behavioral paralysis', because none of the options can ever offer *absolute* certainty. The anxious thought "What, if this medication has side effects?" makes side effects more likely.[1] Catastrophizing makes pain worse[2] and life hell.[3]

Cognitive deficiency or ***denial*** occurs when an important aspect of a situation is ignored or negated. An angrily yelled "I AM NOT EMOTIONALLY DISTRESSED AT ALL"[4] is an obvious example.

Demanding and ***commanding*** can be recognized by the use of "should" or "ought". They focus on how things *should* be instead of on either how to improve a situation or how to make the best of it. "Doctors should have more time for migraine patients" is wishful thinking that only produces anger and disappointment, but doesn't generate any extra time for and with the doctor.

Dichotomous reasoning is also called 'black-and-white' thinking. It wrongly assumes that things are always 'either-or' (black or white) and not both (black *and* white) or something in between (gray) or something different (colorful). "MIGRAINE IS NEUROLOGICAL, NOT PSYCHOLOGICAL." is an example, which asserts one statement by negating the other, although both may be true.

Disqualifying the positive is behind the behavior to shoot down new ideas for arbitrary and invalid reasons. "THAT THERAPY CAN'T BE GOOD, BECAUSE I'VE NEVER HEARD OF IT BEFORE." The problem here is, that the speaker might even have convinced himself, that his grumpy and dismissive reasoning was reasonable.

---

[1] Fillingim RB et al "Sex-related psychological predictors of baseline pain perception and analgesic responses to pentazocine" Biol Psychol 2005;69(1):97-112
[2] Campbell CM et al "Situational versus dispositional measurement of catastrophizing: associations with pain responses in multiple samples" J Pain 2010;11(9):876-84
[3] Holroyd KA et al "Impaired functioning and quality of life in severe migraine: the role of catastrophizing and associated symptoms" Cephalalgia 2007;27(10):1156-65
[4] Cottrell et al. "Perceptions and Needs of Patients with Migraine: A Focus Study Group" J Fam Pract 2002; 51(2): 142-147

Jumping to conclusions describes how distressed minds often process information in haste and without questioning whether an idea is logical and stringent. "Last night I ate a tomato, today I have a migraine attack, therefore I know, without any doubt, that the tomato triggered the migraine attack." This omits the option that the attack was sparked by something else (e.g. the hunger before dinner) or not 'triggered', but due.

Labeling expresses the habit to use a buzzword or a phrase in a thought or discussion without being aware of its meaning or the ramifications. An example is the phrase "MIGRAINE IS GENETIC" that gets copied from book to book and from website to website, without explanation as to what it means. The consequence is that laypeople are forced to come up with their own interpretation, which is not necessarily what the original scientific author meant to say.

Mind reading occurs when a person believes that they know what other people are thinking or feeling without asking. "If I go to the emergency room, they'll think that I'm a drug-seeker." This delusion burdens people with the need to fulfill non-existent demands.

Minimization is the term for turning something important into a minor issue. For example in a report about possible side effects of Botox®: "... cases that required feeding by 'nasogastric tube' (a hose through the nose into the stomach) have been rare." This is indeed a minor issue for the doctor, but a major issue for the affected patients.

Overgeneralization means uncritically extending the validity of a fact beyond sensible limits. A typical migraine example is the statement "CITRUS FRUITS ARE TRIGGER FOODS" based on someone's report that his or her migraine attack was allegedly triggered by an orange. Even if that could be proven, that does not mean that *all* citrus fruits are potential migraine triggers for *all* migraineurs. It is not always easy to spot overgeneralization, because absolute words (all, everybody, always, nobody) are often not expressed but clearly implied. In my experience very few things in life are always true or always false, so never say never ever again!

Prophesying or *fortune telling* is predicting a typically grim future as in "I bet I'll have a migraine attack during my daughter's wedding." Pessimistic predictions burden the soul with premature negative feelings and tend to come true as 'self-fulfilling prophecies'. Why would you not imagine a positive future scenario to lift the spirit?

Reasoning with Emotions as in "...BECAUSE I HATE MEDICATION" is unhelpful when mature thinking is required to weigh up facts and make rational judgments in order to find a way out of the dark.

One can make it a habit to observe one's own thinking to identify cognitive distortions. The goal is <u>not</u> *the extinction of wrong ideas*, which could easily lead to being rigid, righteous and judgmental. Instead, it is about making sure that the majority of thoughts and statements become part of this *magic alphabet*:

ADVANTAGEOUS, BENEFICIAL, COMPASSIONATE, DEPENDABLE, ENCOURAGING, FUNNY, GENEROUS, HELPFUL, INSPIRING, JOLLY, KIND, LIBERATING, MOTIVATING, NICE, POSITIVE, REASSURING, SUPPORTIVE, TRUSTWORTHY, USEFUL, VALUABLE, WORTHWHILE, X-HILARATING, YIPPEE OR ZESTY — Wouldn't you like that?

The half empty glass

Have you heard of PLWES (Post Lottery Win Euphoria Syndrome)? That is a severe psychiatric disorder of a constant state of elation and euphoria, caused by an overly exciting and lucky life event. The affected patients are stuck in happiness and can't shake off their positive memories. Have you never heard of it?

Have you at least heard of PTSD (Post Traumatic Stress Disorder)? Following life-threatening or otherwise traumatic events, sometimes people don't recover fully from the extreme stress of the experience.[1] Typical examples are soldiers, crime victims or disaster survivors, whose nervous systems remain altered in a state of hypervigilance (= over-alertness, constantly looking for threats, over-responsiveness to sensory stimuli, increased brain arousal).

Due to the hypervigilance, patients with PTSD struggle with relaxation and sleep[2], which sooner or later leads to emotional turmoil (neuroticism)[3] and behavioral problems, for example hostility[4] or alcoholism[5]; but also migraine[6] and other pain issues.[7]

When you look at brain activity and hypervigilance, you will find quite a few similarities between migraine and PTSD.

---

[1] D'Souza D "Post-traumatic stress disorder--a scar for life" Br J Clin Pract 1995;49(6):309-13
[2] Westermeyer J et al "Quality of sleep in patients with posttraumatic stress disorder" Psychiatry (Edgmont) 2010;7(9):21-7
[3] Cox BJ et al "Neuroticism and self-criticism associated with posttraumatic stress disorder in a nationally representative sample" Source Behav Res Ther 2004;42(1):105-14
[4] Kubany ES et al "Relationship of cynical hostility and PTSD among Vietnam veterans" J Trauma Stress 1994;7(1):21-31
[5] Gruden V et al "PTSD and alcoholism" Coll Antropol 1999;23(2):607-10
[6] Peterlin BL et al "Post-traumatic stress disorder, drug abuse and migraine: new findings from the National Comorbidity Survey Replication (NCS-R)" Cephalalgia 2011;31(2):235-44
[7] Frayne SM et al "Medical care needs of returning veterans with PTSD: their other burden" J Gen Intern Med 2011;26(1):33-9

In contrast, there are no similarities between migraine and PLWES (post lottery win euphoria syndrome), because there is no such thing as a disorder of too much happiness in the brain, of course. The interesting question is: Why not?

The answer is quite sobering: Happiness has no value for survival on the savannah. If there were ever any jolly jokers amongst our early ancestors, who were merrily frolicking or blithely gallivanting across the sun-burnt open plains, bubbly and boisterous, exultant and exuberant, with a blissful smile and sunshine on their faces, lost in beautiful daydreams whilst enjoying being tickled by the high grass, ALL of them were killed; by lions, hyenas, wild dogs, snakes or scorpions, you name it. And so they missed out on procreation and passing on a copy of their happy genes to the next generation. Logically, the ones with the best chance of survival and reproduction in that kind of neighborhood were the anxious, nervous, cranky, highly vigilant cowards. In other words: It was us who survived.

Bad is stronger than good

Our brain's obsession with potential threats to our survival is called *negativity bias*.[1] It ensures that any piece of information that might be the tiniest bit threatening ('negative') to a hunter-gatherer, grabs our subconscious attention[2] within milliseconds[3] and gets the highest priority on every level of information processing.[4] The negativity bias makes our body reactive and clips our capacity for clever consideration[5]. It even gives neutral information a negative spin.[6] Think of the sentence "You never know, what's gonna happen." Doesn't it sound a little concerning? It's a completely neutral statement. That what's going to happen may well be positive, but our brain tends to find uncertainty negative. Thus the negativity bias makes even tranquil brains prone to producing negative emotions,[7] which trigger negative thoughts when we're distressed.

---

[1] Baumeister RF et al "Bad Is Stronger Than Good" Rev Gen Psychol 2001;5(4):323-370
[2] Ito TA et al "Negative information weighs more heavily on the brain: the negativity bias in evaluative categorisations" J Pers Soc Psychol 1998;75(4):887-900
[3] Smith NK et al "May I have your attention, please: electrocortical responses to positive and negative stimuli" Neuropsychologia 2003;41(2):171-83
[4] Huang YX et al "Temporal course of emotional negativity bias: an ERP study" Neurosci Lett. 2006;398(1-2):91-6
[5] Gordon E et al "An "integrative neuroscience" platform: application to profiles of negativity and positivity bias" J Integr Neurosci 2008;7(3):345-66
[6] Yang W et al "Time course of affective processing bias in major depression: An ERP study" Neurosci Lett. 2011;487(3):372-7
[7] Watters AJ et al "Negative biases and risk for depression; integrating self-report and emotion task markers" Depress Anxiety 2011;28(8):703-18

It is no surprise then that negative thinking (pessimism) in turn increases the stress response,[1] and voilà, another vicious cycle that drives severely affected patients deeper into despair: Stress promotes pessimism, pessimism nurtures stress.

God meant really well, when he even installed a specialized organ into each hemisphere (= half) of our human brain, which not only scans all the incoming information for negative content, but also stores negative events as memories. This threat-detection organ is called amygdala (= Latin for almond) and it makes sure that we remember negative stuff well.[2] Since human brains don't have a similar organ for positive information, bad memories are stronger than good ones.[3] In essence, our human brain is like Velcro for negative experiences and like Teflon for positive ones:[4] Bad stuff sticks, good stuff slips off. No wonder that we're grumpy.

We must admit, the negativity bias did work for us as a species, since we did survive the savannah and meanwhile have lions, bears and other predators well under control. The downside is, that although we now live in a world with very few natural dangers and almost unlimited possibilities, we are still slaves to a pessimistic savannah-brain, which constantly overestimates risks and underestimates opportunities, possibilities and resources.

Learning helplessness

Two dogs were strapped into harnesses for an experiment. Both had a panel in their respective cage that operated an off-switch, but only for dog A was the 'panel-switch' connected. The researcher pressed a button and both dogs, A and B, received a painful electric shock for 30 seconds. Of course, both dogs tried to do something about the pain and it didn't take long until they pressed the panels. Dog B couldn't switch the power off, his panel-switch was disconnected. In contrast, dog A succeeded; and so with every trial, dog A got faster at pressing the panel and switching the power off; it got literally *empowered*. But what about dog B?

---

[1] Williams LM et al "'Negativity bias' in risk for depression and anxiety: brain-body fear circuitry correlates, 5-HTT-LPR and early life stress" Neuroimage 2009;47(3):804-14
[2] Botzung A et al "Component Neural Systems for the Creation of Emotional Memories during Free Viewing of a Complex, Real-World Event" Front Hum Neurosci 2010;4:34
[3] Moscovitch DA et al "Retrieval properties of negative vs. positive mental images and autobiographical memories in social anxiety: outcomes with a new measure" Behav Res Ther 2011;49(8):505-17
[4] Hanson R "Buddha's Brain: The Practical Neuroscience of Happiness, Love, and Wisdom" New Harbinger Publications 2009

The B-dog soon learned that its panel-pressing had no effect and so it gave up trying. The electric shocks were inescapable and dog B was howling helplessly in that situation.

A second experiment yielded an interesting result. Both dogs were without harnesses inside their little pens when the researcher pressed his button and sent the electric shock through the metal floor plate of the respective pen. Dog A ended the pain by jumping over the fence, problem solved. But what about dog B?

The B-dog endured the whole period of the shock whining and howling and never even tried to jump out of the pen. During the first experiment it had learnt that 'it was helpless' and never 'questioned' that, even though it wasn't in a harness anymore and *could* have jumped over the fence just like dog A did. But dog B did not jump—it *suffered* instead.

Two thirds of the B-dogs showed this learned helplessness, a lack of fighting spirit after experiencing powerlessness in a helpless situation.[1] The decisive mechanism in learning helplessness is the acceptance of the belief that the helplessness is *a quality of the victim*, instead of recognizing that it is a *quality of one special circumstance*, but not of every situation.

We could also say that dog B was so discouraged and miserable, that it developed a *victim-attitude* ("The world is hostile towards me"). During the second experiment it found its victim-status confirmed ("I knew it, oh my God, here we go again"). So dog B was trapped in suffering and despair, when it could have ended the pain by jumping over the little fence of the pen. But dog B didn't even try anymore.

Feeling helpless versus being helpless

How can you not feel helpless during a full-blown migraine attack? Hours of agony and misery do break the spirit and inevitably make you feel helpless to the assault. Unless some medication brings relief, the attack seems inescapable and many migraineurs suffer like dogs. In that sense, a migraine is like the first experiment for dog B in the harness. The inescapable migraine attack is somehow similar to the electric shocks for the helpless dog. However, there is a difference between migraineurs and dogs.

---

[1] Seligman ME et al "Failure to escape traumatic shock" Journal of Experimental Psychology 1967;74(1):1-9

Humans can protect themselves from the effect of learned helplessness with a sharp rational mind, which makes them aware that you may *feel* helpless during a migraine attack, but that doesn't mean that you *are* always helpless against migraine.

This insight, based on knowledge and critical thinking, offers an escape route from the prison of helpless suffering. The understanding that the helpless feeling belongs to the agony and misery *during* an attack makes it possible to explore several options to solve the migraine problem in the phase *between* attacks.

Worry, pessimism and cognitive distortions don't make that task easier, but the human mind is strong enough to overcome negative thoughts and feelings, when there is a clear goal in sight. Think of a marathon runner, who is sick with pain and exhaustion at kilometer 35 (mile 22) and still keeps on fighting to make it to the finish line. Why does he keep going? He knows the pain and exhaustion will be over soon and triumph is achievable.

However, what would happen, if you told the hurting runner that there *is* no finish line, that he *can't* reach his goal, that all his effort is in vain? It would be reasonable for him to be discouraged and give up, because his situation is hopeless. But is it, really?

Factually his situation hasn't changed at all. All that has changed is how he *judges* his circumstances (sick with pain *and* hopeless), because you've told him there was no finish line and he believes that. *You* made him feel hopeless, *you* made him give up. Of course, he is too exhausted and hurting too much. The tired marathon runner doesn't have the astuteness to dismiss your discouraging message and keep running until there is sufficient compelling evidence one way or the other.

So, if there is discouraging information about migraine and the finish line, that indeed could turn temporary feelings of weakness into learned helplessness; that indeed could stimulate a victim attitude; that indeed could foster pessimism and hopelessness; that indeed could make you give up and sink into despair and depression.

Isn't it amazing that there are all these psychological brain mechanisms that make us distressed, simple, anxious, grumpy, pessimistic and helpless; but decisive is, what we *believe* to be true: Unhelpful beliefs are the shackles and chain of migraine and pain.

The deathblow for hope

Let's have a quick look at what messages migraineurs get dished up about migraine and their 'finish line'. The important aspect in *this* chapter is not, what is true and what is false, but what is *helpful* and *en*couraging, and what is *not helpful* and *dis*couraging.

"MIGRAINE IS A PRIMARY HEADACHE"[1]
directs the attention to one symptom of an attack, during which migraineurs typically feel pretty helpless, unless they buy medication; so it's encouraging drugs, it's not encouraging migraineurs.
"MIGRAINE IS SWELLING AND INFLAMMATION OF BLOOD VESSELS AROUND YOUR HEAD."
Well, what can you do about swelling and inflammation other than taking drugs? Breathing exercises definitely can't help you with that, right?
"MIGRAINE IS GENETIC"
suggests that you can't escape, because you carry your genes with you in every cell of your body. Do you find the idea of migraine allegedly being inescapable helpful or encouraging? I don't.
"MIGRAINE CAN'T BE CURED"
is quite a party stopper and leaves no doubt: "There is no finish line for you. You should give up now." Who has a benefit from this disheartening message? Certainly not the patient.

In fact, hopelessness is a popular dark cult in some circles of severe migraineurs. One book author goes so far to instruct her readers to watch out for the word 'cure'. If a book promises a 'cure', the reader is commanded to make a note of the author and not waste any more time reading anything by that offending person.

In other words, if anybody dares to challenge the dark cult of hopelessness, that person is to be censored and ostracized, perhaps even defamed (*"make a note of the author..."*). This kind of appeal is reminiscent of what secret services in totalitarian dictatorships do in order to silence critical voices and to squash resistance at its roots. It is certainly not an appropriate behavior for an author, who pretends to be on the migraineur's side.

Let me make that crystal clear: No matter how helpless and hopeless *someone* might feel in a situation, nobody has the right to drag *others* down into the dungeon of despair, into the hell of hopelessness,[2] into the prison of chronic migraine — nobody.

---

[1] http://ihs-classification.org/en/02_klassifikation/02_teil1/
[2] Pompili M et al "Psychiatric comorbidity and suicide risk in patients with chronic migraine" Neuropsychiatr Dis Treat 2010;6:81-91

The typical argument that the hopeless come up with is: "I DON'T WANT TO GET MY HOPES UP, BECAUSE I'LL BE DISAPPOINTED, WHEN THE ADVERTISED 'CURE' DOESN'T WORK." Constant hopelessness as a protection against potential disappointment? You gotta be kidding! What if the advertised 'cure' would have worked for you? What if you've missed out on an opportunity to halve the frequency of your migraine attacks? Or does hopelessness provide a form of safety?

"THIS ONLY GIVES PEOPLE FALSE HOPES" is another down-turner. Certain approaches to migraine therapy can be *false*, for example when they don't solve the problem. Relying solely on medication can be *false*, for instance when the interval between attacks slowly starts shrinking and the frequency of attacks gradually increases.[1] This could explain why too many migraineurs become dependent on drugs, a horribly *false* strategy.

Getting lost in learned helplessness, which is common in migraine,[2] is *false* because it increases the emotional load and sabotages constructive attempts to reclaim a normal life. Spreading misleading and discouraging information is *false*, because it stops patients from seeking and finding a solution for their specific situation with migraine and getting help on every level. Denying the 'psychological' factors in migraine is *false*, because it is the emotions, beliefs and behaviors that decide whether someone becomes symptom-free or a 'difficult' patient who depends on drugs and doctor's mercy. Not addressing the underlying brain dysfunctions[3] is *false*, because it forces migraineurs in pain to overuse medication and thereby creates additional problems. Immature, emotion-focused coping behaviors like 'acting out' ("LOOK, HOW MUCH I'M SUFFERING, HOW HELPLESS AND HOPELESS I AM!") in order to get sympathy[4] and attention[5] is *false*, because it accelerates the sensitization[6] and chronification[7] through operant conditioning (= learning by reward).[8] — In contrast, hope can *never* be false.

---

[1] Beau-Salinas F et al "Drug dependence associated with triptans and ergot derivatives: a case/non-case study" Eur J Clin Pharmacol 2010;66(4):413-7
[2] Sheftell FD et al "Migraine and psychiatric comorbidity: from theory and hypotheses to clinical application" Headache 2002;42(9):934-44
[3] Gómez-Beldarrain M "Orbitofrontal dysfunction predicts poor prognosis in chronic migraine with medication overuse" J Headache Pain 2011;12(4):459-66
[4] Romano JM et al "Sequential analysis of chronic pain behaviors and spouse responses" J Consult Clin Psychol 1992;60(5):777-82
[5] Gil KM et al "Social support and pain behaviour" Pain 1987;29(2):209-17
[6] Hölzl R et al "Implicit operant learning of pain sensitisation" Pain 2005;115(1-2):12-20
[7] Borkum JM "Chronic headaches and the neurobiology of somatization" Curr Pain Headache Rep 2010;14(1):55-61
[8] Treisman GJ et al "A behaviorist perspective" Adv Psychosom Med 2011;30:8-21

How to break concrete

We have seen how discouraging messages can ...

- create unhelpful beliefs ("There is no finish line for migraine"),
- induce hopeless feelings ("I'm so hopeless and depressed")[1] and
- promote helpless behaviors ("There is nothing I can do myself").

One would think that it is easy to replace the pessimistic messages with encouraging information, e.g. "There are fabulous therapies for migraine". That should lift the spirit instantly, restore hope and motivate severely affected migraineurs to make their way to those tremendous therapies. You would certainly expect that thousands of cheerful patients now sing and dance in the streets, animated by the anticipation that their awful ailment will be alleviated soon. The good news will spread over the internet like a roaring bushfire and so it's merely a matter of weeks and months until the majority of them are either migraine-free or at least drastically improved.

Unfortunately, it is not that easy and pleasant and the reason for that is another mechanism in the way the human mind operates. It's called the *confirmation bias* and describes a type of selective attention, a bias towards confirming evidence.[2] Human minds tend to look out for and pay attention to the kind of information that confirms their existing beliefs and convictions. At the same time we are inclined to ignore or dismiss messages that contradict our current opinions, without much consideration as to whether that is reasonable or true or helpful.[3] The most important aspect seems to be that the new information mustn't contradict or question our current view of the world. That way our mind prevents our brain from wasting energy on 'stupid' new ideas that lead nowhere anyway; a useful mechanism in the stable environment of the savannah, where until recently[4] we used to hunt and gather. In our savannah past it was probably important to secure established solutions[5] and behaviors and conserve precious energy.

---

[1] Joiner TE Jr "Negative attributional style, hopelessness depression and endogenous depression" Behav Res Ther 2001;39(2):139-49
[2] Madey SF et al "Effect of Temporal Focus on the Recall of Expectancy-Consistent and Expectancy-Inconsistent Information" J Pers Soc Psychol 1993;65(3):458-468
[3] Mercier H et al "Why do humans reason? Arguments for an argumentative theory" Behav Brain Sci 2011;34(2):57-74
[4] Wynn T "Archaeology and cognitive evolution" Behav Brain Sci 2002;25(3):389-402
[5] Munro GD et al "The dark side of self-affirmation: confirmation bias and illusory correlation in response to threatening information" Pers Soc Psychol Bull 2009;35(9):1143-53

For our life in a modern world, which changes constantly and rapidly, in which we face new challenges all the time, more mental flexibility and openness to new solutions would be beneficial. Yet we're stuck with an outdated savannah-brain and a rather rigid mind, which is still reluctant to explore unfamiliar possibilities.

Therefore we tend to feel quite uncomfortable whenever new information challenges our good old familiar beliefs, and we end up arguing vehemently against knowledge that could be helpful, if only it didn't contradict our current preconceptions.

The confirmation bias is well known in medicine.[1] Doctors are trained to keep questioning their first impressions of a clinical case[2] and to remain open for signs and symptoms that point towards a different diagnosis. It is easy to imagine how a doctor's rigid reluctance towards new information could lead to fatal decisions, for instance in the emergency department (At the funeral: "I was convinced it was just the appendix").[3] In contrast to the popular myth of divine descent, the majority of medical doctors have human savannah-ancestors too and so they're just as prone to cognitive errors as their patients:[4] confirmation bias, negativity bias, cognitive distortions and so on.

Patients with severe migraine often have *particular* difficulties embracing new and encouraging information about innovative and 'revolutionary' therapies. Firstly, they get repeatedly hammered with the same depressing messages in books, magazines, websites and TV-programs: Repetition makes the confirmation bias stronger.[5] So the most aberrant nonsense can quickly become 'common knowledge', simply by frequent repetition in the media. Secondly, the brain area that would have the power to overrule the confirmation bias is the PFC (the prefrontal cortex), which is probably not the strongest player in a brain team with a hopeless and depressed migraineur as the 'head coach'.[6]

So what can be done to crack the nasty 'mind-concrete'?

---

[1] Mendel R et al "Confirmation bias: why psychiatrists stick to wrong preliminary diagnoses" Psychol Med 2011;20:1-9
[2] Eli I "Reducing confirmation bias in clinical decision-making" J Dent Educ 1996;60(10):831-5
[3] Pines JM "Profiles in patient safety: confirmation bias in emergency medicine" Acad Emerg Med 2006;13(1):90-4
[4] Groopman J "How Doctors Think" Mariner Books 2008
[5] Jonas E et al "Confirmation bias in sequential information search after preliminary decisions: an expansion of dissonance theoretical research on selective exposure to information" J Pers Soc Psychol 2001;80(4):557-71
[6] Grimm S et al "Imbalance between left and right dorsolateral prefrontal cortex in major depression is linked to negative emotional judgment: an fMRI study in severe major depressive disorder" Source Biol Psychiatry 2008;63(4):369-76

The confirmation bias isn't concerned about the quality of the competing messages and so we can save the time to discuss that. Also, it doesn't really matter, whether the new information is backed by research, since there is always a casual phrase to dismiss scientific evidence as dubious or invalid, once a competing idea has taken root in our savannah-brain. For example, if I wanted to communicate the message **"There are some fabulous therapies for migraine available"**, this would conflict with the already established belief "MIGRAINE CAN'T BE CURED", a message which can be found almost everywhere and which has been repeated many times.

A *logical* response would be: "That's awesome, tell me more about it. Perhaps I can finally end my migraine saga." But in many people and especially in severe migraineurs the confirmation bias, supported by pessimism and determined hopelessness, lures the mind into defense mode and dismisses the promising message like so: "IF IT WAS TRUE, THAT THERE ARE FABULOUS THERAPIES FOR MIGRAINE, THEN THAT WOULD BE ON THE FIRST PAGE OF EVERY NEWSPAPER. AND SINCE THAT IS NOT THE CASE, YOUR STATEMENT ABOUT FABULOUS MIGRAINE THERAPIES CAN'T BE TRUE." Sound familiar?

At first the argument sounds incredibly compelling, but it is only logical if the *assumption* "WOULD BE ON THE FIRST PAGE OF EVERY NEWSPAPER" were true. This, however, is completely *bizarre*: Neither medical nor therapeutic stories are *ever* on newspapers' title pages, positive stories are seldom newsworthy and the old myth "MIGRAINE CAN'T BE CURED" was *never* on page one either.

This demonstrates that, after a belief has conquered the mind, it turns into concrete, which cannot be cracked with logic, because the mind has no problem to defend established beliefs with irrational, illogical or otherwise whacky arguments, no matter how unhelpful the defended idea is. We need something better than scientific progress, compelling arguments and brilliant logic.

A solution could be, *not* to make a decision whether the new idea is better or true, but to keep in mind that either idea could turn out to prompt 'wrong' decisions. It could be an error to make decisions based on the old idea ("Migraine can't be cured") and it could be an error to base decisions on the new idea ("There are fabulous migraine therapies").[1] Now we need the PEDMIN strategy.

---

[1] Friedrich J "Primary error detection and minimization (PEDMIN) strategies in social cognition: a reinterpretation of confirmation bias phenomena" Psychol Rev 1993;100(2):298-319

PEDMIN stands for 'Primary Error Detection and MINimization' and means: in order to reduce the risk, it would be good to find out, which of the two possible *errors* has the more negative consequences: What is my loss, in case my decision turns out to be wrong (= the 'error')? Let's play it through.

In the *first error scenario*, the idea "Migraine can't be cured" is true, but a migraineur commits the *error* of seriously trying those fabulous migraine therapies. The risk is some waste of time, some waste of money and a few disappointing experiences, in case the fabulous therapies don't help at all. Of course, it could also lead to worthwhile improvements, but the PEDMIN strategy is not about opportunities, it is about increasing safety by avoiding true disasters in case we were misled by incorrect information.

In the *second error scenario*, the idea "There are fabulous migraine therapies" is indeed true, but our test patient erroneously follows the statement "Migraine can't be cured" and doesn't explore any of the fabulous therapies. The potential risk is lifelong migraine attacks, the chance of additional headaches from medication overuse and finally chronic daily headaches. In addition a rich selection of migraine comorbidities are waiting to be acquired, with major depression at the top of the list. The impact on family, social life and workplace will be substantial and quality of life will go down the drain.

With this PEDMIN strategy, the insecure brain can make up its mind, which of the two risk-scenarios it is willing to accept. That way the nasty belief-concrete—mixed from confirmation bias, pessimism and hopelessness—can be cracked and unfriendly, illogical arguments with a potential for conflict can be avoided.

The PEDMIN strategy also frees the migraineur from the unpleasant role of the critical customer, who needs to question and rigorously scrutinize the 'fabulous therapy', which is not a good starting point for the desired therapeutic partnership. Since the underlying and accepted hypothesis is "an error is possible and can not be ruled out", the pressure is off anyway. It has become a free decision, which every patient can make, no matter how severe the migraine is, how strong their confirmation bias, pessimism or hopelessness are and how distressed, neurotic or alexithymic the 'difficult' patient is. What risk are you willing to take?

Welcome to the dead end

Frequent severe migraine attacks, constant worry, a brain in emergency mode, a heavy emotional burden, hopeless feelings, helpless behaviors and pessimistic beliefs; all these factors together transform a normal migraineur into a very 'difficult' patient. During this transformation, patients migrate from family doctors via neurologists to specialized headache centers.

We already know that neurologists find many migraineurs 'difficult'. Wouldn't it be interesting to know how the expert doctors in a specialized *headache center* experience their migraine patients? Of course, all these general descriptions are neither representative for all migraineurs, nor do they refer to one person; but they give us ideas, how personalities develop under the weight of long-term treatment-resistant migraine.

In my experience, many people are a bit reluctant to look at personality factors, perhaps out of the fear of ending up with some 'psycho label'. Yet, this is not about tagging migraineurs as nutcases, this is about finding out what their *unmet needs* are.

One article[1] describes severe migraineurs as "deliberate, hesitant, insecure, detailed, perfectionistic, sensitive to criticism and emotionally deeply frustrated". They were said to "lack warmth" and to have "difficulty making social contacts".

A second article[2] lists "rigid, compulsive, perfectionistic, ambitious, competitive, chronically resentful, unable to delegate responsibility" and "troubled relationships with their parents, protected themselves from intimacy and attempted to dominate their environment".

A third article[3] portrays severe migraineurs as "orderly, overly conscientious, meticulous in appearance" and "they showed hostility, irritability, withdrawn social behavior, and transitory and prolonged depression".

All three authors merely write about their personal impressions from the position as experienced migraine doctors. They were not trained in psychology or psychotherapy and no standardized assessment tools was used to create personality profiles. So it is up to us to examine these lists, if we want to get a better idea, what makes a very 'difficult' migraine patient tick.

---

[1] Touraine GA et al "The migrainous patient: a constitutional study" J Nerv Ment Dis 1934;80:1-204
[2] Wollf HG "Personality features and rections of subjects with migraine" Arch Neurol Psychiatry 1937;37:895-921
[3] Friedman AP et al "Migraine" in Headache, diagnosis and treatment, Philadelphia: FA Davis 1959:201-49

This is how I would group the collected adjectives:

A	B	C
hesitant	hesitant	deliberate
insecure	insecure	orderly
sensitive to criticism	sensitive to criticism	overly conscientious
lacking warmth	lacking warmth	ambitious
emotionally deeply frustrated	troubled relationships with their parents	perfectionistic
protect themselves from intimacy	withdrawn social behavior	unable to delegate responsibility
chronically resentful, hostility	difficulty making social contacts	rigid
depression	irritability	compulsiveness

When I now look at the emerging list in column A, I can't help myself but think of *emotionally hurt*. This can be interpreted in at least two directions:

A1.) 'Difficult' migraineurs are emotionally hurt, because it feels to them that they are left alone with the horrible attack symptoms, especially with the crippling head pain; OR

A2.) Amongst the migraineurs, who don't do well and end up in a specialized headache center, there are some who've experienced some form of trauma. This speculatory interpretation is in accordance with studies [1] that show a high prevalence of childhood maltreatment in migraine patients who ended up in a headache center. Those patients reported:

• 21% physical abuse	• 25% sexual abuse	• 38% emotional abuse
• 22% physical neglect		• 38% emotional neglect

58% reported *at least one* form of childhood maltreatment, 26% reported *more than one*. Of those 58% of migraineurs, who *did* report childhood abuse, 43% also experienced abuse in adulthood. Physical abuse, emotional abuse and emotional neglect were found to be risk factors for migraine *chronification*.[2] *Emotional* abuse was also related to an earlier *onset* of migraine.

---

[1] Tietjen GE et al "Childhood maltreatment and migraine (part I). Prevalence and adult revictimization: a multicenter headache clinic survey" Headache 2010;50(1):20-31

[2] Tietjen GE et al "Childhood maltreatment and migraine (part II). Emotional abuse as a risk factor for headache chronification" Headache 2010;50(1):32-41

In addition a strong link between *multiple pain conditions* and multiple forms of *childhood maltreatment* was discovered.[1] This is not too surprising, considering that there is a substantial overlap between *physical* and *emotional* pain mechanisms in the brain,[2] to the extent that analgesics (painkillers) have been found to be useful in the treatment of *emotional* pain.[3]

The experience of abuse or neglect is connected to migraine by the typical *hypervigilance* of a traumatized and distressed brain. We've discussed hypervigilance already in clinically diagnosed PTSD. We can safely declare: One possible explanation for persistent migraine is, when a bit of PTSD hits a slightly unstable brain with a weak-ish prefrontal cortex (PFC).

This also shows how so-called 'psychological' factors and so-called 'biological' mechanisms are linked. They're better seen as two sides of the same coin and it would be smart to look at both sides in every case; but *especially* when migraine patients *begin* deteriorating. Medicine's narrow-minded insistence on the failed pharma-medical model in these cases is a cruel continuation of the physical and emotional abuse and neglect that many migraineurs have had to endure already. When dollars can be made with drugs, mercy and compassion have no seat on the money train.

Column B of our personality table makes me think of **low self-esteem**, which we've already mentioned. The lack of emotional stability and of social amenability can be interpreted in two ways:

B1.) After their long tale of woe, migraine patients at headache centers are simply 'pissed off' with the world and prefer to be left alone. Their trust in other people has been crushed by too many disappointing interactions with non-migraineurs, who just don't understand that migraine is not 'just a headache'. The listed insecurity and hesitation merely show the lack of trust; OR

B2.) General timidity and somewhat guarded social contact could also indicate an insecure 'attachment style'. A study done with migraineurs at a headache center found: The attachment style is the *most significant* predictor of disability in episodic migraine.[4]

---

[1] Tietjen GE et al "Childhood maltreatment and migraine (part III). Association with comorbid pain conditions" Headache 2010;50(1):42-51
[2] Eisenberger N et al "Why rejection hurts: a common neural alarm system for physical and social pain" Trends Cogn Sci 2004;8(7):294-300
[3] DeWall CN "Hurt feelings? You could take a pain reliever…" Harv Bus Rev 2011;89(4):28-9
[4] Rossi P et al "Depressive symptoms and insecure attachment as predictors of disability in a clinical population of patients with episodic and chronic migraine" Headache 2005;45(5):561-70

A feeling of safety

What is an attachment style? After birth, it takes an antelope baby about fifteen minutes of training, until it has a fair chance to outrun a lion. In contrast, a human baby is utterly vulnerable and defenseless for many years and its survival depends entirely on its parents. Therefore a baby has a vested interest in attaching itself to its mother (or whoever the primary caregiver is) by forming a tight emotional bond. Only a reliable attachment to a dependable and responsive mother can guarantee safety, security and survival.

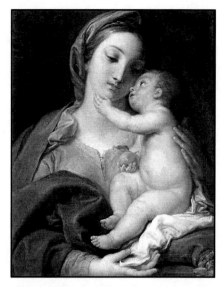

As we all know, young infants can be quite distressed, when they're separated from their mother, but also when the mother doesn't provide the emotional security, which the needy human bundle requires. Rumor has it that the quality of this early attachment has a bit of an influence on that child's development, well-being, health and resilience, even much later in life.[1]

Several patterns of attachment have been described,[2] which also form a person's first blueprint for how relationships work. If the interactions between mother and child meet the little critter's needs, there is a fair chance that a *secure attachment style* develops and the child (and the ensuing adult) tends to feel rather safe and secure in life and relationships.

If the childcare misses the mark, it is more likely that the developing mind and brain learn an *insecure attachment style*, tend to feel unsafe and insecure and later struggle to develop a healthy self-confidence and trust in close relationships.[3]

The many statements in migraine land along the lines of "THE WORLD IS A HOSTILE PLACE FOR MIGRAINEURS", could be seen as a clue for a universal feeling of un-safety derived from an *insecure attachment*.

---

[1] Kidd T et al "The association between adult attachment style and cortisol responses to acute stress" Psychoneuroendocrinology 2011;36(6):771-9
[2] Bretherton I "The Origins of Attachment Theory: John Bowlby and Mary Ainsworth" Dev Psychol 1992;28(5):759ff.
[3] Mikulincer M et al "Attachment security in couple relationships" Fam Process 2002;41(3):405-34

On the other hand, you could also argue that experiencing the world as hostile, reflects of the 'biological' reactivity that certain migraineurs are plagued with. Moreover, some would categorically *discount and dismiss any* idea of *any* involvement of 'psychological' mechanisms in the chronification of migraine, because migraine is solely A GENETIC NEUROLOGICAL DISEASE and nothing else, right?

Attachment theory gives a *reasonable* explanation for the resistance, petulance and hostility, frequently reported and observed in very 'difficult' migraineurs. People, especially men, who missed out on the experience of a nurturing secure attachment, sometimes develop a *dismissive-avoidant* style[1] that can translate into angry-dismissive behaviors and correlates with depression.[2]

An insecure attachment style is not only a strong risk factor for disability, but it also seems to occur very frequently in migraineurs and other headache sufferers.[3] Additionally and not surprisingly, a connection between maternal care behavior and activation of the PFC (prefrontal cortex) has been discovered.[4]

"ARE YOU SAYING THAT I'M PSYCHOLOGICALLY DAMAGED AND MY MOTHER IS TO BLAME FOR THAT?" In my experience some patients with a chronic illness, especially those with chronic pain, tend to mistake psychological explanations as an attack on their integrity as *real* sufferers. Unfamiliar with the strange psycho-jargon and mind-body connections ("psychophysiology"), they become defensive and angry.

Nowadays we are fairly comfortable to openly discuss issues as long as they're labeled 'medical'. "I can't eat that, I have irritable bowel syndrome" is almost a fashion statement in some circles. Yet, we're unwilling to consider emotional factors. "My irritable bowel is probably related to my fearful-avoidant attachment style, since I felt emotionally neglected as an infant" would be quite a puzzling disclosure at a dinner party.

In both cases, the speaker reveals troubles with bowel pain, frequent farting and diarrhea or constipation, but it's the *emotional* side of IBS that is too embarrassing to be discussed, perhaps too painful to be contemplated. Therefore, we understandably prefer dealing with IBS and the like as 'medical' problems over facing and resolving our emotional traumas and refining our coping skills.

---

[1] Bartholomew K et al "Attachment styles among young adults: a test of a four-category model" J Pers Soc Psychol 1991;61(2):226-44
[2] Bifulco A et al "Adult attachment style I: Its relationship to clinical depression" Soc Psychiatry Psychiatr Epidemiol 2002;37(2):50-9
[3] Savi L et al "Attachment styles and headache" J Headache Pain. 2005;6(4):254-7
[4] Ramasubbu R et al "Neural representation of maternal face processing: an fMRI study" Can J Psychiatry 2007;52(11):726-34

And so the main culprit for the "psychological damage" may *not* be the nervous mother, who indeed didn't manage to nurture her child's confidence and stress-resilience perfectly. The *main* evil may well be our modern society's preference for a convenient and quick pharmacological symptom-fix over a process of healing, resolution, restoration and rehabilitation.

This also answers the question of who is to *blame*: We are all to blame. So what? What is that good for? I can't remember a single case of severe migraine or IBS that magically recovered after ten sessions of *therapeutic blaming*. Denial, resentment, hostility, guilt, shame and blame are not really famous for their healing potential.

There is a solution for the severe migraineur's dilemma between the unhelpful obsession with pharma-medicine and the uncomfortable and scary 'psycho'-field: *Neuroscience*, the discipline that looks at the nervous system (brain), can explain how the development of the personality (mind) is connected to self-regulation (stress-resistance), recovery (resilience) and stress or pain (health).[1] In regard to the quality of attachment, neuroscience research shows, that successful coping with *manageable* early life challenges, *empowered* and *encouraged* by a secure attachment[2] to a dependable, nurturing and supportive mother promotes:

- healthy development of the prefrontal cortex[3]
- higher stress resistance, lower stress-reactivity[4]
- better regulation of emotions[5] and arousal[6] as well as
- greater resilience[7] (= recovery from stress) and
- better coping skills.[8]

Regarding the reported *hostility* of 'difficult' patients: Research revealed that the personality trait agreeableness (= opposite of hostility) relates to how effectively the left and the right side of the prefrontal cortex (PFC) communicate.[9] Isn't that interesting?

---

[1] Friborg O et al "Resilience as a moderator of pain and stress" J Psychosom Res 2006;61(2):213-9
[2] Muris P et al "Behavioral Inhibition as a Risk Factor for the Development of Childhood Anxiety Disorders: A Longitudinal Study" J Child Fam Stud 2011;20(2):157-170
[3] Katz M et al "Prefrontal Plasticity and Stress Inoculation-induced Resilience" Dev Neurosci 2009;31:239-299
[4] Hänsel A et al "The ventro-medial prefrontal cortex: a major link between the autonomic nervous system, regulation of emotion, and stress reactivity?" Biopsychosoc Med 2008;2:21
[5] Waters SF et al "Emotion Regulation and Attachment: Unpacking Two Constructs" J Psychopathol Behav Assess 2010;32(1):37-47
[6] Lyons DM et al "Develpmental cascades linking stress inoculation, arousal regulation, and resilience" Front Behav Neurosci 2009;3:32
[7] Maier SF et al "Behavioral control, the medial prefrontal cortex, and resilience" Dialogues Clin Neurosci 2006;8(4):397-406
[8] Maier SF et al "Role of the medial prefrontal cortex in coping and resilience" Brain Res 2010;1355:52-60
[9] Hoppenbrouwers SS "Personality goes a long way: an interhemispheric connectivity study" Front Psychiatry 2010; 22;1:140

Neuroscience not only provides the missing explanations as to how the symptoms of migraine are linked to developmental influences, personality traits and dysregulated brain areas; *applied neuroscience* (aka neurotherapy) also has the tools to restore and renormalize brain function, which often leads to freedom from migraine or at least to a drastic reduction in symptoms. The rehabilitation of the migraine brain is one of the core components of the migraine revolution and will be discussed thoroughly later in this book. First, we need to get a firm grip on the psycho terror.

So far in this book we have seen how the current treatment regime drives predisposed patients into chronification by creating disempowering beliefs and endorsing unhelpful behaviors.

Emotions, beliefs and behaviors are not only decisive determinants for the deterioration into very 'difficult' patients, but they are also crucial components of the constructive cooperation which we'll need for our victory over the tyranny of migraine. Recognizing the entire history of the problem enables migraineurs to make better decisions in the future. In simple words: You have to understand precisely *what* needs to be done and *why* it needs to be done. Then you won't be a helpless, suffering victim anymore, but your own revolutionary rehabilitation manager. Okay?

Let's wrap up our examination of the personality profile of patients at the dead end of their migraine journey. Column C of our table lists the following descriptions:

> deliberate, orderly, overly conscientious, ambitious, perfectionistic, unable to delegate responsibility, rigid, compulsiveness

This can be interpreted in two ways:

C1.) Migraineurs try to make the most of the time between attacks and so they appear a little tense to non-migraineurs, who don't understand anyway. Beyond that, the list has no meaning; OR

C2.) Severe migraineurs, on average, don't feel very good about themselves. Self-esteem, self-confidence, self-worth and self-efficacy (= the opposite of helplessness) are rather low-ish. So they 'try hard' to *compensate* for that by 'doing things very well'[1] and by seeking external reassurance[2] and approval.

---

[1] Martinius J "Psychological sequelae of child abuse" Monatsschr Kinderheilkd 1986;134(6):333-5
[2] Shaver PR et al "Attachment style, excessive reassurance seeking, relationship processes, and depression" Pers Soc Psychol Bull 2005 Mar;31(3):343-59

The subconscious hope is, to silence the nasty inner voice that says the exact opposite:[1] "You are not good enough" or "You don't deserve ..." The sad thing is, it never works, because no achievement in the present or future can ever heal the pain from the past. And so these compensatory behaviors lead not only to further disappointment,[2] but also to a lot of self-imposed pressure and extra stress. A better strategy is to resolve the traumas of the past and leave the feelings of unworthiness behind.

Over the years many studies have tried to identify a specific psychopathology or a typical personality as a potential cause of migraine. They usually find what we've already discussed in this and previous chapters: anxiety, depression, hostility,[3] neuroticism, hypervigilance, insomnia, childhood trauma, insecure attachment styles, high achievement motivation and so on. Yet, no single psychological 'cause' of migraine has been determined, which just goes to show that the underlying idea is misguided.

None of the 'psychological' factors directly 'causes' migraine, but they co-occur with migraine, intensify the impact, accelerate the chronification and so the deterioration into very 'difficult' patients. Once they've hit rock bottom, it becomes indeed very 'difficult' to help them; not because of the severity of the migraine, but because of the weight of the psycho-baggage that they've accumulated on their journey downhill. This is what I call the psycho terror in migraine land. If we beat the psycho terror, we can end the tyranny.

A tale of two women

On a lighter note, do you remember Clare from the beginning of this chapter? Let me remind you:

> "Clare has her first migraine attack at the end of a particularly stressful week. After a weekend of intense pain and being sick, Clare decides to limit her workload to a reasonable amount and informs her boss on Monday. She begins a regular exercise program on Tuesday and sticks with it. As a result, she never has another migraine attack ever again. This is how Clare deals with problems."

Well, she is not really a 'difficult' patient, is she?

---

[1] Gilbert P et al "Criticizing and reassuring oneself: An exploration of forms, styles and reasons in female students" Br J Clin Psychol 2004;43(Pt 1):31-50

[2] Irons C, et al "Parental recall, attachment relating and self-attacking/self-reassurance: their relationship with depression" Br J Clin Psychol 2006;45(Pt 3):297-308

[3] Bag B et al "Examination of anxiety, hostility and psychiatric disorders in patients with migraine and tension-type headache" Int J Clin Pract 2005;59(5):515-21

That is exactly my point. Why does Clare *not* turn into a 'difficult' patient? Is there anything that we can learn from her? How is she different from a 'difficult' patient with severe migraine? Stories are fun, let's have another one, shall we?

> At the end of a very stressful week, **Daisy** has her first migraine attack. After a weekend of intense suffering, Daisy is shattered, scared and worried. How can she possibly keep her job, now that she has fallen victim to an inherited neurological disease with swollen inflamed blood vessels? What will her boss think? What if she has another migraine attack during the week and is forced to call in sick? Daisy knows, the only way out is to find the right doctor."

What is the difference? Clare's report reads like a technical description or a timetable, whereas Daisy's story sounds like a drama or a soap opera. Both women have their first migraine attack, but their reactions are different. Daisy is overwhelmed by fear and worry and puts all her hope in a doctor whom she hasn't even met.

In contrast, Clare doesn't sound emotionally shaken at all. Apparently she comes to the conclusion, that the episode was initiated by an unfortunate ratio between too high a workload and lack of exercise. In other words, she attributes the migraine to the situation and not to herself (that's also what dog A did, judged by its behavior). Then Clare simply makes the decision to limit her workload and informs her boss. She doesn't hesitate, she doesn't ask her boss for permission, she doesn't worry whether her boss will like it or not and she doesn't catastrophize. Clare simply does, what she thinks needs to be done in order to solve the problem. Dog A did the same on page 96: It jumped out of the pen.

In contrast, after her first migraine attack, Daisy diagnoses herself with an INCURABLE GENETIC DISEASE and thereby attributes the cause of the problem to herself (just like dog B). She spends time and energy on worrying and catastrophizing and, without any need, restricts her options to dreaming of a knight in medical white armor, who shall protect her from the evil by slaying the migraine dragon and rescuing her from her tower of sorrows. And so Daisy has a fair chance to stay passive like dog B, who didn't jump out of the pen, but kept on suffering instead.

Do you think I'm being harsh on poor Daisy and, most of all, it's unfair? You are so right: It *is* unfair, because Daisy has the cumulative disadvantage that might make things difficult.

Of course, both stories are made up and we don't really know what's going to happen. Let's stick to the cliché to fully understand the mechanisms that might drive Daisy to becoming a very difficult migraine patient with anxiety and depression while Clare has a fabulous life without migraine. At any point we're allowed to feel sorry for Daisy and her cumulative disadvantage, but only if we think that our sympathy will *help* her to get rid of the migraine.

	Clare	Daisy
her mother is/was	calm, balanced	nervous, restless
attachment style	secure	insecure: fearful-avoidant
her default brain state	relaxed alertness	hypervigilance
her prefrontal cortex	normal	weak-ish
mood regulation	strong: emotionally balanced, more laughter than tears	weak: emotionally vulnerable, more tears than laughter
her body's default state	relaxed, takes a punch	tense, prone to pain
her overall health	strong health, recovers quickly from illness	rather weak-ish, many little health problems
mother's parenting style	reassuring, encouraging	protective, controlling
mother's attitude	"Give it a crack, Clare!"	"Be careful, Daisy!"
her personality	high levels of confidence & self-worth, does things well enough, but not more than that	low levels of confidence & self-worth, ambitious, pedantic, perfectionistic
her own explanation for the migraine attack = attributional style	"Last week the workload was too high AND not enough exercise" = situational, temporary	"I have fallen victim to an incurable genetic neurological disease" = personal, permanent
coping style	rational: solution-focused	emotional: emotion-focused
preferred coping behavior	facing and solving problems	fearfully avoiding and worrying
active or passive coping?	active	passive
likes dogs?	yes, dog A	feels sorry for dog B, hates dog A + the researcher
thoughts about the future?	"Let's see what happens"	"Oh my God, you never know what's gonna happen"

Looking at the table, you can see how Daisy's disadvantage mounts up. She may have been born with a timid temperament, because her mom's body chemistry was 'anxious' during the pregnancy. We don't know that, but we *do* know that children born to mothers with an anxiety disorder or migraine, have a higher risk of developing migraine. This shows in the *acoustic startle response* (a brainstem reflex of fright to a sudden loud noise) which is more reactive in these children.[1] Applied to our cliché story, we could say that her brain was 'primed for fear' from the very beginning.

That doesn't mean she was doomed at birth, but I'd say she was well prepared to miss the exit. If you consider the two columns as roads, one exit point could have been the *causal attribution*, which is Daisy's own explanation for her first migraine attack. The current regime is to dish up stories of migraine as an "INCURABLE GENETIC DISEASE" with "BLOOD VESSEL SWELLING AND INFLAMMATION" as the key elements. So she went with it and concluded that she can't do anything about it and that she is *helpless*. She is like dog B, who can only hope that someone in a white coat has mercy and stops the suffering. For dog B the white-coated hope was the researcher, for Daisy it is one of the many doctors that she will consult during her deterioration into a 'difficult' patient with severe migraine.

After the causal attribution—for which she received reassurance from websites, books and doctors—the *confirmation bias* almost guarantees that she'll find plenty of further endorsement and evidence for her beliefs and she'll defend that theory like a lioness defends her cubs.

Since Daisy is of a fearful-avoidant nature, she is also totally into the *concept of avoiding* migraine triggers. That concept is logically appealing and is right up her fearful-avoidant alley. The academic version of the expression "right up her alley" is *regulatory fit* and it means that a person's attention tends to follow their mood state. In someone fearful-avoidant like Daisy the attention system of the brain responds well to any information regarding 'avoiding dangers', but tends to miss and dismiss messages relating to 'seizing opportunities'.[2] Although *she* hasn't done anything 'wrong', Daisy's road quickly turns into a railway track. Unfair, huh?

---

[1] Duncko R et al "Startle reactivity in children at risk for migraine" Clin Neurophysiol 2008;119(12):2733-7
[2] Glass BD et al "Regulatory fit effects on stimulus identification" Atten Percept Psychophys 2011;73(3):927-37

Now that she is on that track, it will be difficult to get her off. Her prefrontal cortex is simply too 'weak' to regulate her emotions,[1] to dampen excessive anxiety,[2] to counteract her negativity bias[3] and to steer her thinking away from worrying and catastrophizing.[4] Daisy gradually loses her 'Self' in anxiety, pessimism and helplessness. She becomes one with her pain and suffering.[5]

In accordance with her favorite coping style (emotional, not solution-focused), Daisy describes her *suffering* in great detail to her internet support-group and receives reinforcement from other migraine *sufferers*. At least she is not alone and others like her share the horrible experience of *suffering* from severe migraine.

Isn't it interesting that patients normally *have* pneumonia or malaria or AIDS; or they *have* a stroke or terminal cancer, but when it comes to migraine, they not only *have* it, but we always express that the patients are *suffering* from it. Why is that?

Not only because of the intense symptoms, but especially due to the 'weakness' of the PFC (prefrontal cortex), migraine is a very emotional problem and so it is very easy to get stuck on the 'track of suffering' like Daisy. Perfectly matching the maladaptive coping of migraineurs, the recommended treatment of the current regime is medication (*passive*) and trigger avoidance (*avoidant*), which is in *stark contrast* to what is known to be helpful in other areas of medicine/therapy: Whether it is epilepsy,[6] chronic pain,[7] arthritis,[8] car accident,[9] face injury,[10] brain damage,[11] lung cancer,[12] breast cancer,[13] heart failure,[14] PTSD (post traumatic stress disorder),[15] or

---

[1] Glotzbach E et al "Prefrontal Brain Activation During Emotional Processing: A Functional Near Infrared Spectroscopy Study (fNIRS)" Open Neuroimag J. 2011;5:33-9
[2] Berkowitz RL et al "The human dimension: how the prefrontal cortex modulates the subcortical fear response" Rev Neurosci 2007;18(3-4):191-207
[3] Li H et al "The neural mechanism underlying the female advantage in identifying negative emotions: an event-related potential study" Neuroimage 2008;40(4):1921-9
[4] Miller EK "The prefrontal cortex and cognitive control" Nat Rev Neurosci 2000;1(1):59-65
[5] Dimaggio G et al "Impaired self-reflection in psychiatric disorders among adults: a proposal for the existence of a network of semi independent functions" Conscious Cogn 2009;18(3):653-64
[6] Westerhuis W et al "Coping style and quality of life in patients with epilepsy: a cross-sectional study" J Neurol 2011;258(1):37-43
[7] Samwel HJ et al "The role of helplessness, fear of pain, and passive pain-coping in chronic pain patients" Clin J Pain 2006;22(3):245-51
[8] Benyon K et al "Coping strategies and self-efficacy as predictors of outcome in osteoarthritis: a systematic review" Musc Care 2010;8(4):224-36
[9] Hall PA et al "Changes in coping style and treatment outcome following motor vehicle accident" Rehabil Psychol 2011;56(1):43-51
[10] De Sousa A "Psychological issues in acquired facial trauma" Indian J Plast Surg 2010;43(2):200-5
[11] Wolters G et al "Coping following acquired brain injury: predictors and correlates" J Head Trauma Rehabil 2011;26(2):150-7
[12] Prasertsri N et al "Repressive coping style: relationships with depression, pain, and pain coping strategies in lung cancer out patients" Lung Cancer 2011;71(2):235-40
[13] Heppner PP et al "Problem-solving style and adaptation in breast cancer survivors: a prospective analysis" J Cancer Surviv 2009;3(2):128-36
[14] Doering LV et al "Is coping style linked to emotional states in heart failure patients?" J Card Fail. 2004;10(4):344-9
[15] Amir M et al "Suicide risk and coping styles in posttraumatic stress disorder patients" Psychother Psychosom 1999;68(2):76-81

multiple sclerosis,[1] major depression,[2] irritable bowel syndrome,[3] panic disorder,[4] stressful life events,[5] generalized anxiety disorder,[6] or headaches [7,8] — those patients, who are engaged in *active* coping strategies, such as facing and solving problems, are always much better off than those, who remain passive, helpless or try to avoid problems. That finding, *active* coping is better for patients, is *especially* true for migraine [9,10,11,12,13] and even for chronic migraine.[14] Everybody knows that. Clare does and even dog A — woof.

What *can* we learn from Clare?

What *is* Clare's secret? How *did* she end the tyranny? I'm not even sure that Clare knows that it was a migraine attack, which spoiled her weekend. She was sick and had intense head pain, but we haven't heard anything about emotional suffering. So she kept her cool and rationally identified the issue. Typical for Clare, she assumed that there is nothing wrong with *herself*, but with the situation leading to the attack: a particularly stressful week, which she is not willing to repeat. Why should she?

The second step was starting a regular exercise program and sticking to it. Clare recognized that the stress-load of that week was too high, which also indicated to her, that her stress-resistance could be improved. And Clare knows that regular exercise can increase the resistance to distress. So that's what she does; increase her own resistance, because *resistance ends the tyranny*! What a freakishly fast migraine revolution. It's okay to be envious of her.

---

[1] Rabinowitz AR et al "A longitudinal analysis of cognitive dysfunction, coping, and depression in multiple sclerosis" Neuropsychology 2009;23(5):581-91

[2] Wang J et al "The moderating effects of coping strategies on major depression in the general population" Can J Psychiatry 2002;47(2):167-73

[3] Wrzesińska MA et al "The assessment of personality traits and coping style level among the patients with functional dyspepsia and irritable bowel syndrome" Psychiatr Pol 2008;42(5):709-17

[4] Hino T et al "A 1-year follow-up study of coping in patients with panic disorder" Compr Psychiatry 2002;43(4):279-84

[5] Hovanitz CA "Life event stress and coping style as contributors to psychopathology" J Clin Psychol 1986;42(1):34-41

[6] Olatunji BO et al "Linking cognitive avoidance and GAD symptoms: The mediating role of fear of emotion" Behav Res Ther 2010;48(5):435-41

[7] Siniatchkin M et al "Coping styles of headache sufferers" Cephalalgia 1999;19(3):165-73

[8] Heath RL et al "Locus of control moderates the relationship between headache pain and depression" J Headache Pain 2008;9(5):301-8

[9] Bornmann M et al "Coping with stress and pain in migraine patients" Schmerz 1989;3(4):195-203

[10] Huber D et al "Personality traits and stress sensitivity in migraine patients" Behav Med 2003 Spring;29(1):4-13

[11] Abbate-Daga G et al "Anger, depression and personality dimensions in patients with migraine without aura" Psychother Psychosom 2007;76(2):122-8

[12] Radat F et al "Anxiety, stress and coping behaviours in primary care migraine patients: results of the SMILE study" Cephalalgia 2008;28(11):1115-25

[13] Radat F et al "The GRIM2005 study of migraine consultation in France. III: Psychological features of subjects with migraine" Cephalalgia 2009;29(3):338-50

[14] Lafittau M et al "Headache and transformed migraine with medication overuse: what differences between disability, emotional distress and coping?" Encephale 2006;32(2 Pt 1):231-7

Who is going to do something about it?

Life is a lot about making decisions. Successful decisions, unsuccessful decisions, smart decisions, stupid decisions; even the refusal to decide anything ("I can't decide") is the result of the decision not to decide. The question is, what is *your* decision?

To start their revolution, migraineurs have to come to the ***conclusion*** that staying on the chronification track is *not working* for them: "I have severe migraine, it's not getting better, I want change ..."; and then they have to make the ***decision***: "... and I'm willing to put the effort in, I'm ready to face the difficulties lying ahead, and I'm going to see it through. I'm gonna do, what needs to be done." Conclusion • Decision • Revolution.

The title of this book is "The Migraine *Revolution*" for a reason. A revolution normally is a bit of an effort and demands 'blood, sweat and tears', which is not for everyone. It is not for people, who are somewhat comfortable on that migraine track, who—as weird as it may sound—feel somewhat *safe and cozy* with their "INCURABLE NEUROLOGICAL DISEASE". It is not for those who secretly enjoy the drama of *acting out* their suffering and despair or who feel pleasantly *powerful* being peeved, petulant, dismissive or hostile.

It's also not for those, who *can't be bothered*, because they are too lethargic or blasé ("It's the doctor's problem, if the medication has side effects, migraine is a medical disease"). All those are free to ***decide*** to stay on the track until "*The Complimentary Migraine Cure Room Service*" comes along, which is not only for free, but always works instantly, without any effort and it tastes like candy. For those of you, who have decided to *stay* on the migraine track, the tale of the two women ends like this:

"Daisy finally finds a fantastic doctor and after the removal of several face muscles and with regular Botox® she is almost migraine-free. Clare was unlucky; she was jogging and enjoying cheery music with earphones, when she got hit by a truck. Now she's in a wheelchair and has severe migraine. And dog A has rabies!" Happy?

If you *don't believe* in this ending and you've come to the conclusion that the current regime *isn't working* for you <u>and</u> you really want *change* <u>and</u> you're willing to face the *difficulties* lying ahead <u>and</u> you're going to *see it through* <u>and</u> you're gonna *do, what needs to be done*, even if it takes effort, blood, sweat and tears, after that decision *you are ready* for the migraine revolution.

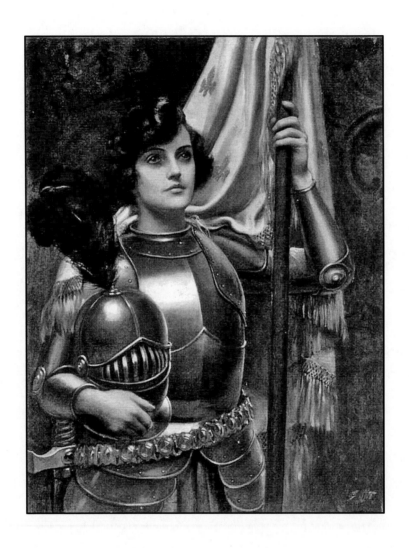

Part II:
Preparing for Battle

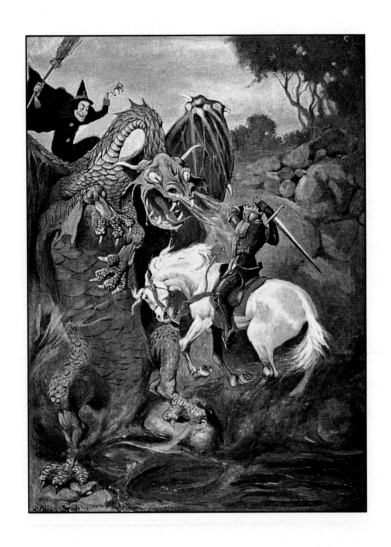

Chapter 6

Dealing with Difficulties

"Difficulties strengthen the mind, as labor does the body."
Seneca

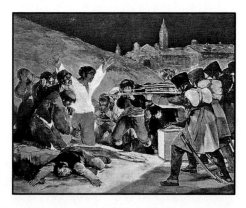

The day had come. The famished people had gathered at the marketplace. The peasants, armed to the teeth with hayforks and scythes, and the laborers, with long crowbars and heavy spanners in their furious fists; they were standing side by side, forming the angry army of the proletarian masses. The air was filled with hatred and rage and the mob's face left no doubt that today was the day, on which they would rise up to bring down the despot; they would unleash their wrath to terminate the tyrant's terror and they would fight to the death to eventually end the unendurable injustice of oppression, to gain their freedom at last.

Bertrand, the schoolteacher and leader of the rebellion, leapt onto a bale of straw and waved a large bread knife above his head like a sword. In a posture worthy of an adored ancient commander and with epos in his voice he addressed the expectant gathering: *"Citizens! ... Comrades! ... Brothers and Sisters! The day has come."* – "**Hooorrraaayyy**" roared the crowd in one voice and went silent again. Bertrand continued: *"Today is the day, on which we'll rise up to bring down the despot."* – "**Hooorrraaayyy**" – *"Today we will unleash our wrath to terminate the tyrant's terror ..."* – "**Hooorrraaayyy**" – *"... today we will fight to the death to eventually end the unendurable injustice of oppression and today we will gain our freedom at last. Follow me to the palace!"* – "**Hoooooorrrrraaaaayyyyy**" General Bertrand hopped off the bale and started marching up the hill towards the palace, closely followed by the angry proletarian army of furious freedom-fighters, cursing and swearing all along the way. Spiteful slogans were bellowed and answered with another roaring "**Hooorrraaayyy**".

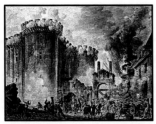 The agitated people were eager to finally change their pitiful fate, to take their destiny into their own hands. They were prepared to sacrifice everything, were ready to risk their lives, because they knew what they were fighting for: A better future for themselves and for their children and a fair opportunity to forge their luck. And so they were utterly determined to finish the reign of that cruel and greedy dictator, determined to end the tyranny.

The bloodthirsty horde reached the top of the hill and approached the palace. A single unarmed soldier was guarding the gate. The guard stepped forward and shouted at the approaching proletarian army: "What is it that you want?" General Bertrand took that as his cue and raised his furious commander voice once again: *"We're rising up to bring down the despot, we're unleashing our wrath to terminate the tyrant's terror, we'll fight to the death to end the unendurable injustice of oppression, to gain our freedom at last."* The rebellious horde exploded in excitement: "**Hoooorrrraaaaayyyyy**".

The guard didn't flinch: "I do understand where you're coming from and I'm so sorry to cause any disappointment, now that you've gone to the trouble of organizing such a promising rebellion, but I'm afraid the honorable despot is out for lunch."

The people were stunned. They just stood there in front of the gate with their jaws dropped and didn't move. Then someone said: "Actually, lunch sounds good. I'm getting a bit hungry."–"Yeah, me too" said a second one. "Huuuuuh, it's starting to rain and I don't have an umbrella."–"I'm getting cold here."–"Let's go home and come back later."–"Later is inconvenient, I have an appointment. What about tomorrow?"–"My mother-in-law is coming, so I can't tomorrow."–"Whatever, let's grab a beer, shall we?"

And while they were discussing which tavern had the best beer, the nimble guard snatched Bertrand's bread knife and swiftly decapitated the rebellion's leader.

"Hey, look at that. The guard killed the teacher."–"So what? You don't wanna go to school at your age or do you?"–"That teacher bloke was a bit of a tosser anyway."–"Exactly."–"Did you understand what he was ranting about earlier?"–"Nah, sorry, I wasn't listening really. I just went with my mates."–"Come on, let's go to the pub."–"Yep."

What makes a revolution tough is not the start, but the expected and the unforeseen difficulties along the way.

A true story

After a long phase of deliberation, a 'difficult' female long-term migraine sufferer with chronic fatigue syndrome and multiple chemical sensitivities decided to give a program with nutritional supplements and bio-identical hormone creams a try. Erica, let's call her, filled out 20 pages of a medical history questionnaire and had the required lab tests done. She received recommendations for 15 different supplements and hormones, but started having trouble tolerating some of the products before she had even acquired all of them. Apparently, she had to substitute the recommended magnesium powder for plain magnesium (???) and felt that the hormone creams made her nauseous. Erica stuck with the program for an entire week and then abandoned it, because it didn't help with her migraine. She then wrote a report and complained about the program advisor being basically a salesperson and that there was no medical professional, who felt a strong sense of responsibility for the patient. In addition, she emphasized that her naturopath, who filled out the required prescriptions, was never enthusiastic about the program. She concluded that the whole thing was a waste of money and warned other migraineurs with immune system problems that this program may not be for them.

What can we learn from this true story? Should we take it as a warning that there are scam artists out there, who take migraine sufferers' money and then obviously don't feel "a strong sense of responsibility for the patient"? Should we join in and protest against this unendurable injustice? Or should we have a factual look at what went wrong in this case, so that we can learn from it? I knew you would choose the second option. Well done!

Bio-identical hormone supplementation can make a lot of sense in *those* cases where the hormone system is out of balance. This alone can be enough in some cases to stop the migraine attacks completely (and that's why we'll look into that later). It is, however, very unfortunate, if you have to buy the therapy before you have the results of the diagnostic tests; because only if the system is out of whack, does the hormone supplementation make sense. Clear?

A patient with multiple intolerances and reactivities *cannot* expect to tolerate herbs, minerals, supplements or creams without any problems. This type of difficulty was *foreseeable*, was it not?

Those adverse reactions to otherwise harmless substances (or even weather), which we call 'reactivity', 'sensitivity' or 'intolerance', are not immune system responses like allergies. Instead they are exaggerated defense reactions of the central nervous system (say brain, if you want) due to a process called *sensitization*. Essentially the nervous system trained itself to a level of mastery to hysterically defend itself against whatever comes along, because it feels 'attacked' or 'threatened'. In Erica's case, the reaction was nausea. The 'nausea center' is located in the brainstem and so nausea is undoubtedly a nervous system response. The immune system can do other funky things, but it can't perform nausea. There were *no signs* of "immune system problems" in Erica so far.

If this highly reactive patient doesn't have the support of an experienced 'reactivity therapist' in her corner to help her sort out these foreseeable tolerance issues, then she has two options: Either she cannot start such a program or she is prepared to sort it out for herself. One way to sort it out for herself is *not* to begin with the recommended dose for 'normal' people. Instead she would take a tiny fraction of that dose, to give her reactive system the opportunity to slowly slowly slowly get used to every single one of the new 'stuffs' (supplements, hormones, whatever). Once Erica tolerates that fraction of the target dose without any further abreactions, she can very very very slowly and gradually increase the dose in tiny tiny tiny baby-steps, because anything else will only trigger her nervous defenses and launch the dreaded reactions (agitation, nausea, ... the sky is the limit). Makes sense?

Erica is a mature adult and she knew about her intolerances. Nevertheless, here she '*diligently*' followed a program for 'tolerant' people. She swallowed untried supplements and smeared new hormone creams onto her skin: all in all up to 15 potential 'threats'. Consequently, she had her usual adverse reactions and ended up as the 'innocent victim', neglected and 'abused'. But who did that to her? Was it the program advisor, who *should* have known that Erica could have extreme reactions to normally benign substances? Or was it her naturopathic doctor, who filled out the scripts as requested by Erica? *Who* treated Erica with no regard or care? *Who should* have known better, but chose to neglect her duty of care. Who abused Erica here, if not she herself?

The intriguing question is: *Why* did Erica act like that? Why did she end up as the disappointed, angry, innocent victim again? The conclusion "I need to go very slowly with unfamiliar substances" is not rocket-science. It's very basic common sense. Yet, Erica ignored this simple principle. Is she *that* stupid?

I don't think she is. She managed to write a coherent report of her experiences and published it as a 'book review' on the internet. So she is smart enough to write, to operate a computer and to navigate the internet. So she can't be too stupid. What else is there?

Erica's story is an example of a well-known human behavior pattern, which is active in every one of us; sometimes more, sometimes less. We tend to seek and create situations, in which we feel the way we used to feel in the past. *Familiarity* is utterly attractive for those parts of our brain that create our subconscious mind. And we are all familiar with the magnetic effect of familiarity, have observed it many times in others, but probably not so much in ourselves.

Have you ever met a woman, who is really 'unfortunate' in that she always ends up with the 'wrong guy'? "I was so sure, that Jim would be different from the abusive bums, I dated previously. But he turned out to be exactly the same kind of pig."

Have you ever met a man, who had his heart broken by a manipulative, emotionally cold, but pretty girl? But then you meet his new girlfriend and how is she? Manipulative, emotionally cold and pretty yet again.

We are attracted to people and circumstances that create that subconscious feeling of familiarity and so the man whose mother was manipulative and emotionally cold is attracted to 'copies' of his mother. The woman with the somewhat abusive father is attracted to somewhat abusive guys, because the subconscious mind is still the same (call it 'inner child', if you want) and it still has the desire to be loved by 'father'.

This human compulsion to repeat and to repair the 'childhood drama' ("but this time I'll succeed") is not restricted to relationships or trauma, but can influence all areas of life. There are several concepts in psychology describing and addressing this mechanism in their way: 'repetition compulsion' or 'life script' or 'maladaptive schema'. The best expression for non-psychologists is 'life-trap'.

Erica is obviously stuck in the life-trap of a '*helpless victim*'. In the true story she didn't manage to take the necessary care of herself, despite sufficient intelligence. Instead she acted out her 'innocence', which I called 'diligence' earlier: She 'diligently' followed the program to the letter without making the obvious adjustments. She basically *made sure* that she would end up ...

- suffering ("... made me quite nauseous")
- troubled ("had trouble tolerating...")
- damaged ("waste of time and money")
- lonely ("nobody advised me")
- vengeful ("be warned ...")

Additionally she did what she could to guarantee the failure of the program by quitting after one week. Balancing hormones is a process that takes several months in men and many months in women, if all goes well. Otherwise it will take longer.

Erica declared the program to be ineffective, because it hadn't stopped her migraine. The goal of hormone supplementation is to correct imbalances in the hormone system, not to stop migraine. If these imbalances are the key drivers in someone's individual situation, then rebalancing the hormone system alone *may* be sufficient to stop the migraine. Otherwise it will make it easier for other therapies to correct other imbalances or deficits. To leave the hormone system out of whack can certainly create a roadblock.

Erica is a mature adult *woman*. She is knows the duration of her cycle and is familiar with the time scale of the hormone system. Based on her experience as a woman and with a bit of common sense she could have guessed *three months* as an appropriate first phase, without consulting an expert. Since she is clearly capable of operating computers and navigating the internet, she could have explored the appropriate time frame herself. Instead she found her role as the *helpless innocent victim* confirmed after one week and published her appalled report. Can you see that she is stuck in a life-trap? She is not stupid, she is stuck and needs help.

This story also shows the limits of insufficiently assisted programs: you just can't do everything without professional help. If you're a talented handy(wo)man, you might be able to build a cute dog shed. But when you need to build a skyscraper, you will appreciate the help of an architect. The same is true for therapy.

The type of therapy that addresses these life-traps directly is *schema therapy* and will be introduced later in this book ('schema' means life-trap in psycho-lingo). When people recognize that their troubles in life tend to end with similar results (the wrong guy again, a failed therapy again etc.) it might be worthwhile to consult with a therapist who knows about life-traps and schema therapy.

Seeing a psychotherapist—I prefer the term 'psychological coach'—does not mean that someone admits being a 'nutcase' or 'crazy'. It only means that they are smart enough to get professional support for one of the most important areas in life: How does my *mind* interact with the world and how can I get the most out of it? In elite sport it has become standard to utilize a mental coach, typically a psychologist specialized in performance improvement techniques, when the athlete wants better results.

In that sense, those severe migraineurs who haven't had much luck with their therapy attempts so far, may want to explore the option to seek support from a 'mind coach' as well, when they want better results from migraine therapies.

We've seen examples of how defensive some people are, when it comes to 'psychological' traits. ==**"I'M NOT A NUTCASE, MIGRAINE IS NEUROLOGICAL"**== displays a lot of fear, based on misinformation, misinterpretation and cognitive distortions. All I can do here is educate and explain: "No, you're not a nutcase, but you're not getting what you need. You are a human being with a human mind inside a human brain, you can't change that. What you *can* change is what your mind and brain have learnt so far. Also, you can acquire skills that you haven't learnt yet and that are missing."

In Erica's case the missing skill is *looking after herself* with kindness, care and love, which could render the frantic defenses of her nervous system unnecessary. Then she could use her energy to end the tyranny of migraine instead of wasting it on pitiful protests against the 'unendurable injustice' towards 'victims' like her.

That would also benefit those patients, who *she* is currently misleading at the end of her report: ==**"If you are a migraine sufferer who also has serious immune system problems be warned that this program may not be for you!"**== What does Erica know about the immune and the hormone system? As we have seen, not enough. She clearly can't look after others either and might have scared suitable candidates off. Shame.

Overcoming obstacles

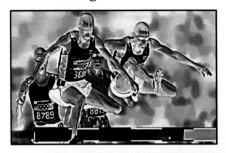

After watching the track and field championship on his divine plasma-TV, God became inspired. "Wow, that 3000m steeplechase, man, what a pearler!" he said to himself and decided to design human life after that model:

"Let there be obstacles, for thou shalt find spirit in the sweat of thy face. Spirit giveth life to he who overcometh what the Lord hath put in hith path."

This leadeth us to the one and only question: *How*? Once you arrive at that question, it's merely a matter of "*spirit*" (= positive motivation) and "*sweat*" (= effort) until you've overcome an obstacle.

Let's say our new friend, the reactive Erica, comes across the advice to try Aspirin for her headaches during a migraine attack. She would say: "I can't take Aspirin, because I have a very sensitive stomach." And then in a more whining voice: "I'VE TRIED ONCE BEFORE AND THE RESULT WAS HELL ..." (drama, victim). Her *causal attribution* (see page 114) leads into a dead end; the pattern is: "I can't, 'cause I am ...." Logically, she can't think of anything but *avoiding*, Aspirin in this case. Since her head pain is too severe to endure without meds, she might end up with an opioid drug and after a while on that stuff, chronification becomes her destiny: abused and victimized by her own stomach.

Had she instead asked the question "*How* can I take aspirin despite prior adverse reactions?" the pharmacist would have given her buffered Aspirin or a combination of paracetamol and Aspirin,[1] which is less irritating for 'sensitive' stomachs. Had she asked "*How?*", a fellow–member on her migraine internet-forum, a nutrionist, could have advised her to eat yogurt before taking the Aspirin, and others could have reported their solutions. Being very 'sensitive' she could have combined certain tricks (a lower dose of buffered Aspirin *and* paracetamol *after* a yogurt etc.). All that may not be the ideal answer, but with some persistence Erica could develop her own stomach-protection strategy, step by step.

---

[1] Stern AI et al "Protective effect of acetaminophen against aspirin- and ethanol-induced damage to the human gastric mucosa" Gastroenterology 1984;86(4):728-33

God didn't create the world in one step either, but he started by asking himself: "How am I gonna do this?" and not with a fearful, whining: "I can't. I've tried once before and the result was hell."

Partly difficult

Finding solutions to problems is not always easy, but it is comparatively simple. The decisive step is to overcome the *feeling* of "I can't, 'cause I am...", which only leads into a dead end. Instead, the question "How am I gonna do this?" is the first step to a solution. However, there are obstacles, which are indeed quite difficult to overcome, because of *conflicting interests*, as you shall see.

People have a personality, which is the sum of their typical thoughts, emotions and behavior patterns. Think of some bigwig bank boss, who is strict, authoritative, loud and slightly belligerent; a *hard-hitting money-maker* with no regard for people's emotions. What happens, when he comes home to his little baby daughter? Is he still the strict, authoritative, loud and slightly belligerent, hard-hitting money-maker? Of course not, he'll change into a gentle, *calm and loving father*. When he's with his mates from high school, he might be a *jovially joking entertainer*. And when he talks to his mom, he might even turn into a *sulky teenager*: "Yes, mom."

Does that guy ("Fred") have a split personality? Yes, of course! If he's healthy, he has several 'sets of personality' for different situations. Additionally, he is still carrying personalities from the past in his brain and mind. For instance, when Fred is in front of the board of directors, he feels a bit like he used to feel in the past, when his strict grandfather treated him with a lot of contempt.

We all hopefully carry a collection of these (sub-)personalities with us. That is normal and healthy. In different schools of psychology these sub-personalities have different names: 'ego states', 'egos', 'parts of self' to name but a few. The most commonly known is probably the 'inner child', which is basically a set of thoughts, emotions and behavior patterns that was 'us' at a certain early age.

What *can* happen and what actually *does* happen is that this inner child still has 'unfinished business', relating to needs that weren't met at the time. I would even say, that everybody has an inner child with partly unmet needs; sometimes more, sometimes less. To some extent, that is what motivates us in life.

The boy who got bullied and beaten in the schoolyard might become a righteous attorney, now fighting for 'justice'. The girl, who felt 'not heard' by her father, might become a professor and can finally force someone (her students) to listen to her 'lectures'.

Children can also be persistent and petulant and here patients might hit an obstacle: It *can* happen, that the adult parts of someone's personality are ready to move on, to change and to try new behaviors in order to end the tyranny; but there is a 'child'–part of their personality that stays persistent in it's demands: "I insist to be 'rescued', I won't do it myself. I want my ... (mommy, daddy?) to solve the problem for me. Otherwise I won't feel loved."

So the adult parts feel sufficiently loved and just want to get rid of the migraine, but that petulant 'child' part of the Self has conflicting interests and sabotages every therapy. Techniques that specialize in dealing with this difficulty are Ego State Therapy or DMNS (= developmental needs meeting strategy). As often in psychology, the names aren't really inviting, but resolving these issues can make all the difference. In some cases it *can* go so far that the 'difficult part' stops driving the brain into attacks after the successful resolution of the internal conflict. This seems less unfathomable, when you imagine the subconscious mind driving the *right* and the conscious mind driving the *left* half of the brain.

Identity theft

The last — I promise — 'difficult' obstacle to ending the tyranny is this one: Migraine has become the *identity*. Imagine a 'difficult' patient with severe migraine, whose entire life revolves around migraine *only*. During pain-free phases he/she sees doctors or is active on internet migraine-forums, writes blogs, you get the idea.

In that situation it *can* and *does* happen that the migraine not only takes over their entire life, but also that the sub-personality "I am a migraineur" suffocates all the other, healthy parts of the Self.

No more 'jovially joking entertainer', no more 'silly sexy seductress'; all that's left are those parts that play a role in the migraine drama: the 'suffering victim' at home, the 'angry patient' in the doctor's office, the 'migraine expert' who writes blogs and articles. To overcome this obstacle, a therapist would help the client to revive and foster the healthy parts and nourish *a new identity*.

Successfully dealing with difficulties

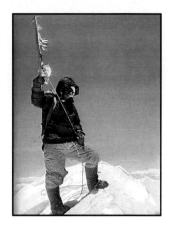

The guy in the photo has just climbed Mt Everest. Evidently he successfully dealt with all the *massive difficulties* that are part of such an ambitious endeavor which makes him one of less than 3500 people who made it to the globe's highest summit. What is truly special about him is that *nobody before him* had ever succeeded. He was one of the two who first conquered Mt Everest: Edmund Hillary and Tenzing Norgay. Hillary took this photo of Tenzing.

All the climbers after them knew that it is *difficult but possible* to reach the summit of Mt Everest (and to return alive) and so, since that day in 1953, many others have dealt with all the difficulties to reach this extraordinary goal, knowing: it is possible.

Would dealing with difficulties be easier for migraineurs, if they knew that it is *possible* to end the migraine tyranny? What do you think? Or do you think it doesn't really matter, so it's no big deal when migraine sufferers get told that "MIGRAINE IS AN INCURABLE GENETIC NEUROLOGICAL DISEASE THAT CAN ONLY BE ALLEVIATED BY MEDICATION "?

What's your opinion? Would migraineurs benefit if someone told them that there are fabulous therapies out there that can help terminate the tyrant's terror (especially as part of a comprehensive rehabilitation program)? Would migraineurs do what needs to be done, overcome the inevitable difficulties and gain their freedom at last? Who is going to *tell* sufferers that *others* have already successfully conquered Mt Migraine?

Good wishes for the mission

We do know what migraine patients *want*: no pain, no other migraine symptoms, no comorbidities, no drug side effects. Everybody wants that and so much more. 'Wanting' is fairly easy and there are practically no limits to what people *wish* for.

If you want to reach the summit of Mt Everest, wishing alone won't make that come true. First, you have to turn the wish into a *vision* and make it your *mission* to realize the vision. Second, you need to plan *goals*, the action steps to approach the summit.

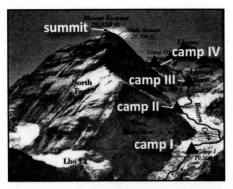
Hillary and Tenzing's *vision* was to conquer Mt Everest and for that they first needed to reach base camp, camp I, camp II, camp III and camp IV before they could attempt to push for the summit. So the camps were the *goals* that allowed them to complete their mission and fulfill their vision.

Good wishes are welcome, but in order to achieve anything you need a *vision*, a strong commitment to the *mission* and well aligned *goals* that lead you to your summit.

The value of goals

It's much easier for us to deal with difficulties and accomplish goals when these are aligned with our personal core *values*. Values are deep-seated, non-negotiable convictions that guide our visions, goals, decisions and actions. A bit like an *inner constitution* in our subconscious mind, telling us what is *right* and *important*.

Let's have a look at your values and convictions so that you can make sure that you pick the right vision for yourself, that you can fully commit to *your mission*, that there are no hidden doubts about the *goals* that you've aligned and that you conquer the right summit for yourself, and not somebody else's peak.

I certainly don't know what your personal values are and I don't need to know, but you do. Therefore, to make it really easy for the both of us, I'll give you two statements each to pick from and so you might get a clearer picture of what your values are, what is right *for you* and important *to you*. Agreed?

Many people and organizations consider effective protection from pain a universal *human right*.[1] What is your conviction?

Everybody has the right to live a life without severe pain.	Pain is a part of life and pain patients should learn to suck it up.

You might want to write the statements that you've picked on a nice piece of writing paper since they represent the core values of the most important person in your life: you.

---

[1] Cousins MJ et al "Pain relief: a universal human right" Pain 2004;112(1-2):1-4

All migraine sufferers have the right to live a life without migraine.	Migraineurs shouldn't be such sissies and also learn to suck it up,.

2.5% of episodic migraineurs develop *chronic* migraine every year.[1] Every fifth migraineur ends up with chronic migraine at some point,[2] strongly assisted by medication overuse.[3]

Migraineurs are entitled to receive protection from becoming chronic.	Migraine is just a bit of a headache

An entire expedition with dozens of people supported Hillary and Tenzing. Their success was the result of a *team effort* as is every successful ascent to the top of a high mountain.

Migraineurs deserve support for the mission to end the migraine tyranny.	Migraineurs don't deserve any support at all.

Studies prove that increased *knowledge* has a positive impact on migraine: In one study, a mere migraine education-program *at least* halved the attack rate in almost half of the participants.[4]

Migraineurs are entitled to a helpful education about migraine.	Migraineurs should be banned from access to any helpful information.

Education, provided by well-informed migraineurs, led to results twice as good as standard treatment only.[5]

Well-informed migraineurs should educate other migraine sufferers.	Well-informed migraineurs should keep their knowledge to themselves.

Supportive *communication* over the internet helped migraine patients significantly: increased social support, decreased stress, decreased catastrophizing, decreased helplessness and depression.[6]

It is important to inform and support all migraineurs via the internet.	Migraineurs should not be informed and supported via the internet.

Whether you already *know* that it's true or whether you *don't believe* it yet: Please <u>*imagine*</u> for a moment that there were indeed therapies available that can actually end the migraine tyranny — especially as part of a complete rehab program. Are you ready?

---

[1] Bigal ME et al "Acute migraine medications and evolution from episodic to chronic migraine: a longitudinal population-based study" Headache 2008;48(8):1157-68
[2] Cady R et al "Cosensitization of pain and psychiatric comorbidity in chronic daily headache" Curr Pain Headache Rep 2005;9(1):47-52
[3] Bigal ME et al "Overuse of acute migraine medications and migraine chronification" Curr Pain Headache Rep 2009;13(4):301-7
[4] Smith TR et al "Migraine education improves quality of life in a primary care setting" Headache 2010;50(4):600-12
[5] Rothrock JF et al "The impact of intensive patient education on clinical outcome in a clinic-based migraine population" Headache 2006;46(5):726-31
[6] Bromberg J et al "A randomized trial of a web-based intervention to improve migraine self-management and coping" Headache 2012;52(2):244-61

Migraine sufferers *must never* find out that they *can* end the tyranny.	All migraine sufferers have the right to be told about effective therapies.

As shareholder companies all medication manufacturers are obligated to maximize their financial profit to enrich their shareholders (= maximization of shareholder value).[1]

It's the drug companies responsibility to inform migraine sufferers about therapies that can end migraine.	It is migraine sufferers' responsibility to inform other migraine sufferers about effective therapies

The off-label use of anti-seizure medication for migraine has a "much higher sales potential" for pharma companies than the FDA-approved use of these drugs for epilepsy.[2] At least one company was fined for pushing a drug into the migraine market of which they knew "it did no good". They plead guilty and paid $34 million.

Drug companies main interest is to help migraineurs end the tyranny.	Migraineurs are obliged to help other migraineurs end the tyranny.

In 2004 the marketing budget of the pharmaceutical industry was close to $60,000,000,000 (= $60 billion) in the US alone.[3] That's a decent sum to spend on spreading misleading migraine myths. Of these $60 billion, "36% was spent on visits to physicians by industry representatives (= 'detailing')". I wonder how doctors show their gratitude?

All doctors are eager to get all migraine patients off drugs and migraine-free.	Only migraineurs are eager to get all migraine patients migraine-free and off drugs.

As you can see, any migraine revolution will be an uphill-battle. In order to better deal with the expected and the unforeseen difficulties along the way, it might be a good idea to turn the conquest of Mt Migraine into a team effort.

Migraineurs get all the support they need from doctors and drugs.	Migraine sufferers of all countries! Unite to bring down the despot!

Today is the day that migraineurs rise up, to terminate the tyrant's terror and so end the unendurable injustice of migraine, to gain their freedom at last ... — "**Hooorrraaayyy**" — ... and return alive.

---

[1] Lazonick W et al "Maximizing shareholder value: a new ideology for corporate governance" Journal Economy and Society 29 (1): 13–35
[2] Edwards J "How Big Pharma Profits From Bogus (and Illegal) Migraine Drugs" CBS news, June 10, 2011
[3] Gagnon MA et al "The cost of pushing pills: a new estimate of pharmaceutical promotion expenditures in the United States" PLoS Med 2008;5(1):e1

Chapter 7

On Top of the Barricades

> "The great enemy of the truth is very often not the lie – deliberate, contrived and dishonest, but the myth, persistent, persuasive, and unrealistic. Belief in myths allows the comfort of opinion without the discomfort of thought."
>
> John F. Kennedy

The cunning old regime has put insidious obstacles in the way of our migraine revolution: *discouraging myths*, cleverly crafted to diffuse any hope to ever end the tyranny. This 'barricade strategy' is working for the regime: Three quarters of migraineurs at least worry that they'll have to put up with the attacks for the rest of their lives.[1] The only aid and succor—so the myths imply—is consuming medication or some suspicious surgery to function as a desperate attempt at a 'migraine prison-break'.

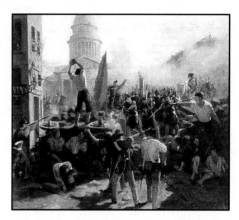

The temptation to accept the myths as truths is great, when you're not well anyway and don't know better either. So let's know better now and get well soon. Let's get on top of the barricades!

"Migraine is genetic"

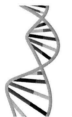

Most people without knowledge of genetics tend to assume that the word 'genetic' means *pre-determined* or 'set in stone', as if the genes were the embodiment of one's destiny; ciphered instructions, encoded in mysteriously twisted strands, the blueprint for our entire life, secretly commanding the health and well-being of our body, mind and brain, as well as the occurrence of migraine attacks.

But the reality is decisively different from this scenario of inexorable doom. The subject has been studied extensively and the findings are confusing at first, but eventually clear.

---

[1] Harris Interactive online poll, cited in Brandes JL "The Migraine Cycle: Patient Burden of Migraine During and Between Migraine Attacks" Headache 2008;48:430-441

If the occurrence of migraine were determined exclusively by the genes, then it would be inevitable that identical twins with identical genes are 100% *concordant*. Concordant means, they *both* would either have or *both* would not have migraine; they couldn't possibly be discordant (= only one of them has migraine).

In 1999 a study showed that in those pairs of monozygotic, identical twins, *where migraine is present*, the concordance rate is only 40%. That means, if you meet a monozygotic 'identical' twin *with* migraine, it is more likely that their sibling is *migraine-free* rather than a migraineur too, *despite* the identical migraine genes.[1]

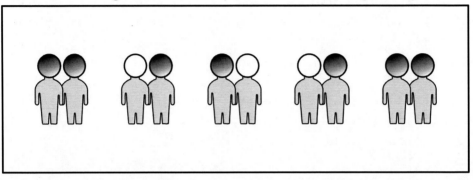

They also studied same-gender, dizygotic non-identical twin pairs and found a concordance rate of 28%.[1] In plain words, despite having the same parents, in *almost three quarters* of these pairs only one of the 'simultaneous siblings' had developed migraine.

Please note that all this excludes *those* twin pairs, where both twins have the genetic 'talent' for migraine and *could* have developed migraine, but neither one actually does have migraine.

Earlier family studies calculated the probability to be a migraineur, when first-degree relatives (parents, siblings, offspring) were migraineurs. This probability is called 'relative risk' in statistics, which does not mean that there is a causal relationship. It measures the increased occurrence in comparison to the population average. And here are the results of a Danish study:

- migraine *with* aura between first–degree relatives: 3.8-fold risk
- migraine *with* aura between **spouses**: no risk increase

This indicates that the occurrence of migraine *with* aura might be influenced by genetic factors. Is that also true *without* aura?

---

[1] Gervil M et al "Migraine without aura: a population-based twin study" Ann Neurol 1999;46(4):606-11

- migraine *without* aura between first-degree relatives: 1.9-fold risk
- migraine *without* aura between **spouses**: 1.5-fold risk (!) [1]

Considering that spouses normally don't have common genes, these numbers support the conclusion that either
- there is some rotten incest going on in the state of Denmark
- or migraine without aura is an infectious disease.

A third possibility is that there is some genetic influence, but personality factors play a role too. The unexpected 1.5-fold rate of migraine between spouses could be explained by the plausible assumption that *personalities* prone to migraine—in the spirit of "like attracts like"—find each other 1.5 times more attractive.

Population-based genetic studies, like this one, are always a bit messy, when potentially many factors are involved, as is the case in the development of migraine. How do you discriminate the effects of 'nature' versus 'nurture', of genes versus 'life'? Is it mom's migraine-gene that you've inherited or was it her nervousness that lead to an insecure attachment[2] and so to a more tense brain state? How can migraine be programmed by genes, when children born to mothers with migraine have a 1.9-fold increased risk of ending up with *asthma* instead?[3] How did they switch the program? Was it perhaps a somewhat altered breathing pattern that interfered with the gene expression (= how the genes are used)? That is impossible, you think? Fact is that the tissue levels of CO_2—a gas that we exhale—can indeed impact on gene expression.[4] Is that even conceivable: Could migraine be less of a 'genetic,' but more of a disorder of faulty breathing? This can't possibly be true. Or can it?

There is one thing that we should always keep in mind. At certain times in history it was *inconceivable* that the earth is not flat or that man could fly to the moon. Once it was *unthinkable* to talk to someone, who isn't there; or to listen to music from an orchestra inside your shirt-pocket. Today there are still educated people out there who would refuse to believe that it is possible to rehabilitate a stroke victim from half-sided paralysis to playing the piano.[5]

---

[1] Russell MB et al "Increased familial risk and evidence of genetic factor in migraine" BMJ 1995;311(7004):541-4
[2] Savi L et al "Attachment styles and headache" J Headache Pain. 2005;6(4):254-7
[3] Chen TC et al "Asthma and eczema in children born to women with migraine" Arch Neurol 1990;47(11):1227-30
[4] Taylor CT et al "Regulation of gene expression by carbon dioxide" Source J Physiol 2011;589(Pt 4):797-803
[5] Adamovich S et al "Recovery of hand function in virtual reality: Training hemiparetic hand and arm together or separately" Conf Proc IEEE Eng Med Biol Soc 2008:3475-8

Looking at the history of science, we all are well advised to be extremely cautious with absolute judgments that we can't prove. "That is unthinkable, inconceivable, impossible!" — "Prove that!"

Genetic studies on twins are more illuminating, since it is clear that monozygotic twins have identical genes, which makes things easier. One study could identify that migraine *with aura* and migraine *without aura* are distinct disorders in Denmark, probably with different genes.[1] In the Netherlands, however, the researchers found no clue for genetic differences between the two migraine types,[2] which is in accordance with the first twin study in 1999: 23% of pairs were discordant for aura; one of the identical twins had aura, the sibling did not.[3] Isn't this weird?

It might be that the question "How strong is the genetic influence in migraine?" turns out to be misguided before an answer is found. The assumption that the genes, at least partly, pull the strings *independently* from other factors and we simply measure how strong the gene's impact is, that assumption may be naïve. It's a bit like trying to understand a book by counting the letters and words. Epigenetics, the science of gene expression, tells us that genes get switched on and off all the time, for instance based on levels of CO_2 or distress[4]. How do you account for that?

We could go on for hours looking at hundreds of studies, but we have a revolution to attend to. Let's cut to the chase, shall we?

You *can not* genetically inherit migraine, migraine symptoms or migraine attacks. At best you can inherit the *genetic disposition* for migraine, which makes it *possible* to develop migraine.[5] I tend to call this the 'talent', because everybody understands that a talent won't come to fruition unless it gets *developed*.

Studies with 30,000 twin pairs tell us that the 'heritability' (= statistical 'genetic risk') of migraine varies from 34% in Australia up to 57% in some groups in Finland.[6] On average it's 45%.

45% only? That's not particularly 'genetic', is it?

---

[1] Russell MB et al "Migraine without aura and migraine with aura are distinct disorders. A population-based twin survey" Headache 2002;42(5):332-6

[2] Ligthart L et al "Migraine with aura and migraine without aura are not distinct entities: further evidence from a large Dutch population study" Twin Res Hum Genet 2006;9(1):54-63

[3] Gervil M et al "Migraine without aura: a population-based twin study" Ann Neurol 1999;46(4):606-11

[4] Karssen AM et al "Stress-induced changes in primate prefrontal profiles of gene expression" Mol Psychiatry 2007;12(12):1089-102

[5] Loder E "What is the evolutionary advantage of migraine?" Cephalalgia 2002;22(8):624-32

[6] Mulder EJ et al "Genetic and environmental influences on migraine: a twin study across six countries" Twin Res. 2003;6(5):422-31

The genetic influence on migraine is best understood the other way round: The lack of 'talent' for migraine is 100% 'genetic'.[1] A lot of people have inherited the genes that provide complete migraine resistance. All the others can possibly develop migraine, when their 'resistance' drops too low. There can be many reasons for that, but it is clear that an estimated 55% of those with a 'talent' for migraine actually *do not* develop any migraine symptoms ever in their lives.

Based on what we know, people with the 'talent' or 'genetic disposition' for migraine can't lose that 'talent'. But they can raise their level of resistance to the degree that they're migraine-free. In a catchy phrase: Resistance ends the tyranny. Makes sense?

The odd phrase **"MIGRAINE IS GENETIC"** is <u>shorthand</u> among experts, who know what it means to them,[2] which is: You need the genetic talent in order to have migraine. Obviously there are plenty of authors (books, articles, websites etc.) who take the phrase and run, spread the word without the meaning. In our information age 'copy & paste' wins over 'learn & think' and the text slays the word.

The slack expression **"... IS GENETIC"** alone indicates a form of slang. It's nothing more than geek-speak, lingo or jargon, meant for a closed circle of insiders only. Clearly, the unique geek-speak did leak from the sleek clique — freaks!

"Migraine can't be cured"

"The tyrant can't be toppled." Who would say that, if not the tyrant's helpers? Dedicated devotees who have found their mission in supporting the despot's dreaded dominion? Who would be keen to systematically *discourage* migraineurs from terminating the tyrant's terror, to gain their freedom at last?

The pharma industry is off the hook. They have no interest in launching a sales-damaging rumor by Chinese whisper like this:
Speaker for Big Pharma: "Migraine can't be cured."
First person in the crowd: "What did they say?"
Second person in the crowd: "They said they can't cure migraine."
Third person in the crowd: "Sorry, what was that?"
First person again: "They said, they have nothing for migraine."

That's not good for sales, is it?

---

[1] Svensson DA et al "Shared rearing environment in migraine: results from twins reared apart and twins reared together" Headache 2003;43(3):235-44

[2] Loder E "What is the evolutionary advantage of migraine?" Cephalalgia 2002;22(8):624-32

If it's not the pharma industry, could it be doctors, who have a vested interest to make a truckload of money with their migraine patients? And so they use their position to dispirit patients?

Well, I don't think so. We know that a majority of migraineurs manage the malady without a medico. The ones who regularly see doctors are often (more or less) anxious, depressive, neurotic, fearful- or dismissive-avoidant, pessimistic catastrophizers with little trust and a strong tendency for emotional coping behavior. Not the kind of patient that makes it easy to conduct profitable conveyor-belt-medicine.

The idea of earning truckloads of money with Botox® or PFO closure-procedures seems far-fetched. Advanced severe migraine, which would typically lead to these desperate treatment attempts, is more prevalent in households with a low income[1] and many patients are out of work by then.[2] And whilst it is conceivable that some doctors with a private practice in a wealthy area can make that kind of concept fly, in general the treatment of migraine is considered rather time-consuming and draining[3] than rewarding and lucrative.

> "Hold on. Are you saying that doctors are not that wild about seeing lots of migraineurs every day? Then why on earth would they not refer them on to other therapies, especially to those evidence-based behavioral methods with maximal scientific blessing that are explicitly mentioned in the treatment guidelines?"

The puzzling info here is that many doctors regularly do make referrals to *behavioral* therapies[4] (= where patients *do* something) in the treatment of migraine; for instance for children,[5] adolescents,[6] pregnant women,[7] for medication overuse[8] or even chronic transformed migraine.[9] Why not in all suitable cases?

---

[1] Tepper SJ "A pivotal moment in 50 years of headache history: the first American Migraine Study" Headache 2008;48(5):730-1

[2] Buse DC et al "Sociodemographic and comorbidity profiles of chronic migraine and episodic migraine sufferers" J Neurol Neurosurg Psychiatry 2010;81(4):428-32

[3] Miller RC "The somatically preoccupied patient in primary care: use of attachment theory to strengthen physician-patient relationships" Osteopath Med Prim Care 2008;2:6

[4] Holroyd KA et al "Behavioral approaches to the treatment of migraine" Semin Neurol 2006;26(2):199-207

[5] Termine C et al "Overview of diagnosis and management of paediatric headache. Part II: therapeutic management" J Headache Pain 2011;12(1):25–34

[6] Baumann RJ "Behavioral treatment of migraine in children and adolescents" Paediatr Drugs 2002;4(9):555-61

[7] Contag SA et al "Contemporary management of migrainous disorders in pregnancy" Curr Opin Obstet Gynecol 2010;22(6):437-45

[8] Andrasik F et al "Behavioral medicine for migraine and medication overuse headache" Curr Pain Headache Rep 2009;13(3):241-8

[9] Grazzi L et al "Behavioral and pharmacologic treatment of transformed migraine with analgesic overuse: outcome at 3 years" Headache 2002;42(6):483-90

I can think of two plausible answers to this question. First, migraineurs *demand* medication, like everybody. That makes sense for those with rare attacks, who respond well to meds; a convenient and simple solution. However, whenever I read the exchanges on internet forums between severe 'difficult' patients, who *don't* do well on drugs, I am amazed by the displayed persistence, with which drugs are discussed (à la "There **must** be one that works").

In contrast, behavioral therapies are barely mentioned, unless a new member inquires about them and the group veterans take that as their cue for failure-reports in the spirit of "I'VE TRIED THAT ONCE AND THE RESULT WAS HELL." Erica is everywhere.

The question is: "Why do doctors push behavioral therapies for 'problem' cases like children, moms-to-be or chronic migraine, but not for everybody suitable?" The second plausible answer is that doctors — typically, usually, in general, on average, blablabla — are *biased* in favor of their own treatments, just like every other therapist, healer, coach, lawyer, butcher, baker, candlestick-maker.

In my experience **A**cupuncturists are biased in favor of Acupuncture, **B**ehavioral therapists are biased in favor of Behavioral therapies, **C**rystal healers are biased in favor of **C**rystal healing, and **D**octors are biased in favor of **D**rugs. Go on with that alphabet, if you want, but human as we are, we all tend to *like* our own stuff more. That's all. (Or do you believe docs get bribed?)

Obviously, doctors have no interest in spreading the morose myth "MIGRAINE CAN'T BE CURED". Who is it then? Who has a *benefit* from placing dark clouds in migraineurs' already overcast sky?

One migraine-book author asserts: "ANYONE WHO PROMISES TO CURE YOUR MIGRAINES IS SELLING SNAKE OIL." Of course, he doesn't provide any *evidence* for his belief, but he connects the already laden term 'cure' to 'promise' and 'snake oil' (= quack medicine). Migraine + cure + promise = snake oil. Wow, that is hard to crack. Does this mean that therapists, who rehabilitate migraine successfully, are inevitably quacks? Or is the 'promise' the snake–oily part here?

The author reasons: "WE HAVE NO MIRACLE CURE OR SECRET FORMULA THAT WORKS FOR EVERYONE, ..." So his logic is: "Because we have no *miracle cure for everyone*, therefore the promise of *any* 'cure' for *anyone* is quackery." We've talked quite a lot about cognitive distortions in chapter 5. Here you see why.

The bar is set very high. That author demands not only a *cure*, but also insists that only a *miracle cure for everyone* warrants any promise. Otherwise he claims the patients for himself and his migraine-management method, a self-serving cognitive distortion.

The word 'cure' in "MIGRAINE CAN'T BE CURED" sums up the issue with the current treatment regime. We typically say "They haven't found a cure for the common cold", which is a viral infection, or "a cure for cancer". Infectious diseases and cancer are typically treated with medication or other passive medical remedies. The infective intruders (virus or bacterium) or the wicked tumor cells are the targets of destructive medical therapies, which can be superbly successful. Think of bacterial pneumonia or the most common form of leukemia in children; they typically get *cured* like that.

In contrast, migraine is *neither* an infectious disease *nor* a cancer *nor* does it present with a comparable target for a similar passive cure. There is no migraine-*germ* or migraine-*cancer*, no ill core, which could be annihilated as a 'cure'.

Migraine occurs, when the patient's body, mind and brain—otherwise healthy—are merely but severely somehow *out of balance* or *dysregulated* and the brain takes the brunt. Therefore adjustments, support and strengthening are needed rather than demolition work.

That's why '*cure*' is simply not an appropriate word, when it comes to effective therapy or successful rehabilitation of migraine. But this is not what they want to point out, when *they* say: "MIGRAINE CAN'T BE CURED." I mean, it's not that they're saying: "Cure is a crap word, but migraine can be overcome!" Instead the message is a stern and stubborn: "MIGRAINEUR, YOU'RE STUCK IN THE TRAP; GET USED TO IT!" Why would you say that? What's the intention or purpose?

It can be a good idea to ask yourself that very question: "What is the probable intention behind someone's statement? What's the purpose of this myth?" As we've learnt in this chapter from that author with his cognitive distortions, he obviously meant to emphasize how valuable his migraine management method is.

In other cases the intention may be 'vengeance' or 'a cry for help' or there may be no conscious intention behind it anymore, but pure hopeless frustration. Perhaps some can't endure the emotional pain of "I personally have lost any hope and faith", and so they display their hopelessness as "MIGRAINE—BY ITS VERY NATURE—IS INCURABLE."

Emotions are a good thing, everybody should have some at the right time and place. However, we cannot allow someone's hopeless frustration or their self-serving interests to define the limits of our possibilities. How dare they clip our options? How dare they bring us down? As much as I feel sympathy for their pain and suffering and as much as I acknowledge their bleak emotions, when it comes to exploring the potential or to seizing opportunities, we need to be driven by *confidence* and guided by *facts.*

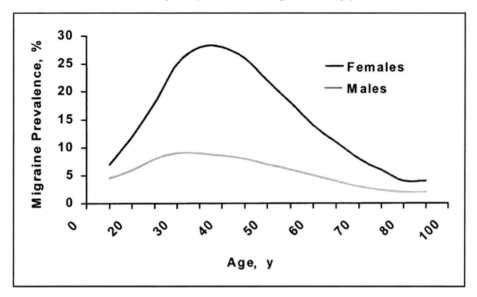

The above graph[1] shows the prevalence of migraine in different age groups. The percentage of women with migraine (black line) shows a pretty steep increase from age 20 to the peak in the early 40s. After that the number decreases steadily.

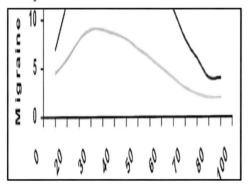

In order to see the men's data better, I've stretched the graph a bit. It shows a similar pattern. The number of male migraineurs rises from 20 to 30 years and then declines. In the *vast majority* of cases, migraine is only present during a certain phase in life.

---

[1] Lipton et al "Prevalence and Burden of Migraine in the United States: Data From the American Migraine Study II" Headache 2001:41(7):646-657

Migraine comes and goes. Women in their prime are the most hard hit. At a time when kids and career clash, women with migraine buckle under their own ambitions and suffer. After that the migraine cloud miraculously starts lifting. With menopause, most become migraine-free. This doesn't look like the footprint of an *'incurable'* disease, does it?

An incurable disease doesn't respond to treatment. Yet, we've seen plenty of favorable treatment responses in this book already (and I haven't even mentioned the really good stuff):

- preventive meds do at least halve the attack rate in up to 50% of patients
- PFO closure (fake or real) did reduce the headache days by a third
- Botox® injections (fake or real) did reduce the rate of attacks by a third
- Education about medication risks reduced the days on drugs from 22 to 6/month

Treatment methods, which are not part of evidence-based medicine are typically called 'alternative' medicine/therapy. Many migraineurs try to get additional help from these methods, be it as true alternative or complementary to medication. An Italian study on *headache clinic patients* found that in the majority of cases a personal suggestion by a friend or a relative was the motivation. Among those 'difficult' patients 40% reported beneficial effects from some alternative treatment.[1]

Aromatherapy, Bowen technique, chiropractic, hypnotherapy, massage, nutrition, reflexology, Reiki and yoga are all endorsed as alternative treatments for migraine by professional organizations in the UK.[2] None of these methods is recognized as 'proven effective' and yet, they get recommended and utilized. It is unlikely that all these methods *never* do anything for anyone; otherwise nobody would ever recommend them privately or officially. The experience is rather the other way round. There is probably *not* a single healing method under the sun, which has *not* helped at least a few migraineurs. If a fake surgical procedure is helpful to some degree, why not aromatherapy? An Indian study reported that 35% of migraineurs in an Ayurveda treatment became *symptom-free*.[3]

---

[1] Rossi P et al "Prevalence, pattern and predictors of use of complementary and alternative medicine (CAM) in migraine patients attending a headache clinic in Italy" Cephalalgia 2005;25(7):493-506

[2] Long L et al "Which complementary and alternative therapies benefit which conditions? A survey of the opinions of 223 professional organisations" Complement Ther Med 2001;9(3):178-85

[3] Vaidya PB et al "Response to Ayurvedic therapy in the treatment of migraine without aura" Int J Ayurveda Res 2010;1(1):30-6

There is no reason to doubt any success-reports from any form of conventional or alternative treatment. It is *characteristic* for migraine that sometimes even quite severe cases suddenly become drastically improved or 'cured' by something: by a therapy method of recognized or of questionable value; or by leaving an abusive partner; or by finding such a one; or by starting an exercise routine and sticking to it; or by changing jobs; or by cosmetic surgery or... .

We only need to peruse the migraine-book reviews on amazon.com to run into an abundance of these stories:

Several people reported that they became *migraine-free* after reading a book about magnesium and following the given advice.

Other people apparently have *healed* their migraine headache and taken charge of their pain by following a 1-2-3 program, which suggests to simply abstain from any abortive or analgesic medication and to follow a strict and very restrictive diet plan, which avoids all suspected 'trigger' foods on the author's list.

Some readers of a competing breakthrough-book *swear by* the special supplement combination, which the author promotes, and claim substantial life-changing relief.

One book promises to forever banish the curse of migraine with various hormone creams and nutritional supplements. We already know from Erica that this approach is not for everyone and still, a decent number of readers report enthusiastically that it *worked* for them to get their life back.

In contrast to all these success stories in amazon reviews: Heavily endorsed self-help books and raving success-reports about medication-withdrawal, diet restrictions or supplements are exceptionally *rare* for pneumonia, leukemia, Creutzfeldt-Jakob disease or Ebola virus. How odd is that?

As we have seen here, migraine is pretty much the *opposite* of an incurable disease. It's quite a capricious, sometimes puzzling condition with symptoms that vary between attacks, between patients and over time. The placebo response rates in treatment trials reach 33% for preventive procedures and up to over 50% for acute amelioration,[1] which serves as a sign of a considerable contribution of the mind to the mechanisms of migraine.

---

[1] Dumitriu A "Placebo effects in neurological diseases" J Med Life 2010;3(2):114-21

This also indicates what is behind the bizarre myth of the allegedly 'incurable' migraine, which is in complete contradiction of reality: The advocates of this atrocious assertion are *migraineurs* themselves and so we need to understand "MIGRAINE CAN'T BE CURED" not so much as a *statement*, but rather as a *symptom*: a symptom of a mind that is not well, inside a brain that is not good.

By its very nature migraine is particularly pliable and can be formed in our favor. We need to stay on top of these evil barricades in order to topple the tyrant and to terminate the terror.

"Migraine is a neurological disease"

What does that mean? What is the intention behind it? What's the purpose? Words are more than just a 'thing'. They represent concepts, emotions, images and memories. Think of the word "nigger". It is 'politically incorrect' or even taboo, because it is packed with concepts, emotions, images and memories which one might not wish to convey. Otherwise, why would you not use it for persons of dark complexion?

Not that the word "nigger" is not used, it gets said a lot. But if your skin is rather pink-ish–beige, you'll probably think twice before shouting it in the South Bronx in New York. Why? Because it contains concepts, emotions, images and memories, which many people find offensive and which may cause some aggravation.

By now it should be obvious that the word 'disease' is an odd choice for migraine. Sure, it's not illegal by itself and nobody in the South Bronx would break your nose for using it. Yet, 'disease' is also packed with concepts, emotions, images and memories that rather cause *aggravation* than provide *explanation*.

And so I'm asking: Why would anyone want to aggravate migraineurs and their already heavy burden of pessimism? What's the intention behind this choice of word that mentally moves migraine into a corner with conditions like pneumonia, leukemia, Creutzfeldt-Jakob and Ebola virus infection? Is it a passion for drama? Is it meant to impress? "I'M ILL WITH A REAL NEUROLOGICAL DISEASE!" Do people in the bus get up and give you their seat? Do the boy scouts mow your lawn? Or do you get concession tickets at the museum, because you are disabled by a 'neurological disease'? What about handicapped parking? Truly 'crippled' by migraine?

The term **'*disease*'** is used for an unfavorable health condition caused or mitigated by a pathological (= sick) process like a viral or bacterial infection, proliferation of cancer cells and stuff like that. We already know that migraine doesn't belong here.

'*Disorder*' is used, when someone is not well, but there is no 'disease' involved. So there is nothing pathological—no cancer, no germ— but things are 'not in order' nevertheless. Having a disorder is not necessarily better than having a disease; disorder is not 'disease light'. It's a different category. Let's take an example:

When people don't sleep well, because their mind is racing, their body is tense and their brain keeps bouncing up instead of calming down, we would suspect too much caffeine or energy drinks with stimulating substances. If that's not the case and the sleep problem persists, it would be called a *sleep **disorder***.

When insomnia occurs with other symptoms, like confusion and swelling of lymph nodes, then it might be a symptom of an infection with a parasite, transmitted by a tsetse fly, called *sleeping sickness* (congo trypanosomiasis), a parasitic ***disease***. That's different from sleeplessness due to mental or emotional distress, isn't it?

Migraine is ***not a disease***, because there is no infection or comparable process; migraine is a ***disorder***, because obviously things are '*not in order*' when you episodically experience the agony, misery and assault of migraine attacks.

Is migraine a *neurological* disorder then? Well, what does that mean? 'Neurology' means 'the teachings of the nervous system' and neurologists are doctors, who treat 'medical' conditions of the nervous system. When you're drunk, your nervous system is also in an unfavorable condition, but that's not a case for a neurologist.

Is migraine then a case for a neurologist? This is where things get a tiny bit tricky. And a good opportunity to clarify concepts.

Fred has high blood pressure, quite high actually. Over the years the once athletic sunny boy has transformed into a fat bigwig bank boss, a hard-hitting money-maker with no regard for his health. Life has taken its toll, has collected the fee for traveling the road to financial success. Now Fred is scared shitless, because his father died early from a stroke, possibly caused by notoriously high blood pressure. Driven by the fear of an early death, Fred is determined and committed to deal with that problem.

Fred's doctor does all the tests to rule out a disease: no thyroid trouble, no tumor in the adrenals (= glands on top of the kidneys) etc. — diagnosis: essential idiopathic hypertension syndrome.

"Okay Fred," the doctor says, "*the test results are clear. You don't have any disease that would explain your high blood pressure. This is called idiopathic hypertension and can lead to stroke and heart attack and other nasty things.*"

Fred already knows what's about to happen; he's read about it on the internet: The doc is going to prescribe blood pressure meds and instruct him to start a blood pressure diary, to document Fred's own regular measurements.

The doctor continues: "*Fred, your father was one of my first patients and since the time he died, we've learnt a lot about the connections between body, mind and brain. High blood pressure is a <u>disorder</u>, a sign that body, mind and brain are not in balance, in your case they're under <u>too much pressure</u> and that shows up as your blood pressure, but also as your body fat and your mood and temper. You barely take time for your family and your little baby daughter. Your life doesn't have a healthy balance and the question is why? That's what you'll need to address on all levels involved: body, mind and brain.*"

"Wow" Fred is surprised. "I thought, you would give me a bunch of prescriptions and send me on my way."

The doctor sat down slowly, looked out the window and said: "*I know. That's what I did to your father.*"

And so they talked for a while about who else could help Fred to revive his former self, sunny and athletic as he used to be. The doctor gave him business cards: a nutritionist to help with the weight loss, a fitness coach for an exercise program, a psychological coach to support Fred's endeavor to sort out priorities, values and goals in life and an expert to improve his breathing and self-regulation (= ability to control thoughts, emotions and bodily responses). In addition the doctor gave Fred a form for more tests: "*Often, when people are out whack for a while, the hormones are out of kilter too. Then it can help to support them as well.*"

"I'm speechless" said Fred, "it's so weird. I *know* that your suggestions are bang on and yet, I *feel* that the 'inner pressure' is trying to resist a change. That's my issue! Thank you so much, doc. But it will take some time and effort to see this through, right?"

"You're spot on, Fred, that's exactly right, and there will be difficulties along the way. Severely high blood pressure is a serious disorder that needs a sincere approach. You deserve better than what your father got, but deserving doesn't mean that you won't still have to earn it. Look at it this way; today we're all spoilt by the ease with which we can cure diseases that would have killed us a hundred years ago. This disease-fighting strategy doesn't work with disorders, where body, mind and brain are out of balance, but we still want the same cures: medication, radiation or surgery. And you can have that, lots of it in fact, but that's not the solution. If you want to overcome a problem, you need to face it and that's what you're going to do, on every level, body, mind and brain."

Conventional medicine is divided into specialty areas. One type of division is based on organ systems of interest. For example, cardiologists are specialized in heart diseases, dermatologists in skin diseases, endocrinologists in diseases of the hormone system, gastroenterologists in stomach and bowel diseases and neurologists are specialized in diseases of the nervous system. In addition there are other specialty doctors for certain techniques (like surgeons or radiologists) or for the diseases of different age groups. Everything is taken care of as long as it is a disease.

When the problem at hand is *not* a disease, but a *disorder*, like idiopathic hypertension or migraine, that system doesn't work well anymore; at least not well for the patient. So what needs to be done is to connect to other therapeutic professionals to add the missing competence and expertise to the 'medical' treatments.

There are some areas of healthcare where that happens: Several professional therapists cooperate to help the patients better than any single one could. However, neurology is not one of the areas where this model of *multi-level therapy* is common and neurologists are not well trained in collaborating with other therapists. Experience shows that it will take some time to get them on board.

The majority of migraineurs don't see doctors at all or not anymore; the next biggest group gets treated by GPs. Neurologists only treat a minority of migraineurs. In that sense, it is not really critical whether we call migraine a *neurological* disorder or not. It's a *disorder*, in which body, mind *and* brain are 'out of order' or 'out of balance' or lacking 'resistance and resilience' or 'sufficient stability': An earthquake affects the entire 'zoo' and not just a single 'cage'.

"Migraine is caused by swelling and inflammation ...

... OF BLOOD VESSELS AROUND YOUR HEAD." You've heard that one, haven't you? That's a bit of a bummer. What can you do about those swollen and inflamed blood vessels other than take medication? It explains that feeling like a 'helpless victim' is completely justified. It's not your fault that you have inherited those nasty blood vessels that swell and get inflamed, right?

Let's start our drill: What's the intention behind it? Who has a benefit from this myth? Is it helping you to end the tyranny?

Imagine, *you* are the creative director of an advertising agency. Your client is a shampoo manufacturer and you have to come up with a campaign to boost the sales of Silkenshine—Hair Care from Mother Nature–with natural Amarula-oil and vitamins.

As a professional communicator, you know what you have to do to really hammer home the two-step message. First: "Normal hair is horrible." Many women respond particularly well to negative messages, tickling their 'defectiveness'. Think of their endless self-criticism: "I'm not good at this, my butt is too big, my boobs are ... etc.". To prove how 'horrible' normal hair is, you organize some images of normal hair under a super research-microscope. That will give your campaign credibility, because it looks somehow scientific.

For the second message you'll have another picture, which shows that the natural Amarula-oil gently smooths the rough nano-structure of every single hair, whilst the vitamins nourish it from the inside. This way you will tell women, that their dreams are about to come true (under the condition they buy your client's product): "Silkenshine will give women what they truly desire: soft, shiny and healthy hair."

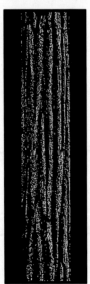
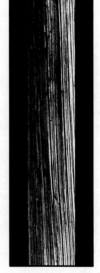

⬅ normal human hair under a microscope: rough nano-structure; simply **horrible**, yuck!

same hair after washing with Silkenshine ➡ now it is **soft, shiny and healthy** thanks to Silkenshine's Amarula-oil and vitamins
SILKENSHINE – Hair Care from Mother Nature
"Because you are naturally beautiful."

Your campaign is amazing. I'm completely sold and can't wait to get my hands on that fabulous Silkenshine shampoo. Now that I've understood how the Amarula-oil gently smooths the rough nano-structure of my horrible hair whilst the vitamins nourish it from the inside, I have no doubt that Silkenshine will give me soft, shiny and healthy hair. *"How did you do that?"*

"The human mind is eager to 'understand' and demands an explanation for everything as to how it works.[1] Once the mind has the impression, it has 'understood' a mechanism, it is happy like a baby after being fed." — It shows that you're an advertising guru.

You continue: "I've given you the *illusion* of an explanation, but that was enough already for your mind to relax. The truth is that you still have no idea how the smoothing is supposed to work and you didn't notice that vitamins do jackshit for hair, since it's dead tissue and can't possibly use vitamins."

"Absolutely! And what the heck is 'nano-structure' anyway?" — "I have no idea either, but you now have a mental concept in your head, which *you can't get rid of*. The images are in your memory and you're somehow still keen on buying Silkenshine. That is a stable idea in your head and it won't disappear, even when I tell you that the images were photos of *tree bark*." — Your client is so lucky to have you as his advertising expert.

Once an explanation sounds good, our mind often can't be bothered to question, whether the reasoning is logical and compelling, whereas it can drive us nuts, when we don't have a clue how things work (Have you ever been to a magician's show?)

"MIGRAINE IS CAUSED BY SWELLING AND INFLAMMATION OF BLOOD VESSELS AROUND YOUR HEAD." Could that be true? Well, let's look at the symptoms of a migraine attack:

- prodromal phase: changes in mood, thinking, speech, self-control, alertness, appetite, water balance, digestion, body temperature, sensory tolerance
- aura phase: visual field disturbances; visual, sound, smell hallucinations; muscle weakness, difficulties with language comprehension and speech
- headache phase: head pain, dizziness, nausea, vomiting, sensory intolerance stuffy or runny nose, as well as continuation of the prodromal symptoms; distinct feeling of being ill, 'illness behavior', social withdrawal;

---

[1] Grimm SR "Explanatory Inquiry and the Need for Explanation" Br J Philos Sci (2008) 59 (3): 481-497

I personally am dumbfounded that anybody would assume that a blood-vessel dilemma outside the brain could cause this amazing diversity of symptoms. When I look at this list, I can't help but think, what all these symptoms have in common is that they originate in the brain itself: mood, thinking, speech, self-control, alertness, appetite, water balance, digestion, body temperature, vision, hearing, smelling, dizziness, nausea, vomiting..., they're all brain functions. Therefore I would have expected that there is some form of 'storm' in the brain responsible for all those symptoms.

In 1873 the English medical doctor Edward Liveing[1] wrote about migraine as an *electrical nerve storm* after he recognized that all those peculiar brain symptoms couldn't possibly be caused by blood vessels outside the brain. Funnily enough, in his time a popular explanation was: Migraine is caused by the *constriction* (= narrowing) of blood vessels; an idea that also still lives on.

The puzzling thing with any blood-vessel theory of migraine is that it doesn't make any sense whatsoever. It neither explains the symptoms *during* the migraine attack, nor the symptoms *between* attacks, nor the breathtaking number of *comorbidities*, with mood disorders (depression, anxiety) — which are clearly brain-related — at the top of the list. Insofar, it also seems entirely irrelevant that research has convincingly *disproven* the so-called vascular theory, the blood-vessel-related inflammatory myth of migraine.[2]

Not even the *migraine headache* is related to vascular constriction and dilation during an attack.[3] That was shown with drug-induced[4,5] as well as with spontaneous[6] attacks utilizing different brain imaging techniques — so what?

That's the cool thing about our human mind: It doesn't really matter that it's unproven, illogical nonsense. Once we've *committed* to an idea, we tend to stick with it, because we want to be *consistent* with prior decisions.[7] I would still buy Silkenshine–Hair Care from Mother Nature, if only it was available. Wouldn't you?

---

[1] Liveing E "On megrim, sick-headache and some allied disorders: A Contribution to the Pathology of Nerve-Storms" 1873
[2] Goadsby PJ "The vascular theory of migraine--a great story wrecked by the facts" Brain 2009;132(Pt 1):6-7
[3] Olesen J et al "Timing and topography of cerebral blood flow, aura, and headache during migraine attacks" Ann Neurol 1990;28(6):791-8
[4] Kruuse C et al "Migraine can be induced by sildenafil without changes in middle cerebral artery diameter" Brain 2003;126(Pt 1):241-7
[5] Schoonman GG et al "Migraine headache is not associated with cerebral or meningeal vasodilatation--a 3T magnetic resonance angiography study" Brain 2008;131(Pt 8):2192-200
[6] Nagata E et al "The middle meningial artery during a migraine attack: 3T magnetic resonance angiography study" Intern Med 2009;48(24):2133-5
[7] Cialdini RB "Commitment and Consistency: Hobglobins of the mind" Chapter 3 in "Influence" Allyn & Bacon 2001:52ff

The appealing idea of Amarula-oil gently smoothing the nano-structure of our 'horrible' hair, making it soft and shiny, as well as vitamins nourishing it from the inside, *resonates* with our desire to be beautiful and loveable. This easily overrides our conscious insight that tree bark photos prove nothing.

If the idea and mental image of migrainous blood vessels, swollen and inflamed, *resonates* with feelings of helplessness and the burning pain of suffering, then we need to remediate those feelings; by learning to seek competent support, as well as by helping ourselves. This will not only extinguish the 'flames' in our head and soften the rough mental images, but also put a shiny smile on our face and nourish the soul from the inside.

"Migraine is neurological, not psychological"

The earthquake lasted only minutes and so George hopped back on his bike and kept on pedaling as fast as he could. Being late on his first day at a new job was not his style. Simple and friendly, George was a diligent worker, a fine young man, who tried hard to make the best of the cards destiny had dealt him. The scars on his skull were barely visible under his curly hair and the regular cycling had helped him to regain his balance. A certain 'narrowness' in thinking was the last obvious left-over from his accident.

The zoo director was standing at the entrance, scrutinizing his wristwatch when George came flying around the corner and exactly at 7:00 he stood straight in front of the director with a winning smile: "Good morning, sir."

"Listen, mate, I know it's your first day, but we are in a bit of a predicament," the director explained. "*The earthquake has opened all the cages and all the animals are running wild all over the place. I gotta race to the dentist, my tooth is killing me and so you have to step up to the plate, rise to the challenge, pull out all the stops and lift your game straight away.*" Since that workshop 'How to motivate employees' the director tended to use a lot of those flowery phrases: "*At the end of the day all that counts is to serve the community and today it's your chance to make a difference.*"

The director was running out of phrases while George was still thinking about what 'predicament' meant; it sounded like the director was in a bit of a pickle: "How can I help, sir?"

The zoo director abandoned the idea of adding more phrases to his speech and instructed George accurately and thoroughly: *"Tidy up the frickin' mess! Catch them frickin' critters and put them back in their frickin' cages! Put together what belongs together and hurry up!"*

The dust, which the fleeing director's car had stirred up, hadn't settled yet, but George was already on the job. He snatched them frickin' critters at a rate per minute that secretaries would lie in a resume was their typing speed.

George had just locked the last cage when his cell phone rang. It was the director: *"Jimmy, how are you travelling, mate? Did you catch any? Did they bite you? What's the damage? How long is …"*

"All done, sir," George butted in. "I'm finished tidying up. I've caught all them frickin' critters and put them in their frickin' cages. I've put together what belongs together, just like you said."

The director was astonished: *"Jimmy, you're incredible. I'm so impressed. How did you manage the Hippopotamus, the Okapi, the Platypus and the Echidna? What groups did you put them in?"*

George didn't understand the question: "Sir, I don't know what an Okapi is. To be honest, I have no idea what those creatures are. I've only tidied up the frickin' mess, just like you said."

"Jimmy," the director hesitated at first to ask the question that had sprung to his mind, but then he needed to know: *"Mate, if you don't know the animals, how on earth could you classify them?"*

"Sir, at first I sorted them by color, but after that huge beast with the nose like a hose stepped on the goorrr-goorrr-bird, I decided to group them by size and weight. That worked like a charm and they're all getting along really well. The young yellow cats with the big paws are getting a good firm hug from those fat flecked snakes of the same weight; and their parents — one has quite a mane — are playing catch with the striped ponies."

George didn't work at the zoo for long. He is currently unemployed and exploring his options for a career in migraine therapy.

We have established that grouping *diseases* by organs works quite well, because when there is a 'sick' target (like germs or cancer cells) for a bit of medical demolition work, it is helpful when the doctor is intimately familiar with that affected organ in sickness and in health. That's why we have cardiologists, dermatologists, gastroenterologists etc. for organs like heart, skin, guts and so on.

We've also seen that sorting by organ doesn't really cut it, when somebody has a *disorder* rather than a *disease*. Patients suffering from a *disorder* are therefore in a bit of a pickle. Medical therapies, still helpful for symptom control, typically don't address the underlying causes, because medicine can't find the *non-organ-based* origins of *disorders* inside their model of *organ-based disease*.

Instead, patients get fed with myths and half-truths to cement their beliefs that their disorder is an organ-based 'medical' problem *just like a disease*. As a result, patients enjoy a good firm hug from pharma medicine and way too many end up in a frickin' mess.

The only alternative on offer is to classify certain symptoms as "*psychological*" and neither doctors nor patients really know what that means. "Psychological" sounds *insane* and reminds everybody at least of absurd movie scenes with couches, if not of mental asylums for crazy people, who think that they're Jesus or Joan of Arc.

As if to make matters worse, medicine has come up with a specialty called psychiatry, which looks after locked-up lunatics as well as lachrymose[1] ladies and languishing lads, laconically loading them with loopy-laden labels from a lavish selection of 'mental' illnesses and 'psychiatric abnormalities'.[2] That's not too inviting for us normal neurotics, whose needs are not crazy. Liters of lithium and electro-shock treatments can't possibly heal a sub-par attachment or a lack of resilience. And so patients with migraine rather opt for more Botox® or the surgical carving of facial muscles than to put up their hands and declare: "I'm a basket case." That's proof that *they're* sane, but these treatments are crazy.

How is it possible that when we're not well, we are left with this 'black-or-white' choice: medical patient or 'psychological' nutcase, drugs or straight jacket? Morbid or mental, ill or sick? How do you sort your beasts, by color or size? Is there no better way?

We live in an era where personality traits like extraversion, and neuroticism can be quantified not only with questionnaires, but also in imaging studies from brain activity patterns[3] or from variations in the thickness of regions in the prefrontal cortex.[4]

---

[1] lachrymose = cries or weeps very easily and often (from Latin 'lacrima'=tear)
[2] Antonaci F et al "Migraine and psychiatric comorbidity: a review of clinical findings" J Headache Pain 2011; 12(2): 115–125
[3] Eisenberger NI et al "Personality from a controlled processing perspective: an fMRI study of neuroticism, extraversion, and self-consciousness" Cogn Affect Behav Neurosci 2005;5(2):169-81
[4] Wright CI et al "Neuroanatomical correlates of extraversion and neuroticism" Cereb Cortex 2006;16(12):1809-19

When personality is 'psychological', but shows up in the brain, does that mean the brain is 'psychological' and not 'neurological'?

Quantitative analysis of electrical brain activity (QEEG) can distinguish between patients with 'mental' depression and normal controls with more than 90% accuracy.[1] How can talk therapy for depression possibly be effective, when depression is 'electrical'? Is electrical brain activity 'organic' or 'mental'? And is depression 'neurological' or 'psychological'? Who can sort that out?

Organic, mental, medical, all these 'creatures' seem to be running wild all over the place and we can't tidy up the mess. When did our narrowness in thinking begin?

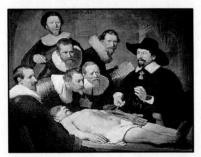

Apparently it happened in the 17th century, at a time when the catholic church had power over life and death. Medical science needed permission to use dead bodies for dissections to study human anatomy. The French universal genius René Descartes ("I think, therefore I am.") struck a deal with the Pope. He promised that he wouldn't have anything to do with the soul, the mind or the emotions, which had to remain under the jurisdiction of Pope and Church. In exchange medicine would take the body as its domain.[2] Essentially, they divided the people like robbers divide their loot.

Today, in the 21st century, conventional medicine still sticks to the bargain and Descartes' declaration: "Anything to do with the soul, mind or emotions, I leave to the clergy. I will only claim the realm of the body." This division of body and mind was confirmed by Isaac Newton, the "father of modern science", who asserted that only physical matter was real, and that was all that really 'mattered'. Organs are matter, mind is not. Organs do matter, mind does not.

This split between body versus mind, real versus fake, medical versus mental, neurological versus psychological is deeply entrenched in our culture and our thinking. We can't even think how *not* to distinguish between 'organic' and 'emotional'; let alone do we have the *words* to think about it differently.

---

[1] Knott V et al "EEG power, frequency, asymmetry and coherence in male depression" Psychiatry Res 2001;106(2):123-40
[2] Pert C "Molecules Of Emotion: The Science Behind Mind-Body Medicine" Simon & Schuster 1999

We're stuck with that concept, whether we like it or not. We cannot erase from our mind, that our body is real, yet our thoughts are not real. What can we do in this predicament?

The answer comes on a platter. Neuroscience, the science of the brain, demonstrates with colorful pictures, sometimes in 3D, that the black-and-white 'sorting' of body versus mind is narrow thinking, a left-over from an 'accident' in the past.

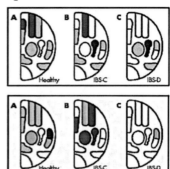

The graphic on the right depicts the different brain activation patterns of healthy controls versus two types of irritable bowel syndrome (IBS) in response to sensory stimulation of the bowel (↑) or of the foot (↓). Even without understanding the details, we can see that IBS-patients' brains process body information differently.[1] IBS—organic or mental illness?

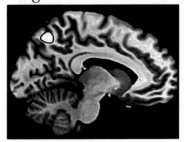

I'm confident that God can forgive us for not sticking to the bargain between medicine and the Church from the 17th century. If he does not, fear of God's anger shows up in brain scans like this one to the left (white area = specific activation).[2] God not only produces a specific activation for fear of his anger, euphoric feelings of God's 'sensed presence' are not untypical in patients with certain epilepsies[3] (That doesn't mean that being religious is a brain disorder).

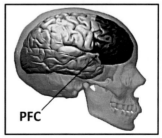

I have mentioned it before, the PFC (= prefrontal cortex, see arrow on the right) is involved in many issues, for example in migraine or depression.[4] Neurotherapy can remediate depression by sprucing up the function of the prefrontal cortex.[5] (Yes, my dear, that also works for migraine.[6])

---

[1] Wilder-Smith CH et al "Brain functional magnetic resonance imaging of rectal pain and activation of endogenous inhibitory mechanisms in irritable bowel syndrome patient subgroups and healthy controls" Gut 2004;53(11):1595-601
[2] Kapogiannis et al "Neuroanatomical Variability of Religiosity" PLoS One 2009; 4(9): e7180
[3] Landtblom AM "The "sensed presence": an epileptic aura with religious overtones" Epilepsy Behav 2006;9(1):186-8
[4] Koenigs M et al "Distinct regions of prefrontal cortex mediate resistance and vulnerability to depression" J Neurosci 2008;28(47):12341-8
[5] Dias AM et al "A new neurofeedback protocol for depression" Span J Psychol 2011;14(1):374-84
[6] Stokes DA et al "Neurofeedback and biofeedback with 37 migraineurs: a clinical outcome study" Behav Brain Funct 2010 2;6:9

The prefrontal cortex is also involved in fibromyalgia,[1] a pain disorder where the entire body tends to hurt.[2] This also explains why so many disorders are comorbid to each other: Fibromyalgia, depression, migraine, irritable bowel syndrome etc. are based on very similar 'weaknesses' in the brain.[3] That's why addressing the brain 'weakness' often yields the desired therapy results.[4]

On the other hand, we mustn't forget 'psychological' factors like any form of childhood maltreatment or an insecure attachment, which are frequent in severe migraine; but are they 'psychological'? When early childhood development is not as smooth and shiny as it could be, the prefrontal cortex doesn't develop perfectly,[5] which later in life can contribute to symptoms all over the place.[6] For research they pick 'maltreatment', but we can assume that sub-ideal childhood factors have an effect even below a 'maltreatment' level.

Neurological or psychological? I don't even understand the question. Neuroscience and neurotherapy prove that this distinction is dated, narrow thinking and a cognitive distortion. In the brain almost everything comes together and the brain doesn't care how we sort its functions, how *we* divide what belongs together. The brain itself never signed the pact that parted body and mind.

Pharma companies have pulled out of drug development for mind-brain disorders and leading neurologists contribute to neuroscientific research.[7] The time has come for patients in a pickle to open the cage of their alleged disease, to tidy up their disorder and sort out the mess themselves. After being firmly hugged for four centuries by an organic-medical concept, we cannot wait until all doctors lift their game and serve the migraine community.

The time has also come to let go of the bizarre idea that 'psycho' means crazy, that 'psychology' stands for 'couch' or that 'psychiatry' equals mental asylum, straight jacket and lithium.

---

[1] Schweinhardt P et al "Fibromyalgia: a disorder of the brain?" Neuroscientist 2008;14(5):415-21
[2] Petrou M et al "Proton MR spectroscopy in the evaluation of cerebral metabolism in patients with fibromyalgia: comparison with healthy controls and correlation with symptom severity" AJNR Am J Neuroradiol 2008;29(5):913-8
[3] Goldenberg DL "Pain/Depression dyad: a key to a better understanding and treatment of functional somatic syndromes" Am J Med. 2010;123(8):675-82
[4] Kayiran S et al "Neurofeedback intervention in fibromyalgia syndrome; a randomized, controlled, rater blind clinical trial" Appl Psychophysiol Biofeedback 2010;35(4):293-302
[5] van Harmelen AL et al "Reduced medial prefrontal cortex volume in adults reporting childhood emotional maltreatment" Biol Psychiatry 2010;68(9):832-8
[6] Arnow BA "Relationships between childhood maltreatment, adult health and psychiatric outcomes, and medical utilisation" J Clin Psychiatry 2004;65 Suppl 12:10-5
[7] Miller G "Is Pharma Running Out of Brainy Ideas?" Science 2010;329(5991):502-504

The accidents of life leave us *all* with some scars and we cannot presume that our experiences so far and the lessons we've learnt are fully sufficient to equip us perfectly for *all* the challenges in an increasingly complex, even crazy world. Again, a dated black-and-white model of mental health versus mental illness leaves no room for us normals who are mentally healthy and still have needs and new things to learn; for example how to *play* the cards well that destiny has dealt us; or how to settle the stirred up dust.

Only the most insane dare to deny that migraine is mainly "all in your head", which only means that the brain is playing catch with itself and so mind and body are also out of balance. And it's not surprising that irritable bowel syndrome is not "all up your ...", but "in your head" too; and so are fibromyalgia and many other disorders, which frequently add to a migraineur's mess. This makes it blatantly mandatory to boost the brain and to mentor the mind.

Nowadays, serious athletes get help from mental trainers, and employers attend psycho-workshops about communication and how to motivate employees. 'Difficult' patients with severe migraine also deserve competent support from a capable psychological coach; anything else would be crazy indeed. If you have severe migraine and want to regain your balance, then you need to step up to the plate, rise to the challenge and pull out all the stops. At the end of the day, all that counts is to snatch your chance to make a difference to your own life and to end the frickin' tyranny.

"Migraine is caused by a chemical imbalance in the brain"

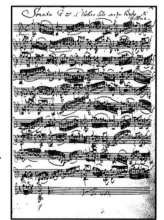

On the right you can see a picture of a manuscript, handwritten by the German composer Johann Sebastian Bach in the early 1740s. Bach died in 1750. Still today, musicians all over the world play this piece although Bach himself didn't record a single album or CD. All he left behind are his manuscripts, which are merely ink on paper. But where is the damn *music*? Is it hidden in the paper? Is the amount of ink the music? Do we sing "Thank you for the ... *paper*"? Or is it even "You can't stop the ... *ink*"? Weird—but we'll find out.

There was a time when people had to write letters in order to communicate over a certain distance. Some people used black ink, some others preferred blue ink and young girls loved their pink ink. So people already knew when a letter arrived and the ink was pink, it probably came from a young girl and not from the city's mayor.

Neurons (= nerve cells) in the brain don't have paper and so they obviously can't write letters (duh). When *neurons transmit* a 'message', they just send their version of neuro-'ink', which we call *neurotransmitters*. The meeting point between one neuron's 'talking' arm (=axon: old Greek for 'axis') and another neuron's 'listening' arm is the legendary *synapse*, a tiny gap or cleft (no touching!).

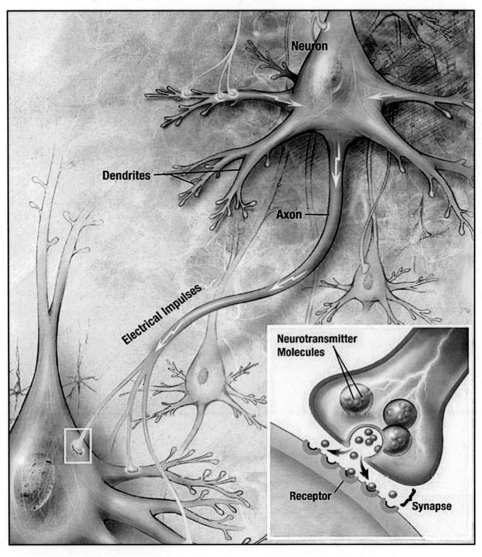

When there is something to 'say', the 'talking' neuron, sends the neurotransmitter molecules to the receiving neuron across the synaptic cleft and into specific 'mailboxes' (receptors), specialized for that one kind of molecule. Like every decent mailbox, the receptor sits next to a gate. When 'mail' comes in (= a fitting neurotransmitter molecule docks onto the receptor), the gate opens magically and one type of charged molecule (ion) will slip from the synaptic cleft through the 'gate' (ion channel) into the cell. These ions change the electric charge inside the cell, which is precharged like a battery anyway.

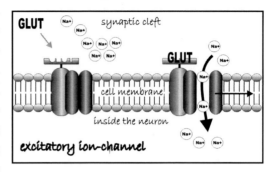

Sodium ions (Na+) have an exciting effect on the receiving cell and so the neurotransmitters, which have a receptor gating the exciting sodium ions, are called *excitatory*. In a way that's cheating, because it's not really the neurotransmitter ('ink'), which determines the effect, but what kind of ion channel ('gate') its receptor typically controls. Glutamate for instance is such a neurotransmitter, which eventually has an excitatory effect, because it's receptor opens a sodium channel.

In contrast GABA's receptor lets chloride (Cl-) into the cell and chloride ions do not excite the cell, quite the opposite. This is called *inhibitory*, because it inhibits the build up of an excitatory charge inside the cell.

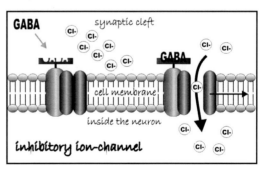

The difference between the overall charge inside this neuron (nerve cell) and the overall charge outside is called 'potential' and measured in Volt. A normal AA battery, which you use for portable electronic devices, has 1.5V (=Volt). A nerve cell doing nothing is precharged to –70mV (=millivolt) or –0.070 Volt.

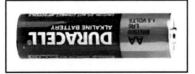

The exciting ions briefly change the potential of the neuron. After that they get shoved back out again and that was it. Nothing happens, because that little change in potential is not enough to motivate this neuron to pass a 'message' on.

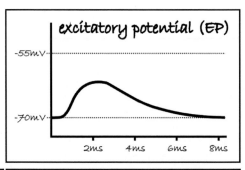

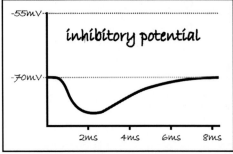

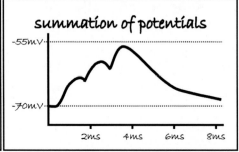

The influx of excitatory and inhibitory ions modulate the overall potential of the neuron *gradually*; so it's no surprise that it's called '*graded potential*'.

The entire procedure reminds me of a referendum and postal votes coming in, for and against something important. However, the 'votes' modulating the graded potential inside the neuron are only valid for a short while and then die off.

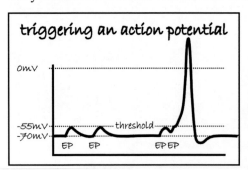

When the exciting signals come in quick succession ('frequent mail') or when many sodium channels get opened at the same time ('lots of mail'), that drives the graded potential up, unless there are too many inhibitory signals, of course.

When the graded potential reaches a threshold, suddenly all hell breaks loose: Many more sodium channels open simultaneously, which leads to a sudden discharge, a 'spark' called '*action potential*'. The advantage of the action potential over the graded potential is that it can travel along an axon ('talking arm') over long distances without data loss. (That's helpful for wiggling your toes, but also inside the brain.)

Having reached the end of the axon with the next synapse, the action potential opens another type of ion channel; this one is for calcium and the calcium-ion influx releases this neuron's neurotransmitter into the next synaptic cleft in order to pass the signal on to the next neuron. And this goes on and on: neurotransmitter → receptor → sodium or chloride ion-channel → excitatory or inhibitory potential → graded potential → threshold → action potential → axon and → calcium channel → neurotrans ….

Congratulations, you've mastered our crash course Neuroscience 101. Time for the final exam:

1.) When a neuron releases the neurotransmitter *Glutamate* into the synaptic cleft, who sits on the next neuron to *receive* it?
a) a Glutamate receptor   b) a GABA synapse   c) George

2.) When Glutamate docks onto the Glutamate receptor, the sodium channel opens and *excitatory* sodium ions enter the neuron, this results in a …
a) smoothing of the hair   b) excitatory potential   c) frickin' mess

3.) When enough sodium ions and their excitatory potential have added up and the graded potential reaches the threshold, what kind of *action* does this *potential* trigger?
a) a pact with the church   b) an earthquake   c) an action potential

Your result: outstanding!

The *intensity* of a neuronal signal translates into the frequency of action potentials, which means how *often* per second the neuron 'fires' its action potentials. These firing frequencies can tell us a lot about the function of the brain, because we have quite a good idea, what they mean.

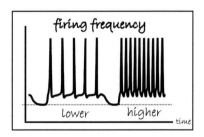

An EEG is a measurement of the electrical activity of the brain from the surface of the scalp and the signal is a mix of all the frequencies in that area (an EEG is an **E**lectro-**E**ncephalo-**G**ram, which means 'electro-brain-recording').

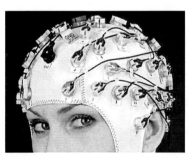

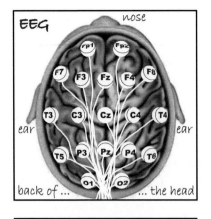

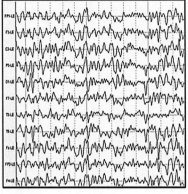

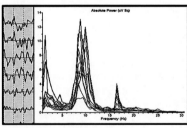

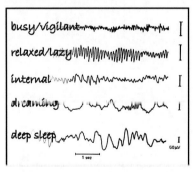

Each of 19 electrodes (= sensors) on the scalp records the electrical chatter in that area. An EEG amplifier with 19 channels (plus a few more for technical purposes) prepares the signal for the computer.

An EEG recording-software converts the signals into wiggly lines. Be aware that actually it's the brain talking and we are eavesdropping.

There are two ways to interpret the information in the EEG traces (= the wiggly lines). A *clinical EEG* is about those patterns, which are characteristic for certain problems. Epilepsy, for example, has typical signatures that can be detected by a trained eye.

In the diagnosis of migraine the clinical EEG is mainly used to rule out nasty stuff; otherwise it is considered to be of limited value.[1]

A second way to make sense of the brain's electrical chatter is filtering and processing this huge amount of data with an appropriate PC software. Since we know what certain frequency bands 'mean', their distribution across the entire cortex (= Latin for 'bark', outer layer of the brain) can tell us a lot.

An excess of 'energy' in the slow band of 0-4Hz (Hertz = cycles per sec.) is a marker for brain injury,[2] for example a forgotten concussion. Even an old and minor brain injury can play a role in migraine.

---

[1] Ambrosini A et al "Migraine - clinical neurophysiology" Handb Clin Neurol 2010;97:275-93
[2] Gilmore PC et al "Correlation of EEG, computerized tomography, and clinical findings. Study of 100 patients with focal delta activity" Arch Neurol 1981;38(6):371-2

On Top of the Barricades

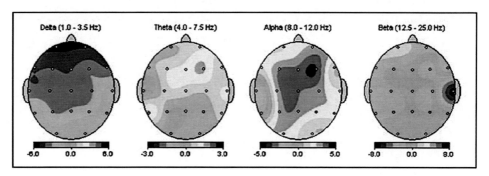

Normally they're pretty colorful, but here in grayscale: The graphic above shows the typical maps of such a brain examination with sophisticated data analysis, called *quantitative EEG* (QEEG).[1]

Apart from a plethora of advanced options to extract a lot of meaning from the brain data, a QEEG normally has one very unique feature: the comparison of an individual's recorded data to a normative database of healthy people (same age, same gender etc.) which gives you an idea how 'abnormal' a brain is.[2]

The patient's symptoms can usually be found in his QEEG analysis as deviations from the average-healthy-brain database. That does not mean that individual differences are always and necessarily a bad thing, but if you have severe problems, you'd wish for a 'normal' brain; stable, flexible and well-balanced.

Migraineurs don't show one type of 'abnormality'; there is no migraine signature ('bug'), which every migraineur has and which could be seen in a clinical EEG. Therefore QEEG is such a valuable tool [3] in the rehabilitation of migraine, because it allows to identify the *individual* 'bug'; the issues of that particular brain, which underlie the symptoms.

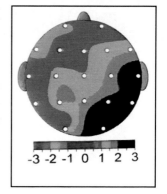

For example, the picture on the right is from the '1Hz-bin' brainmaps of a female migraineur (it only shows the distribution of the 28Hz-activity). The most 'deviant' area (here in black) matches the location of her migraine headache precisely.

---

[1] Sand T "Electroencephalography in migraine: a review with focus on quantitative electroencephalography and the migraine vs. epilepsy relationship" Cephalalgia 2003;23 Suppl 1:5-11
[2] Bjørk M et al "Quantitative EEG power and asymmetry increase 36 h before a migraine attack" Cephalalgia 2008;28(9):960-8
[3] Bjørk MH et al "Interictal quantitative EEG in migraine: a blinded controlled study" J Headache Pain 2009;10(5):331-9

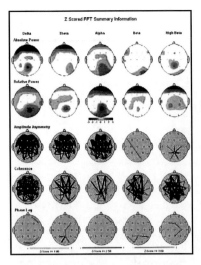

Please note that this was a very simplified description of QEEG. To give you an idea what I mean: Alone the four overview-summary sheets of a typical QEEG report contain 25 color-coded brain maps—each.

QEEG is recorded from the scalp and it still represents the entire brain. How can that be? The brain is organized in networks and even if you can't see some deep structure directly, their activity still shows up on the surface. Think of our puddle puppy from chapter 3; when the puppy crawls under a blanket you can't see it anymore, but somehow you can still visualize it by watching the moving shape of the blanket, right?

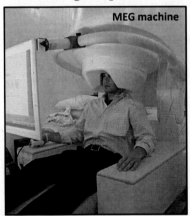

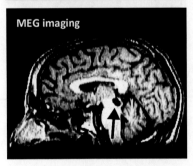

In research,[1] however, scientists want to measure the electrical activity directly, even deep in the brain. That can be done with MEG (= Magnetoencephalography).[2] MEG can detect minuscule magnetic fields, created by the graded potential of at least 50,000 neurons; but you need a kind of bunker, shielded from all the ambient electromagnetic 'pollution' in our environment; this makes it expensive.

To measure deep brain activity in clinical practice for diagnostic and even therapeutic purposes, we can also use LoRETA[3], a groovy technique that calculates 3D images from a QEEG recording, like a 3-dimensional QEEG. LoRETA stands for <u>Lo</u>w <u>R</u>esolution <u>E</u>lectromagnetic <u>T</u>omography.

---

[1] Image with permission from NIMH, National Institutes of Health, Department of Health and Human Services
[2] Image with permission from NJ Ray et al "Using magnetoencephalography to investigate brain activity during high frequency deep brain stimulation in a cluster headache patient" Biomed Imaging Interv J 2007; 3(1): e25
[3] Puskás S "EEG source localization using LoRETA (low resolution electromagnetic tomography)" Ideggyogy Sz 2011;64(3-4):110-8

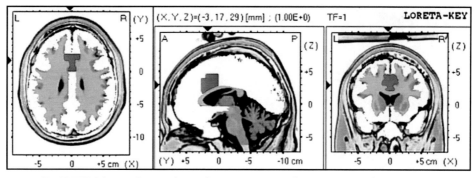

LoRETA[1] analysis has been part of a comprehensive QEEG assessment for some years and several studies have been done on migraineurs between attacks[2,3] and even one during an attack.[4]

Additionally, professional neurotherapists now use LoRETA for targeted brain-biofeedback therapy[5,6] to directly normalize those dysfunctional deep brain structures that cause trouble.

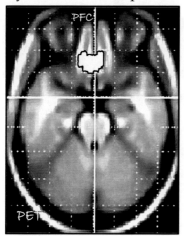

PET is short for Positron Emission Tomography and measures the glucose consumption of active brain areas. For that, a slightly radioactive substance gets attached to glucose and injected. Where the brain is active, the marked glucose gets metabolized (= burnt) and the radioactive particles ('positrons') are emitted and caught by the machine. From that signal a computer creates a picture in slices (tomos= old Greek for slice). In this example the white fleck shows an area of persistent *underactivity* in a part of the PFC[7] in migraineurs in the drug-withdrawal phase after becoming chronic with medication-overuse headache.

---

[1] Pascual-Marqui RD et al "Assessing interactions in the brain with exact low-resolution electromagnetic tomography" Philos Transact A Math Phys Eng Sci 2011;369(1952):3768-84
[2] Clemens B et al "Three-dimensional localization of abnormal EEG activity in migraine: a low resolution electromagnetic tomography (LoRETA) study of migraine patients in the pain-free interval" Brain Topogr. 2008;21(1):36-42
[3] Coutin-Churchman P et al "Vector analysis of visual evoked potentials in migraineurs with visual aura" Clin Neurophysiol 2003;114(11):2132-7
[4] Keeser D et al "Preliminary EEG and Low Resolution Electromagnetic Tomography (LoRETA) measurements results of a migraine patient: An Electrophysiological Evaluation" poster presentation 2011, Technical University Munich
[5] Congedo M et al "Low-resolution electromagnetic tomography neurofeedback" IEEE Trans Neural Syst Rehabil Eng 2004;12(4):387-97
[6] Cannon R et al "Differentiating a network of executive attention: LoRETA neurofeedback in anterior cingulate and dorsolateral prefrontal cortices" Int J Neurosci 2009;119(3):404-41
[7] Fumal A et al "Orbitofrontal cortex involvement in chronic analgesic-overuse headache evolving from episodic migraine" Brain 2006;129(Pt 2):543-50

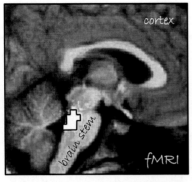

No radioactive stuff is required for an fMRI[1] (= functional Magnetic Resonance Imaging), because its signal stems from spinning water molecules. It typically shows the difference in oxygen consumption in active areas in comparison to a baseline. The example shows the '*Mayhem in the Brainstem*' during a migraine attack.

When neurons burn glucose with oxygen they also produce a certain amount of heat.[2] The more the neurons work, the more heat a brain area generates. To measure the activity in the 'exposed' parts of the prefrontal cortex (PFC), we use thermoimaging.[3]

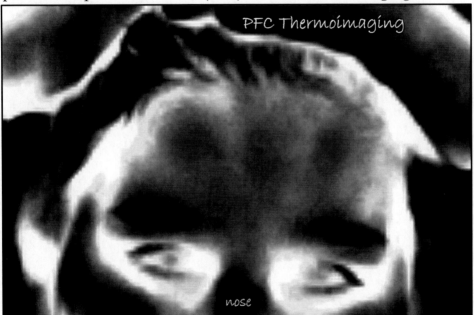

This example[4] shows a forehead during a migraine attack with a lot of heat radiating from the temples and eyes (white) and a sluggish PFC (grey). Thermoimaging of the PFC is a valuable tool in clinical practice, because it reliably identifies underactive zones in the PFC from a comparably quick 'snapshot', without the need for a hospital appointment or radioactive injections.

---

[1] Stankewitz A et al "Trigeminal nociceptive transmission in migraineurs predicts migraine attacks" J Neurosci 2011;31(6):1937-43
[2] Trübel HK et al "Regional temperature changes in the brain during somatosensory stimulation" J Cereb Blood Flow Metab 2006;26(1):68-78
[3] Shevelev IA et al "Thermoimaging of the brain" J Neurosci Methods 1993;46(1):49-57
[4] Image courtesy of Jeff Carmen PhD

Diffusion Tensor Imaging (DTI) is not a functional examination, but it so beautifully depicts fiber connections that it says a lot about the collaboration and cooperation in the brain. DTI is based on MRI technology and complicated calculations. This image here was rendered in color by Thomas Schulz based on a dataset from two universities.[1] I converted it to grayscale, sorry.

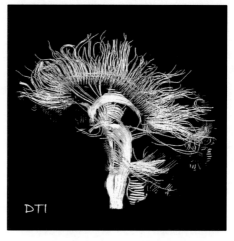

Congratulations, you've now mastered our crash course 'Introduction to brain scanning'. Time for the final exam:

1.) What's the name of the examination that *quantifies* the electric activity of the brain with *EEG* sensors on the scalp?
a) UNICEF			b) RSVP			c) QEEG

2.) Which technique portrays the activity deep in the brain from a QEEG recording in *low resolution* slices, like a *tomography*?
a) CLARE			b) LoRETA			c) ERICA

3.) What kind of 'snapshot' shows the 'sluggish' areas of the *PFC* as cooler (e.g. darker grey on the forehead) in a *thermal image*?
a) PFC Thermoimaging	b) musical score sheet	c) dissection

Your result: supernatural!

Although the human brain accounts for only 2% of its owner's body weight, it demands 20-25% of the total oxygen consumption at rest[2] for its estimated 85-120 billion[3] neurons (nerve cells). Each neuron has 1,000 to 10,000 connections to other neurons, which puts the total number of connections in the ballpark of roughly 100,000,000,000,000 (100 Trillion). More than 100 substances are known to act as neurotransmitters. They are either abundant in the neurons or get synthesized (= put together) when needed. Lack of chemicals is thus mostly the *result* of insufficient neuronal activity.

---

[1] Brain dataset courtesy of Gordon Kindlmann at the Scientific Computing and Imaging Institute, University of Utah, and Andrew Alexander, W. M. Keck Laboratory for Functional Brain Imaging and Behavior, University of Wisconsin-Madison
[2] Grande Covián F "Energy metabolism of the brain in children" An Esp Pediatr 1979;12(3):235-44
[3] Herculano-Houzel S "The human brain in numbers: a linearly scaled-up primate brain" Front Hum Neurosci 2009;3:31

Despite the many substances ('inks') that its neurons produce, the brain is first and foremost an organ of *information processing* and *communication*, talking to the world, but mostly to itself. It creates our mind and operates our body, sometimes to our mind's delight, sometimes less so. Neurotransmitters and other chemicals are essential, but the brain's 'language' is best characterized by the properties of its electrical signals: frequency, power, phase, coherence, symmetry and synchrony to name but a few.

It is misleading to talk about 'chemical imbalances' as a cause of migraine. The 'chemical imbalances' in any brain are rarely a cause, rather an *expression* of the underlying dysregulation. For example, habitual overbreathing leads to a reduction of tissue CO_2 levels, which can impede the synthesis of the neurotransmitter serotonin.[1,2] Then you have a chemical imbalance, which in turn can interfere with the regulation of breathing.[3] Simply swallowing serotonin won't do the trick because 95% of serotonin activity is in the gut[4] and the still low CO_2 wreaks havoc there too.[5] Get it?

It does the brain a grave injustice to treat it as if it only needs a chemical leg-up. The relative failure of antidepressant medication to produce better effects than placebo proves this point.[6] The myth of 'chemical imbalance' is not more than clever drug advertising.[7]

Johann Sebastian Bach left us his music in the form of score sheets; and although paper and ink were essential for that, it is the written *language* of music that holds his compositions for eternity. Conductors who can understand that 'code' on the score sheet can "read the music" and improve the orchestra's performance.

If the orchestra in your head plays out of tune with migraine crescendos, the key might be an expert, who does a brain recording, can read the brain's music and improve its performance; because your brain's orchestral harmony will help you end the tyranny.

---

[1] Hoes MJ "Pharmacotherapy of the hyperventilation syndrome" Ann Med Psychol 1983;141(8):859-74

[2] Carlsson A et al "Effect of hypercapnia and hypocapnia on tryptophan and tyrosine hydroxylation in rat brain" Abstract Acta Physiol Scand 1977;99(4):503-9

[3] Hodges MR et al "Contributions of 5-HT neurons to respiratory control: neuromodulatory and trophic effects" Respir Physiol Neurobiol 2008;164(1-2):222-32

[4] Kim DY et al "Serotonin: a mediator of the brain-gut connection" Am J Gastroenterol 2000;95(10):2698-709

[5] Bharucha AE et al "Hyperventilation alters colonic motor and sensory function: effects and mechanisms in humans" Gastroenterology 1996;111(2):368-77

[6] Ioannidis JP "Effectiveness of antidepressants: an evidence myth constructed from a thousand randomized trials?" Philos Ethics Humanit Med 2008;3:14

[7] Lacasse JR et al "Serotonin and depression: a disconnect between the advertisements and the scientific literature" PLoS Med 2005;2(12):e392

Chapter 8

Know your Tyrant

> "If you know the enemy and know yourself,
> you need not fear the results of a hundred battles."
> Sun Tzu

I may be wrong, but I think it might help to truly understand a problem before attempting to solve it. Of course, one can simply try the *currently popular solutions* without studying the issue, but once that strategy has failed, one might want to reconsider.

We've talked about suffering from migraine as "the tyranny" throughout this book. That's cute, but who is the 'tyrant'? Who or what is responsible for all the symptoms and sorrows? And most of all…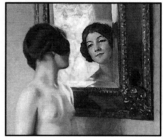

What the heck is migraine?

There is an abundance of pressing and unanswered questions: What's going on in the brain during a migraine attack? What happens in between that leads to attacks? Why does migraine have so many comorbidities? Why is it that so many people *don't* have migraine despite apparently having the genetic disposition? How is it possible that so many treatments and therapies are somewhat effective in migraine, even if they have nothing in common? Why is the placebo effect so strong in trials of migraine medications?

A comprehensive model of migraine has to have plausible answers to all these questions. Additionally, it would be nice if there was some form of proof or validation for that concept. What we don't want anymore, are weird migraine myths and pseudo-scientific nonsense like "Silkenshine's natural Amarula-oil smooths the rough nano-structure of your horrible hair".

Unfortunately, medical research hasn't yet come up with compelling answers to all these questions. They're busy promoting drugs. You and I are just an unorganized bunch of rebels at the forefront of a revolution. We can't possibly put together a convincing and helpful theory of migraine. Or can we?

What happens during a migraine attack?

As mentioned earlier, Dr. Edward Liveing[1] wrote about migraine as an 'electrical nerve storm' in 1873 already. The expert term for 'nerve storm' is seizure: abnormal, unproductive activity of groups of neurons in the form of excessive, synchronous discharges. Think of a seizure as *sneezing neurons*, that'll do.

When we hear the word seizure we all think of epileptic seizures or fits with convulsions and loss of consciousness, called grand mal (= French for 'big bad'). A grand mal occurs, when large parts of the brain have a seizure (= neuron's 'sneezing attack'), including those areas that normally operate muscles (motor cortex). It is easy to imagine how the neurons in the motor cortex have a 'sneezing fit' and that results in convulsions of the body.

Apart from the frightening and spectacular grand mal, which is a "generalized, tonic-clonic motor seizure", there are many other forms of epilepsy: simple partial, complex partial, absence, tonic, atonic, clonic, myoclonic and so on. Depending on the 'sneezing' brain area, different symptoms ensue.

If the sneezing/seizing neurons are close to the surface of the skull, the raw EEG shows a spike or a sharp wave, which is a diagnostic marker for epilepsy. Conversely, if the seizure activity is *deep in the brain*, it won't show up in the EEG signal.

There is growing evidence for this covert seizure activity in *many other disorders*, which also respond to anti-seizure medication[2] (e.g. PTSD,[3] depression,[4] alcoholism, panic and affective disorders[5]) *without* surface-EEG signs, just like in some forms of epilepsy.[6,7]

Many other clues support Edward Liveing's notion of migraine as a form of seizure, for instance the *same gene markers* for migraine and epilepsy[8] on chromosomes 12 and 14 or the *progression* of cases from migraine with aura to occipital epilepsy.[9]

---

[1] Liveing E "On megrim, sick-headache and some allied disorders: A Contribution to the Pathology of Nerve-Storms" 1873
[2] Ettinger AB et al "Use of antiepileptic drugs for nonepileptic conditions: psychiatric disorders and chronic pain" Neurotherapeut 2007;4(1):75-83
[3] Fiszman A et al "Traumatic events and posttraumatic stress disorder in patients with psychogenic nonepileptic seizures" Epilepsy Behav 2004;5(6):818-25
[4] Bob P et al "Subclinical epileptiform process in patients with unipolar depression and its indirect psychophysiological manifestations" PLoS One. 2011;6(11):e28041
[5] Grunze HCR "The effectiveness of anticonvulsants in psychiatric disorders" Dialogues Clin Neurosci 2008; 10(1):77–89
[6] Drake ME et al "Interictal quantitative EEG in epilepsy" Seizure 1998;7(1):39-42
[7] Belcastro V et al "Migralepsy, hemicrania epileptica, post-ictal headache and ictal epileptic headache" J Headache Pain 2011;12(3):289-94
[8] Millichap JJ et al "Shared Loci for Migraine and Epilepsy on Chromosomes 14q12-q23 and 12q24.2-q24.3" Neurology 2012;78(15):1190-1
[9] Dainese F et al "From migraine to epilepsy: a threshold mechanism?" Neurol Sci 2012;33(4):915-8

Let's have a look, *what else* epilepsy (= seizure disorder) and migraine have in common:

Commonalities	epilepsy	migraine
episodic attacks	yes	yes
multitude of variations and variants	yes: generalized/partial, simple/complex, absence tonic, clonic, atonic, myoclonic ...	yes: with/without aura, with/without headache, abdominal, retinal, basilar, hemiplegic ...
precipitating factors	stress, sleep deprivation, skipped meals, flickering lights, hormonal fluctuations ...[1]	stress, sleep deprivation, skipped meals, flickering lights, hormonal fluctuations ...
prodrome and/or aura	yes, but not always[2]	yes, but not always
headaches	40-60%[3,4,5]	very often (but not always)
nausea/vomiting	can occur[6]	occur frequently
vertigo	can occur	occurs frequently
common mechanisms	yes[7]	
treatment with anti-epileptic drugs	yes[8]	yes
treatment with electrical stimulation	yes[9,10]	yes[11,12,13]
treatment with neurotherapy	proven effective even in intractable cases[14]	highly effective even in intractable cases[15]

---

[1] Haut SR et al "Chronic disorders with episodic manifestations: focus on epilepsy and migraine" Lancet Neurol 2006;5(2):148-57
[2] Maiwald T et al "Are prodromes preictal events? A prospective PDA-based study" Epilepsy Behav 2011;21(2):184-8
[3] Verrotti A et al "Peri-ictal and inter-ictal headache in children and adolescents with idiopathic epilepsy: a multicenter cross-sectional study" Childs Nerv Syst 2011;27(9):1419-23
[4] Bernasconi A et al "Lateralizing value of peri-ictal headache: A study of 100 patients with partial epilepsy" Neurology 2001;56(1):130-2
[5] Karaali-Savrun F et al "Seizure-related headache in patients with epilepsy" Seizure 2002;11(1):67-9
[6] Bianchin MM et al "Migraine and epilepsy: a focus on overlapping clinical, pathophysiological, molecular, and therapeutic aspects" Curr Pain Headache Rep 2010;14(4):276-83
[7] Rogawski MA "Common pathophysiologic mechanisms in migraine and epilepsy" Arch Neurol 2008;65(6):709-14
[8] Beyenburg S "Current pharmacotherapy of epilepsy in adults" Bull Soc Sci Med Grand Duche Luxemb 2005;(3):263-81
[9] Englot DJ et al "Efficacy of vagus nerve stimulation for epilepsy by patient age, epilepsy duration, and seizure type" Neurosurg Clin N Am 2011;22(4):443-8
[10] Pop J et al "Acute and long-term safety of external trigeminal nerve stimulation for drug-resistant epilepsy" Epilepsy Behav 2011;22(3):574-6
[11] Cecchini AP et al "Vagus nerve stimulation in drug-resistant daily chronic migraine with depression: preliminary data" Neurol Sci 2009;30 Suppl 1:S101-4
[12] Reed KL et al "Combined occipital and supraorbital neurostimulation for the treatment of chronic migraine headaches: initial experience" Cephalalgia 2010;30(3):260-71
[13] Simopoulos T et al "Implanted auriculotemporal nerve stimulator for the treatment of refractory chronic migraine" Headache 2010;50(6):1064-9
[14] Tan G "Meta-analysis of EEG biofeedback in treating epilepsy" Clin EEG Neurosci 2009;40(3):173-9
[15] Walker JE "QEEG-guided neurofeedback for recurrent migraine headaches" Clin EEG Neurosci 2011;42(1):59-61

In a blunt summary: Episodic migraine and epilepsy (episodic seizures) have the same *precipitating factors*, the same *phases*, the same *genes*, the same *mechanisms* and the same *treatments*.

There is even a form of migraine that shows *involuntary muscle contractions* that are so typical in a grand mal seizure: Cyclic vomiting syndrome (= involuntary stomach muscle contractions) is classified as a form of migraine.[1]

Allegedly it was the American poet J. W. Riley[2] who said:

> "When I see a bird that walks like a duck and swims like a duck and quacks like a duck, I call that bird a duck."

When I see migraine, an episodic disorder of the brain, that can get prompted like a seizure, shows all the characteristics of a seizure and responds to the same treatments as a seizure, I call that disorder a seizure. A migraine attack must be a seizure, period.

How can a seizure produce migraine symptoms?

Sneezing neurons ('microseizures') can also be found in completely healthy brains without migraine, epilepsy or any other episodic disorder.[3] Whether symptoms occur, depends on the number and location of sneezing neurons.[4]

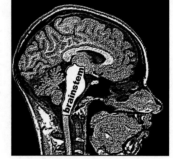

When you think that the human brain looks a bit like a cauliflower, then the stalk is the equivalent to the brainstem. During migraine attacks, a number of imaging studies have found excessive activity in the brainstem,[5,6,7,8,9,10,11,12,13] often referred to as the '*migraine generator*'.[14,15,16]

---

[1] Yang HR "Recent concepts on cyclic vomiting syndrome in children" J Neurogastroenterol Motil 2010;16(2):139-47
[2] Heim, Michael (2007). Exploring Indiana Highways. Exploring America's Highway. pp. 68;
 found on http://en.wikipedia.org/wiki/Duck_typing#cite_note-0
[3] Stead M et al "Microseizures and the spatiotemporal scales of human partial epilepsy" Brain 2010;133(9):2789-97
[4] Dudek FE "Microseizures in human neocortex: a role for ultra-small seizures?" Epilepsy Curr 2009;9(5):151-2
[5] Weiller C et al "Brain stem activation in spontaneous human migraine attacks" Nat Med 1995;1(7):658-60
[6] Diener HC "Positron emission tomography studies in headache" Headache 1997;37(10):622-5
[7] Bahra A et al "Brainstem activation specific to migraine headache" Lancet 2001;357(9261):1016-7
[8] Cao Y et al "Functional MRI-BOLD of brainstem structures during visually triggered migraine" Neurology 2002;59(1):72-8
[9] Afridi SK et al "A positron emission tomographic study in spontaneous migraine" Arch Neurol 2005;62(8):1270-5
[10] Afridi SK et al "A PET study exploring the laterality of brainstem activation in migraine using glyceryl trinitrate" Brain 2005;128(Pt 4):932-9
[11] Denuelle M et al "Hypothalamic activation in spontaneous migraine attacks" Headache 2007;47(10):1418-26
[12] Stankewitz A et al "Trigeminal nociceptive transmission in migraineurs predicts migraine attacks" J Neurosci 2011;31(6):1937-43
[13] Stankewitz A et al "Increased limbic and brainstem activity during migraine attacks following olfactory stimulation" Neurology 2011;77(5):476-82
[14] Tajti J et al "Neuropeptide localization in the "migraine generator" region of the human brainstem" Cephalalgia 2001;21(2):96-101
[15] Fox AW. "Time-series data and the "migraine generator" Headache 2005;45(7):920-5
[16] Hamada J "Pathophysiology of migraine--migraine generator" Rinsho Shinkeigaku 2008;48(11):857-60

Okay, but what does the brainstem do anyway? In simple summary, the brainstem has two main functions: one is to transmit signals from the body to the brain and vice versa; the other function is to keep us alive, awake and alert:

the brainstem is involved in ...	a typical migraine attack symptom is ...
nausea[1]	nausea
vomiting[2]	vomiting
appetite[3]	food cravings or lack of appetite
gastro-intestinal functions[4]	constipation or diarrhea
regulation of body temperature[5]	feeling chilly or hot
regulation of urination[6]	frequent urination
regulation of alertness[7]	tiredness, drowsiness
head/neck movement reflexes[8]	stiff neck, neck pain
regulation of sound sensitivity[9,10]	increased sound sensitivity
regulation of visual sensitivity[11,12]	increased light sensitivity
defensive behavior[13] ('freeze'-response)	immobilization, social withdrawal
processing pain-related information[14,15]	head pain, increased pain sensitivity

As you can see, a 'nerve storm' in the brainstem could potentially cause a variety of symptoms, just like the ones seen during a full-blown migraine attack.[16] What a coincidence!

The area of the brainstem, likely to be responsible for the subjective experience of the migraine headache, is the *Periaqueductal Gray* (PAG).[17,18,19] It is the job of the PAG ('the bouncer') to stop unwanted pain-provoking signals from entering any further.

---

[1] Sanger GJ et al "Treatment of nausea and vomiting: gaps in our knowledge" Auton Neurosci 2006;129(1-2):3-16
[2] Andrews PL et al "The neurophysiology of vomiting" Baillieres Clin Gastroenterol 1988;2(1):141-68
[3] Ahima RS et al "Brain regulation of appetite and satiety" Endocrinol Metab Clin North Am 2008;37(4):811-23
[4] Browning KN et al "Plasticity of vagal brainstem circuits in the control of gastrointestinal function" Auton Neurosci 2011;161(1-2):6-13
[5] Humphreys RB et al "Effects of anesthetic injected into brainstem sites on body temp. and thermoregulation" Physiol Behav 1976;17(4):667-74
[6] Fowler CJ et al "The neural control of micturition" Nat Rev Neurosci 2008;9(6):453-66
[7] Sturm W et al "On the functional neuroanatomy of intrinsic and phasic alertness" Neuroimage 2001;14(1 Pt 2):S76-84
[8] Nardone R et al "Trigemino-cervical reflex abnormalities in patients with migraine and cluster headache" Headache 2008;48(4):578-85
[9] Bear MF et al "Neuroscience-Exploring the Brain" 3rd edition 2007 Lippincott Williams & Wilkins, p. 363
[10] Weber H et al "Central hyperacusis with phonophobia in multiple sclerosis" Mult Scler 2002;8(6):505-9
[11] Bear MF et al "Neuroscience-Exploring the Brain" 3rd edition 2007 Lippincott Williams & Wilkins, p. 287
[12] Debenedictis CN et al "Brainstem tumor presenting with tearing, photophobia, and torticollis" J AAPOS 2010;14(4):369-70
[13] De Oca BM et al "Distinct regions of the periaqueductal gray are involved in the acquisition and expression of defensive responses" J Neurosci 1998;18(9):3426-32
[14] Tracey I et al "Imaging attentional modulation of pain in the periaqueductal gray in humans" J Neurosci 2002;22(7):2748-52
[15] Raskin NH et al "Headache may arise from perturbation of brain" Headache 1987;27(8):416-20
[16] Tajti J, et al "Where does a migraine attack originate? In the brainstem" J Neural Transm 2012;119(5):557-68
[17] Knight YE et al "The periaqueductal grey matter modulates trigeminovascular input: a role in migraine?" Neuroscience 2001;106(4):793-800
[18] Haas DC et al "Headache caused by a single lesion of multiple sclerosis in the periaqueductal gray area" Headache 1993;33(8):452-5
[19] Gee JR et al "The association of brainstem lesions with migraine-like headache: an imaging study of MS" Headache 2005;45(6):670-7

In migraineurs the PAG is not quite up to scratch[1] even between attacks,[2,3] which is in accordance with the known tendency of migraineurs to develop other pain issues.[4]

As mentioned earlier (see chapter 1), various alterations (= damage) have been found in the brains of migraineurs; for example *iron contamination* in the brainstem, especially in the PAG.[5] The meaning of such iron pollution of brain areas is not quite clear, but researchers use *iron injections* into the brain to provoke seizures in laboratory animals.[6] Iron deposits in the brain seem to *promote* epileptic activity[7] and are a diagnostic marker for degeneration in the brain.[8] In short: not good.

Where does the head pain come from?

Let's have another look where some of the attack symptoms come from (and where they obviously don't come from):

migraine attack symptom:	obvious source:	therefore unlikely source:
nausea/vomiting	'nerve-storm' extending to the nausea/vomiting circuits in the **brainstem**[9]	rotten food; swelling and inflammation of the stomach lining
dizziness/vertigo	'nerve-storm' affecting the 'equilibrium pathways' through the **brainstem**[10]	rollercoaster; swelling and inflammation in the inner ear
runny or stuffy nose, teary or dry eyes	'nerve-storm' involving the facial nerve (trigeminus) at the **brainstem**[11,12]	hayfever; swelling and inflammation of nose and eyes

---

[1] Welch KM et al "Periaqueductal gray matter dysfunction in migraine: cause or the burden of illness?" Headache 2001;41(7):629-37
[2] Moulton EA et al "Interictal dysfunction of a brainstem descending modulatory center in migraine patients" PLoS One 2008;3(11):e3799
[3] DaSilva AF et al "Interictal alterations of the trigeminal somatosensory pathway and periaqueductal gray matter in migraine" Neuroreport 2007;18(4):301-5
[4] Ahn AH "Chronic pain and migraine" Headache 2007;47(8):1259-61
[5] Kruit MC et al "Iron accumulation in deep brain nuclei in migraine: a population-based magnetic resonance imaging study" Cephalalgia 2009;29(3):351-9
[6] Sharma V et al "Iron-induced experimental cortical seizures: electroencephalographic mapping of seizure spread in the subcortical brain areas" Seizure 2007;16(8):680-90
[7] Campbell KA et al "Epileptogenic effects of electrolytic lesions in the hippocampus: role of iron deposition" Exp Neurol 1984;86(3):506-14
[8] McNeill A et al "Neurodegeneration with brain iron accumulation" Handb Clin Neurol 2011;100:161-72
[9] Hashimoto I et al "Hyperexcitable state of the brainstem in children with post-traumatic vomiting as evidenced by brainstem auditory-evoked potentials" Neurol Res 1984;6(1-2):81-4
[10] Lin KY et al "Brainstem lesion in benign paroxysmal vertigo children: Evaluated by a combined ocular and cervical vestibular-evoked myogenic potential test" Int J Pediatr Otorhinolaryngol 2010;74(5):523-7
[11] Barbanti P et al "Unilateral cranial autonomic symptoms in migraine" Cephalalgia 2002;22(4):256-9
[12] Hirata H et al "A novel class of neurons at the trigeminal subnucleus interpolaris/caudalis transition region monitors ocular surface fluid status and modulates tear production" J Neurosci 2004;24(17):4224-32

migraine attack symptom:	obvious source:	therefore unlikely source:
tiredness, drowsiness	'nerve-storm' affecting the arousal regulation circuits in the **brainstem**[1]	night out; swelling and inflammation or pinching of the 'sleep'-nerve
gastro-intestinal complaints (constipation, diarrhea)	'nerve storm' activating the dorsal vagal complex in the **brainstem**[2]	spicy food; swelling and inflammation or pinching of the 'poop-nerve'
head pain	'nerve storm' in the PAG, ("pain"-modulating center) in the **brainstem**[3]	hangover; swelling and inflammation of blood vessels; pinched nerves

The question "Where does the head pain come from?" is a bit tricky, because the underlying assumption is that every pain has to "come from" somewhere, supposedly from the outside world and as an attack on our body; insult, injury or inflammation, right?

We've seen that nausea, vertigo and other symptoms *do not* "come from" the outside world, but are obviously caused by seizure activity ('nerve storm') in the brainstem. Unfortunately we can't measure that directly, because sticking needle electrodes into the brainstem of a migraineur is too dangerous.

The "pain"-modulating centers in the brainstem are dysfunctional, also between attacks, and a migraineur's overall heightened "pain" sensitivity[4,5,6] increases even further as the next attack approaches.[7] German researchers have already shown, how a migraineur's brain *behaves differently* for that to occur.[8]

The PAG in the brainstem normally stops random neural noise[9] from falsely activating the pain matrix in the brain. During the migraine-seizure the PAG fails more or less completely, which results in the experience of very severe to moderate head pain.[10]

---

[1] Kayama Y et al "Brainstem neural mechanisms of sleep and wakefulness" Eur Urol 1998;33 Suppl 3:12-5
[2] Browning KN et al "Plasticity of vagal brainstem circuits in the control of gastric function" Neurogastroenterol Motil 2010;22(11):1154-63
[3] Centonze V et al "Migraine, daily chronic headache and fibromyalgia in the same patient: an evolutive "continuum" of non organic chronic pain? About 100 clinical cases" Neurol Sci 2004;25 Suppl 3:S291-2
[4] Nicolodi M et al "Visceral pain threshold is deeply lowered far from the head in migraine" Headache 1994;34(1):12-9
[5] Drummond PD "Photophobia and autonomic responses to facial pain in migraine" Brain 1997;120(Pt10):1857-64
[6] Fernández-de-las-Peñas C et al "Generalized mechanical pain sensitivity over nerve tissues in patients with strictly unilateral migraine" Clin J Pain 2009;25(5):401-6
[7] Sand T et al "Thermal pain thresholds are decreased in the migraine preattack phase" Eur J Neurol 2008;15(11):1199-205
[8] Aderjan D et al "Neuronal mechanisms during repetitive trigemino-nociceptive stimulation in migraine patients" Pain 2010;151(1):97-103
[9] Freeman WJ "Random activity at the microscopic neural level in cortex ("noise") sustains and is regulated by low-dimensional dynamics of macroscopic cortical activity ("chaos")" Int J Neural Syst 1996;7(4):473-80
[10] Lambert GA "The lack of peripheral pathology in migraine headache" Headache 2010;50(5):895-908

The impact of all these findings on treatment options and patient information is rather negligible, because the pharma lobby and their vassals continue to come up with new stories about swelling and inflammation: If it's not the blood vessels outside the brain, what about the meninges (the 'skin' around the brain)?[1]

Migraineurs are understandably vulnerable to those stories, because they seemingly confirm that the pain is 'real' and not 'made up'. Evidence for that is the typical throbbing nature of the headache, which reinforces the torturous image of how the rhythmical pulse in the blood vessels, driven by the stoically pumping heartbeat, is relentlessly hammering against already sore and inflamed tissue; be it vessel walls or brain skin or whatever.

And so it also doesn't matter that the rhythm of the pain throbbing was found *not* to correspond with the rhythm of heartbeat and pulse.[2] Yet, the drama stories make the headlines in migraine land. It's time for a revolution, don't you think?

The fact that the often debilitating head pain is the result of a dysfunction in the brainstem doesn't make it less 'real'. Pain is always 'real', because it's a *real experience* created by a network in the brain, which many refer to as the 'pain matrix'.[3]

In chronic pain patients (like migraineurs) this pain matrix shows persistent, frequency-specific overactivation in QEEG[4] and LoRETA,[5] more evidence for a constant brain dysfunction, which culminates in brainstem seizures (attacks, 'nerve storm').

The obsession, with which some experts still explain the phenomenon of migraine as a form of inflammation or irritation of nerve endings with all kinds of nasty substances, is merely a sophisticated version of the dreaded sentence: "It's just a headache."

We do understand that all those who earn their income from drugs try to insist on biochemical causes for the head pain, but in the context of all the other migraine symptoms, their stories simply don't make sense. We've learned from *Judge Judy* (a TV show): "If it doesn't make sense, then it can't be true." And Judge Judy knows best: Her cases are real and her rulings are final.

---

[1] Levy D. "Migraine pain, meningeal inflammation, and mast cells" Curr Pain Headache Rep 2009;13(3):237-40
[2] Ahn AH "On the temporal relationship between throbbing migraine pain and arterial pulse" Headache 2010;50(9):1507-10
[3] Iannetti GD et al "From the neuromatrix to the pain matrix (and back)" Exp Brain Res 2010;205(1):1-12
[4] Stern J et al "Persistent EEG overactivation in the cortical pain matrix of neurogenic pain patients" Neuroimage 2006;31(2):721-31
[5] Prichep LS et al "Evaluation of the pain matrix using EEG source localization: a feasibility study" Pain Med 2011;12(8):1241-8

What about the cortex and the aura?

Now that we've established that the *'body symptoms'* of a migraine attack—like pain, nausea, vertigo...—are caused by the 'nerve storm' in the brainstem, let's have a look at the *'mind symptoms'* like irritability, difficulties with concentration, comprehension and speech, problems with color perception, object/face recognition, as well as the sensory abnormalities that we call *aura*.

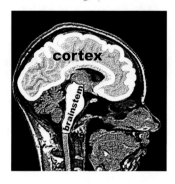

When the brainstem is out of sorts, we can rightfully expect ramifications in the cortex. The brainstem may not have all the sophisticated cognitive functions, which we humans are so proud of. Yet the control 'button' for wakefulness and overall responsiveness of the brain lies in the hands of the brainstem[1,2] and so it greatly influences the functions of the cortex: We perform best, when we're not drowsy, but alert, yet not too hyped up.[3,4,5]

What are the functions of the cortex? Let's have a look:

function of the cortex:	possible migraine symptom:
concentration, focused attention	lack of focus, distractibility
impulse control	impulsive behaviors, restlessness
mood regulation	mood problems, irritability, anger
motivation, approach behaviors	feeling blue, avoidance behaviors
language expression	low motivation to talk, loss of fluency
voluntary movement coordination	clumsiness, even paralysis
touch and other body-senses	odd body perceptions, tingling, numbness
hearing	auditory disturbances, phonophobia
smelling	smell disturbances, osmophobia
face and object recognition	struggle identifying/naming faces/objects
language comprehension	difficulty comprehending
vision	visual disturbances, photophobia

Do any of these symptoms sound familiar to you?

---

[1] Steriade M "Arousal: revisiting the reticular activating system" Science 1996;272(5259):225-6
[2] Loughlin SE et al "Locus coeruleus projections to cortex: topography, morphology and collateralization" Brain Res Bull 1982;9(1-6):287-94
[3] Usher M et al "The role of locus coeruleus in the regulation of cognitive performance" Science 1999;283(5401):549-54
[4] Aston-Jones G et al "Role of locus coeruleus in attention and behavioral flexibility" Biol Psychiatry 1999;46(9):1309-20
[5] Aston-Jones G et al "An integrative theory of locus coeruleus-norepinephrine function: adaptive gain and optimal performance" Annu Rev Neurosci 2005;28:403-50

The difference between 'common' migraine and 'classical' migraine is the occurrence of an aura. In the vast majority of cases that means a visual aura (see chapter 1 for details). The mechanism thought to be responsible for the aura is called cortical spreading depression (CSD).

Cortical Spreading Depression[1]

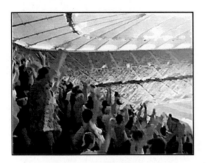

Have you ever seen 'The Wave' or 'The Mexican Wave' in a sports stadium? The spectators stand up, raise their arms, cheer enthusiastically and sit down again; and since they do that in vertical rows, the crowd generates a visual effect like a wave on the ocean (when everybody takes part).

Cortical Spreading Depression (CSD) is a bit like a Mexican wave in the Cortex. Row by row neurons (nerve cells) 'jump up' and sneeze, only to sink back in exhaustion afterwards, barely able to function. This creates a wave of disruption, which causes the signs of an aura:[2] visual symptoms in the visual cortex, auditory symptoms in the auditory cortex and so on.

Typically CSD starts at the back of the brain in area 17 of the visual cortex, where the neuron density is highest. From there the CSD wave travels at a speed of 2-6 mm per minute along the gray matter, initiating massive migration of ions like sodium, potassium, chloride and calcium in and out of the neurons. Additionally the cells take up water and release amino acids (e.g. Glutamate and Aspartate) like crazy. Simply put: Chaos in the Cortex.

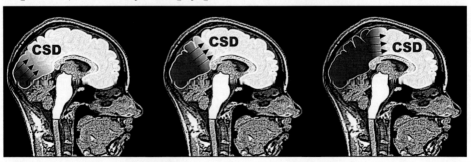

---

[1] Lauritzen M et al "Clinical relevance of cortical spreading depression in neurological disorders: migraine, malignant stroke, subarachnoid and intracranial hemorrhage, and traumatic brain injury" J Cereb Blood Flow Metab 2011;31(1):17-35

[2] Hadjikhani N et al "Mechanisms of migraine aura revealed by functional MRI in human visual cortex" Proc Natl Acad Sci 2001;98(8):4687-92

So it's no surprise that the affected neurons can be severely disabled for a while. It requires a lot of energy and therefore an increase in blood flow to restore everything back to normal.

Cortical Spreading Depression (CSD) can also occur after a traumatic brain injury or different forms of stroke. It may even be, that it is a self-protective mechanism, because it promotes cell growth and increases tolerance for low-oxygen conditions.[1]

There are drugs that can suppress CSD to some degree. This means that they can pretty much avert the aura.[2] Unfortunately these 'CSD-stoppers' cannot prevent migraine *without* aura or headaches;[3] just the aura. This confirms that CSD indeed produces the experience of aura, but—of course—not the headache nor any of the other symptoms of migraine.

In a 'CSD-stopper' drug-trial the 'inactive' placebo pill reached 73% of the effect of the 'active' aura-stopping drug (with fewer side effects).[2] How is that even possible?

As we have heard in chapter 3, the placebo-effect is particularly strong in migraine. In trials of medications for the treatment of attacks up to 50% of patients who received an 'ineffective' placebo pill reported substantial pain relief.[4] In other words, *half the patients unknowingly managed to relieve their migraine headache themselves* without chemicals. How can that be?

Simply put and undeniably, the brains of migraineurs—in principle—*do* have the ability to inhibit aura or prevent migraine attacks or even relieve migraine headache during an attack. This ability can be 'awakened' by the placebo effect, which is believed to be based on a 'vague hope' or 'positive expectation',[5] in other words *a different mind-set*. Or even more bluntly: The mind can stop the brain from having a migraine attack. Is that cool or what?

Patients who respond well to placebo often think that this proves that they've 'made up' their symptoms, that they have faked them.[5] This shows that there are *severe* misconceptions in play.

---

[1] Lauritzen M et al "Clinical relevance of cortical spreading depression in neurological disorders: migraine, malignant stroke, subarachnoid and intracranial hemorrhage, and traumatic brain injury" J Cereb Blood Flow Metab 2011;31(1):17-35
[2] Goadsby PJ et al "Randomized, double-blind, placebo-controlled, proof-of-concept study of the cortical spreading depression inhibiting agent tonabersat in migraine prophylaxis" Cephalalgia 2009;29(7):742-50
[3] Hauge AW et al "Effects of tonabersat on migraine with aura: a randomised, double-blind, placebo-controlled crossover study" Lancet Neurol 2009;8(8):718-23
[4] Speciali JG et al "Migraine treatment and placebo effect" Expert Rev Neurother 2010;10(3):413-9
[5] Kaptchuk TJ et al "'Maybe I made up the whole thing: placebos and patients' experiences in a randomized controlled trial" Cult Med Psychiatry 2009;33(3):382-411

It's all in your head

Most of the symptoms of migraine are felt in the head and we've identified the mechanisms that create these symptoms. The *Chaos in the Cortex* is responsible for the experience of an aura, the *Mayhem in the Brainstem* contributes headaches and other body symptoms. Brainstem and Cortex are parts of the brain and located in your head. So if someone tells you that "I think your migraine is all in your head", you can smile and reply: "Of course, where else could it possibly be?"

The word 'mind' stands for e.g. *thoughts, beliefs and emotions*, all of which are intangible (= you can't touch them). 'Mind' is considered to be a function of the brain[1] and as 'real' as vision, hunger, pain and pleasure. All these phenomena exist in our brains only. When we die, our body is still there, but our mind, vision, hunger, pain and pleasure are gone. Clear?

Therefore it is not entirely *wrong* to say that mind, vision, hunger, pain and pleasure are '*made up*' by the brain, but it is *unfortunate*, because the phrase 'made up' also implies *dishonesty*. And so it feels to migraine patients as if they were being accused of *faking* their symptoms, because you can't see or touch the experience of pain like you can see a broken bone or a bleeding wound.

In the same spirit people assume that 'real' medicine helps with 'real' problems. If now a 'fake' medicine (placebo) leads to symptom improvements, that allegedly proves that the problem was 'fake' too. Does this sound familiar?

The trouble comes from labeling (see page 92) the intangible aspects of an experience as '*made up*', '*fake*' or '*not real*' and thereby ignoring the underlying 'real' brain activity. The experience of a visual aura is the result of a 'Mexican wave' in the visual cortex. Is the wave 'real' and the experience 'not real'? How odd is that?

It is important to understand that the brain generates the mind and the mind can change the brain. Isn't that unreal?

The truly interesting question is: **How** does the placebo effect stop aura and headache and even prevent migraine attacks? **How** can the mind's hope of getting the 'real' treatment (and not the placebo, please) initiate a change in the brain that is more powerful than the chemical effect of 'real' medication?

---

[1] A. Damasio "Self Comes to Mind: Constructing the Conscious Brain" 2010, Pantheon publisher

The placebo effect in the brain

What we call 'placebo effect' is the sum of changes in the brain initiated by a ritual or context that allows the mind to develop a certain level of *hope* or *positive expectation*.[1] These changes can be found and measured in neurotransmitters, hormones, immune regulators and in activity in various brain areas.[2,3,4] In brain scans you can even see this enhanced self-regulatory activity:[5]

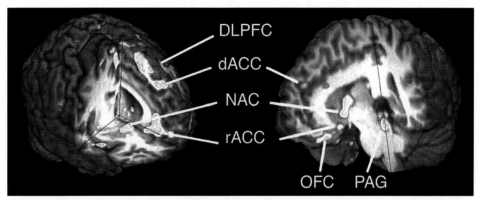

The improved self-regulation ("placebo response") is based on *empowering beliefs*[6] and *positive emotions:*[7] The mind's *hope* or *expectation* of a reward (e.g. pain relief) stimulates pathways that utilize the 'joyful' neurotransmitter dopamine and strongly activates areas in the *prefrontal cortex*.[8,9] Once the PFC is fully awake, it can rein in the naughty pain network, remind the PAG ("pain signal bouncer") to do its job and reduce seizure activity overall.

This is not a small effect. In fact, for pain relief it is stronger than morphine, the strongest analgesic drug. And we have already learnt that the specific effect of Botox® (if there is one at all) in the treatment of chronic migraine is minute at best, compared to the placebo effect, elicited by the patient's beliefs and commitments.[10]

All this reveals the impact of the mind on brain function and especially on the decisive player in self-regulation: the PFC.

---

[1] Benedetti F "The placebo response: how words and rituals change the patient's brain" Patient Educ Couns 2011;84(3):413-9
[2] Kong J et al "Placebo analgesia: findings from brain imaging studies and emerging hypotheses" Rev Neurosci 2007;18(3-4):173-90
[3] Benedetti F "Mechanisms of placebo and placebo-related effects across diseases and treatments" Annu Rev Pharmacol Toxicol 2008;48:33-60
[4] Enck P et al "New Insights into the Placebo and Nocebo Responses" Neuron 2008;59:195–206
[5] Zubieta JK et al "Neurobiological mechanisms of placebo responses" Ann N Y Acad Sci 2009;1156:198-210
[6] Zubieta JK et al "Belief or Need? Accounting for individual variations in the neurochemistry of the placebo effect" Brain Behav Immun 2006;20(1):15-26
[7] Flaten MA et al "The relation of emotions to placebo responses" Philos Trans R Soc Lond B Biol Sci 2011;366(1572):1818-27
[8] Petrovic P et al "A prefrontal non-opioid mechanism in placebo analgesia" Pain 2010;150(1):59-65
[9] Meissner K et al "The placebo effect: advances from different methodological approaches" J Neurosci 2011;31(45):16117-24
[10] Solomon S "Botulinum toxin for the treatment of chronic migraine: the placebo effect" Headache 2011;51(6):980-4

Researchers have found that they can even *stop* a placebo response by interfering with the function of the prefrontal cortex (with magnetic coils).[1] This confirms that the PFC (prefrontal cortex) plays the decisive role in the placebo response in general,[2] in *maintaining stability* in the brain[3] and in preventing and ending headaches[4] and pain.[5] What a pity that it's 'wobbly' in migraineurs.

The prefrontal cortex and migraine

What is a prefrontal cortex good for anyway? Let's have a look and see whether there are symptoms in migraine patients that relate to a dysfunction of the prefrontal cortex:

function of the prefrontal cortex:[6]	dysfunction, potential symptom:[6]
concentration, focused attention	lack of focus, distractibility
mood regulation	mood problems, irritability, anger
short-term memory	poor short-term memory, forgetfulness
behavioral flexibility	rigid behaviors, rituals
language expression	low motivation to talk, loss of fluency
fine motor coordination	poor coordination, clumsiness
planning and decision making	poor planning, indecisiveness
impulse control	impulsive behaviors, restlessness
regulation of body arousal	nervous body symptoms (e.g. indigestion)
social behavior	social withdrawal
constructive coping behaviors	emotional coping behaviors
novelty seeking / approach behavior	avoidance behavior
inhibition of physical 'pain'	increased 'pain' sensitivity
modulation of emotional 'pain'	suffering

Isn't that interesting? All of the listed symptoms can be found in migraineurs; some in the premonitory phase of an attack, some all the time (e.g. in 'difficult' patients). And what about the famous *neuroticism* (= tendency to experience negative emotions)? Voilà, neuroticism too is linked to glitches in the prefrontal cortex.[7,8]

---

[1] Krummenacher P et al "Prefrontal cortex modulates placebo analgesia" Pain 2010;148(3):368-74
[2] Fricchione G et al "Placebo neural systems: nitric oxide, morphine and the dopamine brain reward and motivation circuitries" Med Sci Monit 2005;11(5):MS54-65
[3] Takaya S et al "Prefrontal hypofunction in patients with intractable mesial temporal lobe epilepsy" Neurology 2006;67(9):1674-6
[4] Iacovelli E et al "Neuroimaging in cluster headache and other trigeminal autonomic cephalalgias" J Headache Pain 2012;13(1):11-20
[5] Petrovic P et al "A prefrontal non-opioid mechanism in placebo analgesia" Pain 2010;150(1):59-65
[6] Siddiqui SV et al "Neuropsychology of prefrontal cortex" Indian J Psychiatry 2008;50(3):202-8
[7] Kim SH et al "Resting brain metabolic correlates of neuroticism and extraversion in young men" Neuroreport 2008;19(8):883-6
[8] Wright CI et al "Neuroanatomical correlates of extraversion and neuroticism" Cereb Cortex 2006;16(12):1809-19

One of a 'difficult' migraine patient's heaviest burdens is the frequently mentioned neuroticism, the tendency to feel anxious, worried, sad, tense and apprehensive. Studies show that neuroticism is the result of insufficient control by the PFC over the amygdala, the 'threat detector' in the brain.[1,2]

When a migraineur's poorly controlled amygdala is overly sensitive, vigilant and nervous, and therefore considers almost everything as a potential threat (à la **"THE WORLD IS A HOSTILE PLACE"**), then it can be expected that the mind in that brain is rather miserable. Additionally this already burdened mind has to cope with regular horrible migraine attacks including excruciating headaches.

The officially recommended coping strategy — trigger avoidance — is *ideal* to further foster fear, vigilance and reactivity, which makes matters worse in all too many cases.

It's already clear, what needs to be done: 'strengthening' of the prefrontal cortex, 'taming' of the amygdala (fearful emotions), 'calming' of the stress response, 'stabilizing' of the brain and 'refining' of the cortical arousal regulation. In addition a bit of support for the miserable mind wouldn't go astray. The overall goal must be to boost *resistance and stability* to end the migraine tyranny. We'll get to that soon, but first we need to put it all together.

The threesome in our head

To keep things comprehensible for us, let's use a fairly simple model of the brain.

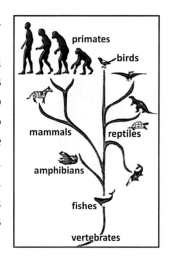

Our brain wasn't constructed from scratch. Over millions of years evolution has added new components and functions to the already established models, in order to secure the survival of the fittest in the struggle for life. Solutions that worked well and that gave an advantage for natural selection were preserved and reused, which makes the brains of different species in parts remarkably similar.

---

[1] Cremers HR, et al "Neuroticism modulates amygdala-prefrontal connectivity in response to negative emotional facial expressions" Neuroimage 2010;49(1):963-70

[2] Drabant EM et al "Experiential, autonomic, and neural responses during threat anticipation vary as a function of threat intensity and neuroticism" Neuroimage 2011;55(1):401-10

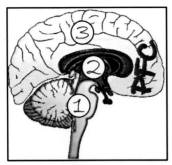
According to the popular model of the *triune brain*[1] ('triune' means 'three in one') the human brain consists of three distinct parts that resemble the brains of other species. In plain words: We have a Lizard, a Horse and a Chimpanzee in our heads. The chunk that makes us human is our uniquely powerful prefrontal cortex.

1) The *reptilian brain* ('the Lizard') essentially consists of the brainstem and a few other pieces involved in movement and locomotion. We already know that the brainstem looks after the body by regulating breathing, digestion, heartbeat, blood flow and blood pressure, as well as various reflexes (blinking, coughing, vomiting etc.). Additionally the brainstem controls sleep and wakefulness (= arousal). Reptilian behavior is largely driven by instincts, rituals, aggression and fear (and not so much by insight, experience, humor, nurturing or loving kindness).

2) The *old mammalian brain* refers to the part that is typical for evolutionarily 'old mammals' like rats, dogs, cats and horses, who require a very different repertoire of behaviors compared to reptiles. A more common name is *the limbic system* (from Latin 'limbus' = girdle). The limbic system includes the amygdala (the 'threat detector') and embodies memory and emotions: As everybody with a mammal as a pet can witness, mammals do have emotions, but regrettably they can't talk about them (just like men).

3) The *neo-Cortex* is the 'new' part of the brain and typical for primates (= apes like us). Especially the *prefrontal cortex* (PFC) is considered so brand-new that, just like other innovative hard- and software, it is still full of bugs and somewhat prone to faults and failures.[2] In humans the PFC grows and matures last,[3] gets a massive overhaul during adolescence[4] and doesn't complete development until the mid-twenties (if all goes well).

"Oh well, that's very interesting" you might think, "but what does that have to do with migraine?". A lot. Bear with me, will'ya?

---

[1] MacLean PD "Evolutionary psychiatry and the triune brain" Psychol Med 1985;15(2):219-21
[2] Goldberg E "The Executive Brain: Frontal Lobes and the Civilized Mind" 2002 Oxford University Press, USA
[3] Gogtay N et al "Dynamic mapping of human cortical development during childhood through early adulthood" Proc Natl Acad Sci USA 2004;101(21):8174-9
[4] Fuster JM "Frontal lobe and cognitive development" J Neurocytol 2002;31(3-5):373-85

These three parts form a team and in a well developed brain the PFC is the team captain, who controls the other two to our advantage.[1] Because we have a PFC, we can behave *reasonably*: When someone steals our parking place, we might swear silently, but we don't get out of the car to beat that bastard up,[2,3] right? And we don't flee from the dentist's waiting room,[4] only because the sound of the drill makes us a tiny bit nervous, right? It is our PFC's control over our instincts[5] and impulses,[6] which allows us to achieve our goals[7] and to get along with other people.[8,9]

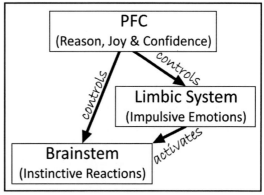

The limbic system and especially the amygdala monitor the environment for threats. When we have to walk through high grass in an area with lions, we want to be extremely awake, attentive and vigilant. For that the limbic system activates the brainstem in order to increase our alertness and reactivity.[10] In this state of hypervigilance we'll react to almost anything with a fright, a "What was that?" and a stress reaction in the body: enhanced breathing, faster heartbeat, higher blood sugar and increased sweat secretion prepare us for plan B, which is running away and climbing a tree.

It has been shown that *stress* plays a major role in migraine; not only as a trigger,[11,12] but also for the attack rate[13,14] as well as for the transformation from episodic to chronic migraine.[15]

---

[1] Price JL "Free will versus survival: brain systems that underlie intrinsic constraints on behavior" J Comp Neurol 2005;493(1):132-9
[2] Peterson CK et al "The role of asymmetrical frontal cortical activity in aggression" Psychophysiology 2008;45(1):86-92
[3] Mobbs D et al "Law, responsibility, and the brain" PLoS Biol 2007;5(4):e103
[4] Masuda A et al "Lesions of the medial prefrontal cortex enhance social modulation of avoidance" Behav Brain Res 2011;217(2):309-14
[5] Murray EA et al "Interactions between orbital prefrontal cortex and amygdala: advanced cognition, learned responses and instinctive behaviors Curr Opin Neurobiol 2010;20(2):212-20
[6] Kim S et al "Prefrontal cortex and impulsive decision making" Biol Psychiatry 2011;69(12):1140-6
[7] O'Doherty JP "Contributions of the ventromedial prefrontal cortex to goal-directed action selection" Ann N Y Acad Sci 2011 Dec;1239:118-29
[8] Clark L "Social and emotional decision-making following frontal lobe injury" Neurocase 2004;10(5):398-403
[9] Wood JN "Social cognition and the prefrontal cortex" Behav Cogn Neurosci Rev 2003;2(2):97-114
[10] Kinomura S et al "Activation by attention of the human reticular formation and thalamic intralaminar nuclei" Science 1996;271(5248):512-5
[11] Wöber C et al "Triggers of migraine and tension-type headache" Handb Clin Neurol 2010;97:161-72
[12] Holm JE et al "Migraine and stress: a daily examination of temporal relationships in women migraineurs" Headache 1997;37(9):553-8
[13] Dodick DW "Review of comorbidities and risk factors for the development of migraine complications (infarct and chronic migraine)" Cephalalgia 2009 Dec;29 Suppl 3:7-14
[14] Sauro KM et al "The stress and migraine interaction" Headache 2009;49(9):1378-86
[15] Bigal ME et al "What predicts the change from episodic to chronic migraine?" Curr Opin Neurol 2009;22(3):269-76

Migraine patients were found to be particularly vulnerable to stress[1] and seem to see themselves that way.[2] One study could even show the lower 'stress threshold' in migraine patients with QEEG (= quantitative EEG, see page 165).[3]

Higher levels of anxiety and a lower threshold for stress make one plausible model for the generation of migraine attacks: The hyped-up limbic system over-activates the brainstem, which then leads to a slow migraine seizure. Case closed, that was easy. However, not every migraine attack is the result of stress and so there must be more to it.

We know that migraine patients tend to have a 'weak' prefrontal cortex (PFC),[4,5,6,7,8] which explains the frequent occurrence of mood disorders,[9] neuroticism,[10] alexithymia,[11] cognitive distortions[12] and excessive negativity bias.[13]

When the PFC is known to be 'weak' anyway, it doesn't come as a surprise to find out that it also doesn't do a good job to control the brainstem, especially the periaqueductal gray (PAG).

We've heard about the PAG already as the 'bouncer' for pain-relevant messages from the body. One could also say that the PAG filters body signals for data which warrant the activation of the pain matrix and the generation of the pain experience, okay?

But the PAG does more than that: When activated by fear, the PAG can even overrule the PFC and initiate instinctive, defensive avoidance-behaviors,[14] e.g. running away and climbing a tree. In migraineurs, the control of the 'terrified' PAG by the 'weak' prefrontal cortex is *dysfunctional* even between migraine attacks. [15,16]

---

[1] Hedborg K et al "Stress in migraine: personality-dependent vulnerability, life events, and gender" SUps J Med Sci 2011;116(3):187-99
[2] Rojahn J et al "Subjective stress sensitivity and physiological responses to an aversive auditory stimulus in migraine and control subjects" J Behav Med 1986;9(2):203-12
[3] Rainero I et al "Quantitative EEG responses to ischaemic arm stress in migraine" Cephalalgia 2001;21(3):224-9
[4] Mongini F et al "Frontal lobe dysfunction in patients with chronic migraine: a clinical-neuropsychological study" Psychiatry Res 2005;133(1):101-6
[5] Kim JH et al "Interictal metabolic changes in episodic migraine: a voxel-based FDG-PET study" Cephalalgia 2010;30(1):53-61
[6] Lev R et al "Orbitofrontal disinhibition of pain in migraine with aura: an interictal EEG-mapping study" Cephalalgia 2010;30(8):910-8
[7] Kim JH et al "Regional grey matter changes in patients with migraine: a voxel-based morphometry study" Cephalalgia 2008;28(6):598-604
[8] Liu J et al "Gender-Related Differences in the Dysfunctional Resting Networks of Migraine Suffers" PLoS One. 2011; 6(11): e27049
[9] Hosokawa T et al "Brain glucose metabolism difference between bipolar and unipolar mood disorders in depressed and euthymic states" Prog Neuropsychopharmacol Biol Psychiatry. 2009;33(2):243-50
[10] Britton JC et al "Neuroticism associated with neural activation patterns to positive stimuli" Psychiatry Res 2007;156(3):263-7
[11] Moriguchi Y et al "Empathy and judging other's pain: an fMRI study of alexithymia" Cereb Cortex 2007;17(9):2223-34
[12] Koechlin E et al "The architecture of cognitive control in the human prefrontal cortex" Science 2003;302(5648):1181-5
[13] Robinson OJ et al "The adaptive threat bias in anxiety: Amygdala-dorsomedial prefrontal cortex coupling and aversive amplification" Neuroimage 2011;60(1):523-529
[14] Mobbs D et al "When fear is near: threat imminence elicits prefrontal-periaqueductal gray shifts in humans" Science 2007;317(5841):1079-83
[15] Moulton EA et al "Interictal dysfunction of a brainstem descending modulatory center in migraine patients" PLoS One 2008;3(11):e3799
[16] Mainero C et al "Altered fMR imaging resting-state connectivity in PAG networks in migraine." Ann Neurol 2011;70(5):838-45

A migraine attack typically begins with symptoms that show that the prefrontal cortex is losing it: fatigue, lack of concentration or moodiness are the most common. These symptoms also occur as a consequence of poor sleep, hunger or around menstruation, which are famous as precipitating factors ('triggers') of migraine attacks. Can you see what these so-called 'migraine triggers' have in common? They all 'weaken' the prefrontal cortex even more and that's why they can precipitate migraine attacks.

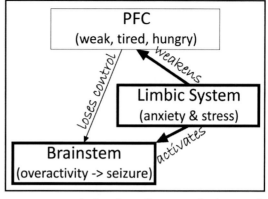

German scientists have shown that after aversive stimulation healthy brains respond with *increased* PFC activity. In contrast, migraine brains showed the opposite behavior, a *decrease* of PFC activity,[1] which is in accordance with our explanation: When the environment is 'nasty', the migraine brain tends to react more and more instinctively and progressively recruits the brainstem.[2] This increasing brainstem activation could be shown with a precision, which allowed the *correct prediction* of the start of the next attack.[3]

There are many potential causes for the 'weakness' of the PFC: insecure attachment experiences,[4,5] early life stress,[6,7] emotional trauma,[8] chronic stress,[9] concussion[10] or traumatic brain injury[11,12] are some of the many sources of a slight PFC dysfunction.

---

[1] Aderjan D et al "Neuronal mechanisms during repetitive trigemino-nociceptive stimulation in migraine patients" Pain 2010;151(1):97-103
[2] Yildirim G et al "Randomised, controlled blink reflex in patients with migraine and tension type headache" J Pak Med Assoc 2011;61(10):978-82
[3] Stankewitz A et al "Trigeminal nociceptive transmission in migraineurs predicts migraine attacks" J Neurosci 2011;31(6):1937-43
[4] Minagawa-Kawai Y et al "Prefrontal activation associated with social attachment: facial-emotion recognition in mothers and infants" Cereb Cortex 2009;19(2):284-92
[5] Viana AG et al "Perceived attachment: relations to anxiety sensitivity, worry, and GAD symptoms" Behav Res Ther. 2008;46(6):737-47
[6] Mueller SC et al "Early-life stress is associated with impairment in cognitive control in adolescence: an fMRI study" Neuropsychologia 2010;48(10):3037-44
[7] V Maletic et al "Neurobiology of depression: an integrated view of key findings" Int J Clin Pract 2007;61(12):2030–2040
[8] Matsuo K et al "Hypoactivation of the prefrontal cortex during verbal fluency test in PTSD: a near-infrared spectroscopy study" Psychiatry Res 2003;124(1):1-10
[9] Garrett JE et al "Chronic stress effects on dendritic morphology in medial prefrontal cortex: sex differences and estrogen dependence" Neuroscience 2009;162(1):195-207
[10] Johnson B et al "Alteration of brain default network in subacute phase of injury in concussed individuals: resting-state fMRI study" Neuroimage 2012;59(1):511-8
[11] Mayer AR et al "Functional connectivity in mild traumatic brain injury" Hum Brain Mapp 2011;32(11):1825-35
[12] Chen AJ et al "Functional reintegration of prefrontal neural networks for enhancing recovery after brain injury" J Head Trauma Rehabil 2006;21(2):107-18

The tyrant's many faces

In this chapter we've discovered that a migraine attack is a form of seizure in the brainstem due to a loss of inhibitory control by the prefrontal cortex. Aggravating and precipitating factors are stress, anxiety, poor sleep, hunger, hormonal fluctuations and in some cases alcohol, because of their 'weakening' effect on the PFC.

Let's apply the triune brain model to summarize our findings: When the smart and happy 'human Ape' (PFC) is confused and loses control over the 'shy Horse' (limbic system) and the 'terrified Lizard' (brainstem), many cognitive, emotional and physical symptoms can ensue. In migraineurs one of these symptoms is migraine attacks, but other disorders are not far away:

glitch	migraine symptom	migraine comorbidity
lame prefrontal cortex (PFC)	lack of concentration and focus, distractibility	Attention Deficit Disorder (ADD/ADHD)
insufficient PFC control over amygdala	mood problems, neuroticism	anxiety, depression, anger, PTSD
weak PFC control over PAG ("the pain bouncer")	headache, neck pain, high pain sensitivity, allodynia	pain disorders, fibromyalgia
unsatisfactory PFC control over arousal regulation	restlessness, reactivity	sleep disorders
PFC: impaired fine motor coordination	clumsiness, impaired motor control	restless leg syndrome
PFC: bad habituation/sensory gating → sensitization	higher sensory sensitivity, more seizure activity	multiple chemical sensitivity syndrome
regulation of body temperature via blood flow	hot or cold flashes	stroke, heart attack, claudication
unbalanced autonomic nervous system	constipation/diarrhea	irritable bowel syndrome

This should make very clear that migraine indeed is not "Just a headache", but rather the tip of an iceberg of woes. I wish parents of kids with migraine as well as 'beginners' would recognize that sooner rather than later, when everything has become 'difficult'.

Answered questions

Let's recap our questions from the beginning of the chapter, so that we know where we are in our understanding of the tyrant:

☑ What's going on in the brain during a migraine attack? A 'Mexican Wave' (cortical spreading depression) creates *Chaos in the Cortex*, because the rattled neurons can't work properly anymore. This causes the aura symptoms. A seizure leads to *Mayhem in the Brainstem*, producing all the other symptoms of a migraine attack. Some people are even lucky enough that the seizure spares the responsible parts of the PAG ('bouncer') and they don't experience any headache at all.

☑ Why does migraine have so many comorbidities? When the PFC loses its cooling, calming and composing influence on the limbic system and the brainstem, then the '*shy Horse*' and the '*terrified Lizard*' go bananas and drive predisposed body systems nuts.

☑ Why is the placebo effect so strong in trials of migraine medications? Positive emotions like hope or expectation of reward not only change the mind-set, but also activate the PFC, which has the power to stop CSD, head pain and even the brainstem seizure. This indicates that the opposite *may* also be true, at least a bit: Negative emotions, e.g. frustration, emotional pain, might be able to *promote* migraine attacks: Perhaps, the true villain is not so much the *alarming* effect of distressing situations, but the *emotional* component (fear of more hurt and frustration) of the stress *response*.

☑ How is it possible that so many treatments and therapies are somewhat effective in migraine, even if they have nothing in common? Every treatment and therapy that manages to instill hope and positive expectations — in principle — has the potential to put an end to migraine. If the mind is convinced that avoiding 'trigger' foods is the kicker, that may well be enough to stop attacks; even if these foods have no effect when they get swallowed without the mind's knowledge (e.g. in so-called "blind" studies). Other minds may be swung by face surgery or injections of sausage-poison, which by itself may have a minuscule effect. Many minds benefit from cognitive behavioral therapy, because it teaches the mind to keep the emotions balanced with levelheaded thinking. And a few rebels wouldn't mind to build up *resistance* and *resilience* to make sure that negative emotions can't hold them to ransom anymore.

Rigid minds may prefer to rely on drugs only and harvest hope and expectation, when they pop a pill. If you know someone who is too narrow-minded to take part in our tyranny-ending revolution, *don't tell them* that triptans are particularly prone to causing medication-overuse headache, that anti-seizure medication can make them *really* stupid and that experts have come to "the conclusion that antidepressants generally do more harm than good by disrupting a number of adaptive processes".[1] Drugs don't end the tyranny.

☑ What leads to attacks? It is clear that the attack symptoms begin when the PFC starts losing it. EEG analyses have found that roughly 36 hours before an attack the PFC slows down significantly, which means, it's not working well anymore.[2] The symptoms before an attack show exactly that: lack of mental sharpness and concentration, moodiness and the like. A LoRETA recording *during* an attack confirmed this scenario: The PFC goes down and the brainstem 'erupts'.[3] What follows are Chaos in the Cortex and Mayhem in the Brainstem, but you know that already.

What's new, is the finding that *several days before* the agony, the brain's 'electrical reactions' (so-called evoked potentials) show the first subtle signs of the oncoming storm.[4,5] Much later — one and a half days *before* the headache phase — the 'dark clouds' can finally be seen in a QEEG as slow, so-called Delta energy, whose amount already flags the intensity of the impending head pain.[5,6]

The trigger food drama

The unexpectedly long duration of this 'brain-weather change' leading up to the 'hurricane in the head', might contribute to an explanation, why so many migraineurs believe in 'trigger' factors and 'trigger' foods whereas medical researchers haven't found a mechanism that could be held responsible for the *'experienced'* immediacy: "Last night I ate a tomato, today I have a migraine attack, therefore I know without any doubt, that the tomato triggered the migraine attack."

---

[1] Andrews PW et al "Primum Non Nocere: An Evolutionary Analysis of Whether Antidepressants Do More Harm than Good" Front Psychol 2012;3:117
[2] Bjørk M et al "Quantitative EEG power and asymmetry increase 36 h before a migraine attack" Cephalalgia 2008;28(9):960-8
[3] Keeser D et al "Preliminary EEG and Low Resolution Electromagnetic Tomography (LoRETA) measurements results of a migraine patient: An Electrophysiological Evaluation" Unpublished poster presentation, Technical University Munich
[4] Siniatchkin M et al "How the brain anticipates an attack: a study of neurophysiological periodicity in migraine" Funct Neurol 1999;14(2):69-77
[5] Sand T et al "Visual evoked potential latency, amplitude and habituation in migraine: a longitudinal study" Clin Neurophysiol 2008;119(5):1020-7
[6] Bjørk M et al "What initiates a migraine attack? Conclusions from four longitudinal studies of quantitative EEG and steady-state visual-evoked potentials in migraineurs" Acta Neurol Scand Suppl 2011;(191):56-63

It is the mind's job to find a cause for the cruel assault. Once the tomato is a suspect, then the *immediacy* and the *intensity* of the torture indeed make it extremely difficult to sit back and say: "I've spent the last 24 hours with **burning lava** in my head and people say, the trigger could have been the tomato I ate. In contrast I am currently inclined to conclude that the evidence for the tomato as the causal factor triggering my woes, is insufficient and I'll continue to eat tomatoes until a thorough statistical analysis of independently recorded data verifies the tomato trigger theory and justifies a tomato ban."

When you're petrified by terror and pain, the normal human reaction is to say: **"OH MY GOD, TOMATOS TRIGGER MIGRAINE ATTACKS."** And I'm not sure that many people will embrace the message that the assault was already *several days* in the making; because now the educated migraineur is in a slight predicament: The knowledge of some study results ("The EEG changes 36 hours before an attack") still can't appease the fear of and doubts about the suspected food triggers and the angst most likely is indeed a precipitating factor.

To make matters really complicated, questions of *habituation* and *sensitization* may play a decisive role in the trigger drama. Explained in simple talk, habituation means *'getting used to it'*. The brain normally reacts weaker and weaker to repetitive stimuli: When any stimulus hits our senses, the prefrontal cortex quickly checks out, whether it's old hat or relevant,[1,2] because we can't allow to be continually distracted by redundant information (Imagine reading a book and someone says "Hello" all the time). So the PFC tells the rest of the cortex that the stimulus is old hat and "Don't worry about it too much. Get used to it".[3,4] Consequently the cortex' electrical reactions get weaker over time (e.g. in the auditory cortex for sound, in the visual cortex for light, in the sensory cortex for touch etc.). This is called 'habituation' or 'sensory gating'.[5,6]

Imagine that someone had a weak-ish or 'wobbly' PFC. Then it could happen, that this person does not habituate well to external stimuli and that he/she ends up overly sensitive to lights, sounds, smells; a bit like someone who hasn't slept in days: tetchy.[7]

---

[1] Goldberg E et al "Lateralization of frontal lobe functions and cognitive novelty" J Neuropsychiatry Clin Neurosci 1994;6(4):371-8
[2] Løvstad M et al "Contribution of subregions of human frontal cortex to novelty processing" J Cogn Neurosci 2012;24(2):378-95
[3] Griffin JP "The role of the frontal areas of the cortex upon habituation in man" Clin Sci 1963;24:127-34
[4] Weiland BJ et al "Evidence for a frontal cortex role in both auditory and somatosensory habituation: a MEG study" Neuroimage 2008;42(2):827-35
[5] Edgar JC et al "Cross-modal generality of the gating deficit" Psychophysiology 2005;42(3):318-27
[6] Lijffijt M et al "P50, N100 and P200 sensory gating: relationships with behavioral inhibition, attention and working memory" Psychophys 2009;46(5):1059-68
[7] Gosselin A et al "Total sleep deprivation and novelty processing: implications for frontal lobe functioning" Clin Neurophysiol 2005;116(1):211-22

That's exactly what goes on in migraine brains. The lack of cooling, calming and collecting influence by the PFC in migraine patients can be seen in experiments that measure the sensory gating/habituation effect ("get used to it") in the brain. In migraine brains, sensory gating[1] and habituation are impaired,[2,3] as if the cortex can't stop asking the PFC "Huh, what was that?"[4] And the effect gets even stronger with anxious overbreathing.[5]

The opposite process to habituation is called *sensitization*: The responses to repetitive stimuli 'potentiate' (= get stronger and stronger) and the migraine brain is prone to that,[6,7] which is not surprising when the habituation is impaired.

"Doesn't it have consequences when the brain's electrical reactions tend to potentiate/escalate even between episodes?" You're probably referring to all sorts of subtle changes in the visual system of migraineurs, e.g. the altered perception of contrast or motion [8,9,10,11] or a certain aversion to flickering lights,[12] which can actually prompt a decent migraine attack[13] (just like a light-sensitive epileptic seizure[14]): The escalating activity spreads *from the visual cortex to the brainstem* via sensitized pathways.[15] Once the traveling escalation has ignited the brainstem-seizure, the visually-triggered migraine delivers the full experience like an attack that was periodically due.

This mechanism of escalating activity in one brain area lighting a 'seizure-fire' in another area, is known in epileptology as 'kindling'. Originally the term 'kindling' was used for sparking epileptic seizures with *electrical* stimulation only.[16]

---

[1] Ambrosini A et al "Reduced gating of middle-latency auditory evoked potentials (P50) in migraine patients: another indication of abnormal sensory processing?" Neurosci Lett 2001;306(1-2):132-4
[2] Siniatchkin M et al "What kind of habituation is impaired in migraine patients?" Cephalalgia 2003;23(7):511-8
[3] Coppola G et al "Habituation and migraine" Neurobiol Learn Mem 2009;92(2):249-59
[4] Demarquay G et al "Exacerbated attention orienting to auditory stimulation in migraine patients" Clin Neurophysiol 2011;122(9):1755-63
[5] Coppola G et al "Changes in visual-evoked potential habituation induced by hyperventilation in migraine" J Headache Pain 2010;11(6):497-503
[6] Wang W et al "Intensity dependence of auditory evoked potentials is pronounced in migraine: an indication of cortical potentiation and low serotonergic neurotransmission?" Neurology 1996;46(5):1404-9
[7] Wang W et al "Interictal potentiation of passive "oddball" auditory event-related potentials in migraine" Cephalalgia 1990;10(5):261-5
[8] McKendrick AM et al "Low spatial frequency contrast sensitivity deficits in migraine are not visual pathway selective" Cephalalgia 2009;29(5):539-49
[9] McKendrick AM et al "Contrast-processing dysfunction in both magnocellular and parvocellular pathways in migraineurs with or without aura" Invest Ophthalmol Vis Sci 2003;44(1):442-8
[10] Antal A et al "Altered motion perception in migraineurs: evidence for interictal cortical hyperexcitability" Cephalalgia 2005;25(10):788-94
[11] Granziera C et al "Anatomical alterations of the visual motion processing network in migraine with and without aura" PLoS Med 2006;3(10):e402
[12] Karanovic O et al "Detection and discrimination of flicker contrast in migraine" Cephalalgia 2011;31(6):723-36
[13] Cao Y et al "Functional MRI-BOLD of visually triggered headache in patients with migraine" Arch Neurol 1999;56(5):548-54
[14] Covanis A "Photosensitivity in idiopathic generalized epilepsies" Epilepsia 2005;46 Suppl9:67-72
[15] Cao Y et al "Functional MRI-BOLD of brainstem structures during visually triggered migraine" Neurology 2002;59(1):72-8
[16] Corcoran ME et al "Kindling of seizures with low-frequency electrical stimulation" Brain Res 1980;196(1):262-5

Later it was found that, due to sensitization, excessive activity in the limbic system can kindle certain epileptic seizures.[1] And so the model expanded to other episodic disorders that might have been *kindled by the limbic system*, e.g. a psychosis[2] (= temporary loss of contact with reality). This also annihilates ancient models of a clear distinction between 'neurological' and 'psychological', because the 'neurological' seizure that caused the 'psychological' psychosis was kindled by emotional tension in the limbic system. Confused?

As I said in chapter 5, the brain doesn't care which of its activities we call 'neurological', 'psychological', 'biological', 'mental' or 'emotional': Helpful beliefs and hope in the mind can *change* the brain and put an end to pain. Who's gonna tell the Pope?

The kindling mechanism also explains how strong scents can prompt a migraine attack in sensitized brains: The smell cortex is seen as belonging to the limbic system and its escalating activity[3] could theoretically kindle[4] a migraine seizure. If that were true, then repeated stimulation with a strong scent would lead odor-sensitized migraineurs to an attack with escalated activity in the *smell cortex*, the *limbic system* and in the *'migraine generator'* in the brainstem. Coincidentally, that's just what German scientists found in an fMRI-study after repeated stimulation with rose odor.[5]

Sensitization is also responsible for the effect that seizures seem to promote more seizures[6] and together with kindling it may be the source of another migraine comorbidity: multiple chemical sensitivity.[7,8] And so it might well be possible that migraine patients indeed end up sensitized to certain foods or substances, as the result of an ever more escalating reaction to something that was once completely harmless (e.g. tomatoes).

Please note, sensitization requires fear and anxiety.[9] It is the *belief* and the *fear* that can turn eating a tomato into a 'trigger.'

---

[1] Adamec RE et al "Limbic kindling and animal behavior-implications for human psychopathology associated with complex partial seizures" Biol Psychiatry 1983;18(2):269-93
[2] Rubin EH et al "Limbic seizures, kindling, and psychosis: a link between neurobiology and clinical psychiatry" Compr Ther 1985;11(7):54-8
[3] Racine RJ et al "Kindling-induced potentiation in the piriform cortex" Brain Res 1991;556(2):218-25
[4] Löscher W et al "The role of the piriform cortex in kindling" Prog Neurobiol 1996;50(5-6):427-81
[5] Stankewitz A et al "Increased limbic and brainstem activity during migraine attacks following olfactory stimulation" Neurology 2011;77(5):476-82
[6] Bertram E "The relevance of kindling for human epilepsy" Epilepsia 2007;48 Suppl2:65-74
[7] Bell IR, et al "An olfactory-limbic model of multiple chemical sensitivity syndrome: possible relationships to kindling and affective spectrum disorders" Biol Psychiatry 1992;32(3):218-42
[8] Gilbert ME "Does the kindling model of epilepsy contribute to our understanding of multiple chemical sensitivity?" Ann N Y Acad Sci 2001;933:68-91
[9] Smock CD "Perceptual sensitization to threat objects as a function of manifest anxiety" Child Dev 1963;34:161-7

It is important to understand that it's not the tomato itself that can trigger an episode in those sensitized patients, but it's their mind's and brain's *escalating reactions* that kindle the attack. Putting tomatoes on a 'trigger food' list, leads vulnerable patients into becoming sensitized to tomatoes. If there were *seizure-promoting substances* in tomatoes, patients with frequent epileptic seizures would have found that out, don't you think?

Yet they haven't. Although there are some discussions and speculations about MSG[1] (a flavor enhancer), artificial sweeteners[2] alcohol[3] and coffee[4] as possibly lowering seizure thresholds, *not a single food* is labeled as 'seizure-trigger' in epilepsy land.[2]

Alone the term 'trigger'—which clearly expresses an immediate effect—*urgently* suggests that sensitization and kindling are involved, just like in those migraine attacks that were 'triggered' by flickering light or strong odors in adequately sensitized brains.

In this context one wonders why in all those years nobody has ever come up with idea to ask experts in rheumatoid arthritis as to which foods might '*trigger*' *inflammation* since allegedly "MIGRAINE IS SWELLING AND INFLAMMATION OF BLOOD VESSELS AROUND YOUR HEAD"?

The only logical conclusion is: There is no such thing as a migraine 'trigger food'. The wicked advice to avoid 'trigger' foods takes advantage of migraine patients' tendency to prefer passive-avoidant coping behaviors and contributes to fear and sensitization, and in the long-term to chronification. It would be sensible to stop talking about 'trigger' food, but we are aware that the current regime asserts: "NO 'SCIENTIFIC DATA' TO THE CONTRARY, FROM A RANDOMIZED CONTROLLED TRIAL OR ANY OTHER SOURCE, WOULD EVER CONVINCE ME OTHERWISE."

Now, after being sensitized, some migraine patients indeed need to avoid certain foods, Chinook-winds and Germany in fall, all of which doesn't necessarily reduce the overall attack rate.

Perhaps it would haven been smarter to suggest therapies that reduce or eliminate migraine attacks by raising the *resistance* to seizures, by increasing the *stability* of the brain, and by *decreasing* sensitization, fear and anxiety; steps that can end the tyranny.

---

[1] Nemeroff CB et al "Monosodium L-glutamate-induced convulsions: temporary alteration in blood-brain barrier permeability to plasma proteins" Environ Physiol Biochem 1975;5(6):389-95
[2] Stafstrom CE "Dietary approaches to epilepsy treatment: old and new options on the menu" Epilepsy Curr 2004;4(6):215-22
[3] Gordon E et al "Alcohol and marijuana: effects on epilepsy and use by patients with epilepsy" Epilepsia 2001;42(10):1266-72
[4] Chrościńska M et al "Caffeine and the anticonvulsant potency of antiepileptic drugs: experimental and clinical data" Pharmacol Rep 2011;63(1):12-8

The unanswered question

☐ <u>Why is it that so many people *don't* have migraine despite apparently having the genetic disposition?</u> This is the question whose answer would completely clarify the concept of the curse and allow us to consolidate the soft ground that is responsible for migraineurs' instability to the wind and weather of life.

One would think that migraine research has put a lot of effort in, to determine why one of two identical twins has migraine and the other one does not. They have the same parents, the same genes and have probably shared much more than just mom's uterus. Discordant twins (one has migraine, the other one does not) would be the perfect study subject for QEEGs, LoRETA, fMRI, PET scans and DTI, as well as for neuropsychological and electrophysiological tests. The differences would probably give us a very good idea what tips a brain over the migraine edge and what makes it stable enough for the wind and weather of life.

"So where are the studies? What did they find?" What studies? Why would they do such a study? It is not very likely that those studies would reveal: "Kevin, the identical twin with migraine has a Botox® deficiency due to his individual temperament" or "Unlike his migraine-free twin-brother Larry, Kevin refused to eat spinach as a child, leading to a severe shortage of triptans, anti-seizure medication and analgesics in his body." Logically, the pharma-financed researchers haven't done such a study.

Are you starting to understand why I've been talking about "the current *regime*" since day one? Are you beginning to comprehend what the patient's role is in this *industry*? Do you get it why I talk about misleading migraine myths as "insidious obstacles"? It doesn't matter whether the current regime is acting out of malice or ignorance or greed: You as the patient are footing the bill. Yes, they're giving you pain relief, but they're taking your 'life'.

Some people who get satisfying pain relief from medication probably think that I'm exaggerating and that it's not right to blame doctors and the pharma industry for making a buck. Dead wrong! As expressed earlier, I'm not *blaming* anybody. Who would benefit from that? Certainly not me. The questions that I'm answering are: "What's going on?" and "What is a better solution?". Instead of "Who's to blame?" we should ask the question: "How can I fulfill my own responsibility to myself better?" Responsible is he who foots the bill. Are you response-able?

I do understand that it's not easy to be critical of the pharma industry when you're a happy customer. That's okay with me. Just be aware what *their* intention is, their self-interest. A study looked at the chronic migraine brain's *sensitization* to painful stimuli and paradoxically found an *increase* in electrical reactions to *decreasing* challenges: These brains *actively kept the pain experience strong*.[1] Alas, the headache-handbook for neurologists recommends for pain sensitization merely "that the patient vigilantly resorts to triptan therapy".[2] Hands up if you believe that more drugs will solve that problem.

What makes the difference?

Since no medical migraine researcher has put discordant migraine twins in a brain scanner or through some other test, we can't answer the last question. Wait a minute! An alternative would be to do some relevant test stuff on a group of young migraineurs and test them again a couple of years later. Some will have lost their migraine and then we'll get closer to an answer. Whadduyathink?

This type of study is called 'longitudinal' and researchers from a university in Kiel, Germany, have actually done that. They've measured a particular electrical potential called CNV. That stands for contingent negative variation, a name that I suggest you forget straight away. Imagine the start of a 100m race. The starter says: "On your marks — set …" and then starts the race with a shot from his pistol. The CNV is an electrical representation of the brain's 'readiness-arousal' between the "set" and the shot. The brain's attentional *eagerness* if you will. This is what they knew already:

- The amplitude of the CNV (the amount of brain 'eagerness') is higher in migraine[3]
- The CNV amplitude habituates ('get used to it') in normal, but not in migraine brains[4]
- Both CNV irregularities get worse **five days before** a migraine attack[5]
- During and shortly after an attack, the CNV of the migraine brain behaves normally[6]
- The source of the higher CNV amplitude in migraine brains lies in the brainstem[7]

---

[1] de Tommaso M et al "Suggestion and pain in migraine: a study by laser evoked potentials" CNS Neurol Disord Drug Targets 2012;11(2):110-26
[2] Burstein R et al "Managing migraine associated with sensitization" Handb Clin Neurol 2010;97:207-15
[3] Kropp P et al "Contingent negative variation--findings and perspectives in migraine" Cephalalgia 1993;13(1):33-6
[4] Kropp P et al "Is increased amplitude of contingent negative variation in migraine due to cortical hyperactivity or to reduced habituation?" Cephalalgia 1993;13(1):37-41
[5] Siniatchkin M et al "Migraine in childhood--are periodically occurring migraine attacks related to dynamic changes of cortical information processing?" Neurosci Lett 2000;279(1):1-4
[6] Kropp P et al "Contingent negative variation during migraine attack and interval: evidence for normalization of slow cortical potentials during the attack" Cephalalgia 1995;15(2):123-8
[7] Bender S et al "Stereotyped topography of different elevated contingent negative variation components in children with migraine without aura points towards a subcortical dysfunction" Pain 2007;127(3):221-33

The German scientists in Kiel measured the CNV in migraine kids and age-matched healthy brats in 1998 and again in 2006. They found that the CNV decreased in healthy adolescents as an effect of *maturation* and that was the same for ex-migraineurs. In contrast, the CNV habituation got worse in those migraine teens whose migraine got worse as well.[1]

This confirmed earlier studies which indicated that these persistent CNV irregularities—especially the lack of normal habituation—represented a disturbance of the normal *development* of the cortex.[2,3] Well, we both know who is responsible for habituation, don't we? Our buddy, the prefrontal cortex. As I've said, the PFC is obviously a little 'wobbly' in migraine brains.

"So, what is it that sabotages the healthy growth and maturation of the PFC in those kids with persistent migraine?"

As we already know, the development of the PFC benefits greatly from the child's *secure emotional attachment* to a dependable, encouraging and supportive 'mother' (= primary caregiver),[4,5,6,7] which promotes resistance[8] and resilience,[9] as well as emotional composure[10] and balance[11] and cognitive control.[12] Disturbances of this crucial process—for whatever reason—are connected e.g. to pessimism,[13] to depression and to migraine disability.[14]

Early life stress[15] (challenges that exceed the child's resistance and resilience at the time) can derail healthy brain development.[16]

---

[1] Siniatchkin M et al "Developmental changes of the contingent negative variation in migraine and healthy children" J Headache Pain 2010;11(2):105-13
[2] Kropp P, et al "Migraine--evidence for a disturbance of cerebral maturation in man?" Neurosci Lett 1999;276(3):181-4
[3] Bender S et al "Lack of age-dependent development of the contingent negative variation (CNV) in migraine children?" Cephalalgia 2002;22(2):132-6
[4] Schore AN "Attachment and the regulation of the right brain" Attach Hum Dev 2000;2(1):23-47
[5] Ramasubbu R et al "Neural representation of maternal face processing: a functional magnetic resonance imaging study" Can J Psychiatry 2007;52(11):726-34
[6] Minagawa-Kawai Y et al "Prefrontal activation associated with social attachment: facial-emotion recognition in mothers and infants" Cereb Cortex 2009;19(2):284-92
[7] Nachmias M et al "Behavioral inhibition and stress reactivity: the moderating role of attachment security" Child Dev 1996;67(2):508-22
[8] Crowley MJ et al "Exclusion and micro-rejection: event-related potential response predicts mitigated distress" Neuroreport 2009;20(17):1518-22
[9] Katz M et al "Prefrontal Plasticity and Stress Inoculation-induced Resilience" Dev Neurosci 2009;31:239-299
[10] Price JL et al "Neurocircuitry of mood disorders" Neuropsychopharmacology 2010;35(1):192-216
[11] Cusi AM et al "Systematic review of the neural basis of social cognition in patients with mood disorders" J Psychiatry Neurosci 2012;37(3):154-69
[12] Kompus K et al "Distinct control networks for cognition and emotion in the prefrontal cortex" Neurosci Lett 2009;467(2):76-80
[13] Gillath O et al "Attachment-style differences in the ability to suppress negative thoughts: exploring the neural correlates" Neuroimage 2005;28(4):835-47
[14] Rossi P et al "Depressive symptoms and insecure attachment as predictors of disability in a clinical population of patients with episodic and chronic migraine" Headache 2005;45(5):561-70
[15] Mueller SC et al "Early-life stress is associated with impairment in cognitive control in adolescence: an fMRI study" Neuropsychologia 2010;48(10):3037-44
[16] Pechtel P et al "Effects of early life stress on cognitive and affective function: an integrated review of human literature" Psychopharmacology (Berl) 2011;214(1):55-70

Emotional neglect or abuse, physical neglect or abuse, *trauma or maltreatment* in general, but even *permanent tension* in relationships can have a detrimental effect on the very vulnerable, immature nervous system and impede maturation of brain and mind.[1,2,3,4,5] Given that almost 60% of patients in headache centers *report* substantial childhood maltreatment, it's about time to lift the ban on this crucial topic and instead encourage migraineurs to face the past that has shaped their brain. It's bad enough that medical doctors can't be bothered to take their patients emotional history into consideration, but we definitely don't need to mistake some destroyed soul's distraught denial as a universal *gagging clause*: **"MIGRAINE IS NEUROLOGICAL, NOT PSYCHOLOGICAL."** Unfortunately the brain doesn't know that it's *not* supposed to write its history of 'psychological' stress and trauma into its 'neurological' structure. Adults denying their laden past are hurting their own kids now.

Statistics show the lifetime prevalence (= rate of occurrence) of *traumatic experiences* is 60% for men and 50% for women. Of these, only 8% of the men, but 20% of the women end up with clinically diagnosed PTSD (= posttraumatic stress disorder).[6] Their *non-recovery from trauma* indicates that women (as girls) were more exposed to events, situations and relationships that softened the young foundation of their resilience and resistance to the thunderstorms of life. If men were similarly affected, our societies would probably have made addressing this issue a top-priority.

Instead the male-dominated medical establishment is quite happy to be annoyed by 'difficult' female patients, to ignore the personal history and to fill them up with medical beliefs and drugs for their allegedly medical syndrome: irritable bowel,[7] chronic fatigue,[8] fibromyalgia,[9] mood disorders, migraine[10] and many more.

---

[1] van der Kolk BA "Childhood abuse and neglect and loss of self-regulation. Bulletin of the Menninger Clinic 1994; 58:145–168
[2] De Bellis MD "Developmental traumatology: the psychobiological development of maltreated children and its implications for research, treatment and policy"Dev Psychopathol 2001;13(3):539-64
[3] Schore AN "The experience-dependent maturation of a regulatory system in the orbital prefrontal cortex and the origin of developmental psychopathology" Develop Psychopath 1996;8:59–87
[4] Liberzon I et al "Paralimbic and medial prefrontal cortical involvement in neuroendocrine responses to traumatic stimuli" Am J Psychiatry 2007;164(8):1250-8
[5] van Harmelen AL et al "Reduced medial prefrontal cortex volume in adults reporting childhood emotional maltreatment" Biol Psychiatry 2010;68(9):832-8
[6] Kessler RC et al "Posttraumatic stress disorder in the National Comorbidity Survey" Arch Gen Psychiatry 1995;52(12):1048-60
[7] Surdea-Blaga T et al "Psychosocial determinants of irritable bowel syndrome" World J Gastroenterol 2012;18(7):616-26
[8] Heim C et al "Childhood trauma and risk for chronic fatigue syndrome" Arch Gen Psychiatry 2009;66(1):72-80
[9] Low LA et al "Early Life Adversity as a Risk Factor for Fibromyalgia in Later Life" Pain Res Treat 2012;140832
[10] Post RM et al "Shared mechanisms in affective illness, epilepsy, and migraine" Neurology 1994;44(10 Suppl7):S37-47

The mother's example shapes the maturing mind's and brain's response patterns;[1,2] and so the high rate of *mood disorders* amongst parents of migraine children is remarkable. An Italian study found, *every second mother* and every fourth father had at least one 'psychiatric' diagnosis (mostly anxiety or depression).[3]

Imperfect attachment, early life stress, neglect, abuse, trauma or moody parents can impair the PFC's maturation and tip a predisposed brain over the migraine edge, but they still don't quite answer the question: "Why does Kevin have migraine, but not Larry?" Despite the lack of studies on discordant twins, I have two answers:

● Trivial and mild *brain injuries* (e.g. concussions) naturally lead to all sorts of minor and major brain dysfunctions.[4] Kevin may have scored one goal too many with a header in kindy soccer,[5] while Larry played defense. And that's just soccer and not gridiron, rugby or footy, let alone boxing and the like.[6] Now, before all the alarmed migraine mothers storm off to snatch their little critters from the sports fields to put them in safe cages, look at this:

● A study observing parental behavior in families with migraine children found the parents more *instructing* and directing towards the affected kid and more *supportive* towards the non-affected sibling:[7] "Dominance of parents and submissive behavior of children were the main features of interactions." Two other studies[8,9] investigated the influence of parent-child interactions on the habituation of the CNV (= the brain's reaction to "set"), a marker for PFC function:

- Parents exerted significantly more control over migraine kids than over their siblings
- The stronger the parent's dominance and control over the child and the more intense the suppression of a child's independence, the greater was the neuroticism in a migraine child and the more pronounced was the loss of CNV habituation (= PFC immaturity)

In other words, the last straw might be the parent's voiced concern: "Be careful, Kevin!" versus "Give it a crack, Larry!"

---

[1] Francis DD et al "Maternal care and the development of stress responses" Curr Opin Neurobiol 1999;9(1):128-34
[2] Korosi A et al "The pathways from mother's love to baby's future" Front Behav Neurosci 2009;3:27
[3] Galli F et al "Psychiatric disorders and headache familial recurrence: a study on 200 children and their parents" J Headache Pain 2009;10(3):187-97
[4] Witt ST et al "Decreased prefrontal cortex activity in mild traumatic brain injury during performance of an auditory oddball task" Brain Imaging Behav 2010;4(3-4):232-47
[5] Colvin AC et al "The role of concussion history and gender in recovery from soccer-related concussion" Am J Sports Med 2009;37(9):1699-704
[6] Marar M et al "Epidemiology of concussions among United States high school athletes in 20 sports" Am J Sports Med 2012;40(4):747-55
[7] Siniatchkin M et al "Migraine and asthma in childhood: evidence for specific asymmetric parent-child interactions in migraine and asthma families" Cephalalgia 2003;23(8):790-802
[8] Gerber WD et al "Slow cortical potentials in migraine families are associated with psychosocial factors" J Psychosom Res 2002;52(4):215-22
[9] Siniatchkin M et al "Role of family in development of neurophysiological manifestations in children with migraine" Prax Kinderpsychol Kinderpsychiatr 2002;51(3):194-208

The Know-Your-Tyrant final exam

Whether you want to or not, here you can test the knowledge that you've acquired in this and previous chapters. If you think "Waah, I'm not good at this kind of stuff", wait and see:

1.) Migraine attacks often have many body symptoms. Why is that?
a) b/c there is Mayhem in the Brainstem (where the body gets regulated) O
b) b/c the inflammation of the head's blood vessels spreads into the body

2.) Many migraineurs experience an aura. What is that?
a) another seizure-like electrical event, called cortical spreading depression O
b) aura is when pinched nerves get annoyed by face muscles that crave Botox

3.) The first phase of an attack is the prodrome. What causes the symptoms?
a) the PFC is slowly losing it and its grip on limbic system and brainstem O
b) the Chimp rides the Horse and catches the Lizard

4.) What is the placebo effect?
a) hope and positive expectations activate the PFC, inhibiting symptoms O
b) when people get deceived into thinking their pain was gone, but it isn't

5.) Why does migraine have so many comorbidities?
a) b/c wobbly PFC = dysregulated brain = the body bears the brunt O
b) b/c the blood vessels in other organs also start swelling

6.) Why do many migraineurs follow the advice to avoid 'trigger' foods?
a) b/c they tend to prefer avoidance-behaviors over confronting problems O
b) b/c 'trigger' foods lead to pinched nerves and blood vessel swelling

7.) What is sensitization?
a) the brain's electrical reactions to repetitive stimuli escalate O
b) when the world's hostility is targeting migraineurs and helpless B-dogs

8.) How can a strong odor prompt a migraine attack?
a) a sensitized smell cortex in the limbic system kindles a brainstem seizure O
b) strong odors or flickering lights create immediate inflammation

9.) What does the loss of habituation of the CNV amplitude show?
a) a problem with the normal development/maturation of the PFC O
b) that migraine disease is *not* psychological or 'all in your head'

10.) What does the amount of Delta energy in the QEEG flag 36 hours ahead?
a) the intensity of the headache of the developing migraine attack O
b) that its time to avoid trigger food, Chinook winds and Germany in fall

That was fabulous. Not a single wrong answer. Well done!

Chapter 9

Thinking about Strategy

"Perception is strong and sight weak. In strategy it is important to see distant things as if they were close and to take a distanced view of close things."

Miyamoto Musashi

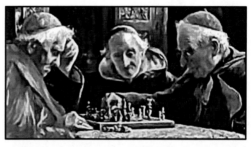

A revolution is a "forcible over-throw of the existing order in favor of a new system"[1]; a radical and courageous change. The most problematic part of that is neither the *force* in 'forcible', nor the *courage* in 'courageous'. Yes, courage and force are required, but the most iffy thing here is the *change* itself. People love talking about their new goals, but experience shows that they usually try to achieve *new* goals in their *old* ways. Yet, *change* is accomplished by doing things *differently*.

What change takes

Change is a skill, that needs to be learnt and practiced, just like walking, swimming or riding a bike. Do you remember how scary it was when you climbed on your first bike? How wobbly and insecure you felt at the beginning? Changing from a migraineur into an ex-migraineur can be just as daring as learning to ride a bike. If it sometimes feels daunting or at least a bit weird, then you're probably on the right track.

Can you also remember your own determination and persistence, which you must have had in your early childhood in order to change from a timid toddler into a proud little pedestrian? During that process you had to deal with so many difficulties and yet, you followed through, didn't you? Changing from a migraineur into an ex-migraineur might take a similar amount of dedication and tenacity. Be prepared for that.

If kids — after several failures and bumping their heads — gave up learning to walk, we'd all be toddlers forever.

---

[1] Oxford Online Dictionary, www.oxforddictionaries.com, 'Revolution'

How many pills for Irene?

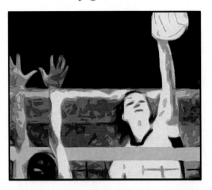

Irene is a world-class volleyball player. To be precise she *was* a world-class volleyball player, but due to an injury she can't play at the moment. During the second set of the season final, she tried to rescue a ball and the point for her team, ran into the umpire's chair and injured her knee. The surgeon did repair some damage, but I don't remember what it was; too much Latin.

Anyway, after a few weeks of limping on crutches, Irene is back to free walking. In fact, it's her first day without the sticks and the surgeon gave her thumbs up for that. Do you think she's back on the team now and she'll play next week?

Of course not, she can barely run, let alone jump. But why? Is she suffering from the mysterious *knee-wobble disease* or the feared *volleyballer's leg-fatigue*? What are the medical treatments for her condition? How many different *medications* will she have to try until she can run, jump and play volleyball again?

In a way Irene is on a similar mission to you. She wants to change from an ex-player into a player on the first team in her club. Similarly, if you suffer from severe migraine attacks, you'd want to change from a migraineur into an ex-migraineur, correct?

There is something else that you have in common with Irene: medication and other passive treatments, although helpful in the short-term, won't make the desired change.

In both cases one could say, there is no *medical condition*; the problem is rather a *lack of condition*, a 'deficit' or a 'weakness'. Irene is lacking strength, stability and stamina. Her body is not fit enough, her mind has lost confidence and her brain has to re-learn the fine motor coordination of a world-class volleyball player.

As a migraineur you might be lacking strength and stamina in your prefrontal cortex as well as stability in your brainstem. Your brain is perhaps not fit enough, your mind probably has lost confidence and your body may be tormented by a nervous system in stress mode. What Irene and you need, in order to make the respective change, is a comprehensive *rehabilitation* program.

Rehabilitation versus treatment

What is the difference? We've talked at length about the distinction between disease and disorder in chapter 7. *Diseases,* like infections or cancer, typically require medical *treatments*. In contrast *disorders,* like migraine, need something to put things back in order. For that 'something' it's better to use the words *therapy* or *rehabilitation*, the latter indicating a comprehensive program.

For example, Irene might also need a few *treatments* from her physiotherapist, but the main part of her program will probably be the exercise *therapy*. So the physiotherapist's treatments are merely a minor part of Irene's entire *rehabilitation* program. Got it?

Now you might think that my distinction between treatment and rehabilitation is a bit pedantic and doesn't really work, since anything can be 'treated' including customers and timber floors.

The point is that *medical treatments* ideally aim at the cause of a disease, e.g. at a bacterium, a bunch of cancer cells or the inflammation in some tissue. If the treatment was chosen well and the target is destroyed, the disease should be over. So we can quickly judge whether the treatment was helpful or not.

We can't apply that same logic to the therapies in a rehabilitation program, because they don't aim at a disease. Instead they usually target one factor of the disorder. Typically a disorder has many components and we can't expect that one single action, measure or therapy fixes all the mechanisms of a complex disorder.

For instance, our injured volleyball player Irene will have to do a whole series of exercises to build up her leg muscles *and* a balance program *and* specific knee stability stuff *and* cardio training at various intensities. Once her coordination has improved and her knee is more stable, she'll start with jumps off and onto a step, fast short-distance runs for agility and squats on a vibrating platform for 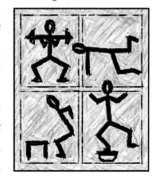 explosive muscle fibers. In addition she'll go swimming, sweat in a sauna, endure different forms of stretching, massage and physical therapy, ultrasound, photonic stimulation and electro-therapy. On top of that she'll utilize EMG muscle biofeedback and will get support from a psychological coach or mental trainer.

Can you imagine the following situation: Irene does a couple of squats with weights on. Her knee starts hurting after a few repetitions, so she stops and says: **"I'VE TRIED IT ONCE, BUT THE RESULT WAS HELL. I'M NOT DOING IT ANYMORE"** (not unlike Erica from chapter 6).

Of course not, that would be stupid. Instead Irene would ask her trainer for advice and he might put a wedge under her heels or correct her movement or reduce the weight or do something else.

Or can you imagine this scenario: Irene diligently does her balancing exercises, but after a week she stops and says: **"IT DIDN'T DO ANYTHING FOR ME: I'M STILL NOT FIT ENOUGH FOR THE NATIONAL TEAM."**

Of course not, that would be stupid. The purpose of the balancing exercises is to improve her balance. That is an important *part* of her program, but it's not enough to make the change from an ex-player into a world-class volleyball player. Got it?

Rehabilitation of migraine

Volleyball injury or migraine, the principles of a successful rehabilitation are the same: Step one is the identification of the underlying weaknesses, deficits and dysfunctions; step two is the correction and normalization of these imperfections with appropriate exercises and therapies. In Irene's case it's about her knee, for migraineurs it's about the brain and the mind.

It is my observation that many migraineurs (like other chronic pain patients) are stuck with the idea that there must be *one* medical treatment (a pill, please) that will do the trick and free them from migraine forever, without effort or side effects.

Unfortunately such a wonder drug doesn't exist, but the idea of the *magic bullet* (the one single treatment that does the trick) lives on and gets transferred to alternative and behavioral therapies. For instance, migraine patients on internet forums report that they've *tried* regular relaxation exercises (or aerobic sport or supplements...), but: **"IT HASN'T WORKED, I STILL HAVE MIGRAINE"**

The purpose of regular relaxation exercises is to improve the ability to relax and to keep cool, calm and collected in stressful situations. Relaxation for the prevention of migraine attacks was found to be quite effective in many studies and meta-analyses.[1]

---

[1] Goslin RE et al "Behavioral and Physical Treatments for Migraine Headache" 1999, Rockville (MD): Agency for Health Care Policy and Research (US)

Thinking about Strategy

Although some migraineurs become attack-free with regular relaxation exercises, this can't be expected in all cases. For severe patients, it's simply not enough, those cases need more.

Despite all my sympathy for the understandable disappointment, the judgment "IT HASN'T WORKED, I STILL HAVE MIGRAINE" is misguided, not helpful and only discouraging for others. Relaxation exercises don't target migraine and therefore cannot be judged like that. A *reasonable* report would be:

> "My hope was that my migraine attacks would stop happening, when I regularly do my relaxation exercises and actually I do have fewer attacks. But the attacks haven't stopped, which means in my case, relaxation home exercises are simply not enough and therefore I'm going to add ... to my program."

On the other hand, it may be that the chosen relaxation exercises really don't fulfill their purpose. Then the report could be:

> "The relaxation exercises on that CD from ... haven't helped me much. I'm still quite tense most of the time, worry a lot and I tend to get frantic when it gets a bit stressful. I'll try a different meditation CD and if that doesn't help me either, I'll start looking for a therapist, who can give me the kind of support that I obviously need."

One important step is to separate the expression of temporary emotions (e.g. disappointment, helplessness, hopelessness) and factual, logical and goal-oriented conclusions from one another. Also, patients should be very careful not to fall victim to their own bad thinking habits (cognitive distortions, see page 90) when evaluating the potential of any therapy. Let me give you an example:

> Daisy, the migraineur from chapter 5, has heard that aerobic endurance sport allegedly is helpful and recommended for the prevention of migraine attacks. She buys jogging shoes and goes for a run with her best friend, a keen jogger. Daisy manages to keep up with her friend, but is quite exhausted after only a 90 minute run, which Daisy's friend called "short and easy". The next morning Daisy wakes up with a migraine attack and concludes: "I must never do that again. Sport is a migraine trigger."

We don't know whether the migraine attack was indeed precipitated by Daisy's first run or whether it was due anyway. We don't know whether it was Daisy's premenstrual week and therefore she was particularly vulnerable—perhaps, perhaps not.

What we do know is that 90 minutes is a bit much for a first training in a long time; and we do know that Daisy is quite ambitious and possibly ran faster than she should have, given that it was her first time. More evidence for that assumption is the fact that she obviously kept up with a well-trained runner.

There is a strong suspicion that Daisy stuffed it up a bit and *perhaps* even sparked a migraine attack herself. Additionally she jumps to exactly that conclusion and over-generalizes from one single stuffed-up jogging experience to sport in general.

What she should have done is clear: Start slowly with a brisk daily walk of 10-20 minutes and take it from there. After a week without incident, Daisy may walk for longer and if that goes well too, she might want to try jogging for 5-10 minutes. Sounds measured and reasonable, doesn't it? Well, that's the way to go.

What are we talking about?

Throughout this book we've talked about migraine as if it was a uniform disorder, but in reality every patient is unique. Some cases are relatively easy to rehabilitate, some others are a bit tricky and some cases can be very problematic, because the cumulative disadvantage has built up to a mountain of troubles.

We can estimate the degree of chronicity by looking at the complexity and the difficulty of a case. The *complexity* describes how bad it is and the *difficulty* denotes the sum of obstacles to a successful rehabilitation:

factors of complexity	factors of difficulty
chronic migraine	mood disorders (e.g. anxiety, depression)
very frequent attacks	bad thinking habits/cognitive distortions
multiple 'functional' disorders[1]	impaired judgment/mental rigidity
'physical' comorbidities	dismissive-avoidant attitudes
high reactivity	helplessness/victim attitude
very high sensitivity	strong medical beliefs
traumatic brain injury	hopelessness
emotional trauma history/PTSD	anger/hostility

---

[1] 'Functional' disorders is a highly disputed label and often applied to irritable bowel syndrome, fibromyalgia, chronic fatigue syndrome, multiple chemical sensitivity, restless leg syndrome and other 'medically unexplained' symptoms; disorders that don't behave like diseases (see chapter 7).

Thinking about Strategy

When you now look at complexity and difficulty together, you get a sense for the degree of chronicity (▲= bad; ▽ not bad):

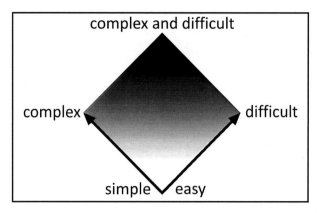

Simple and easy cases may even become migraine-free with a few lifestyle changes only. In contrast, very complex and difficult cases will probably need a lot of professional support to reduce the mountain of problems to an acceptable level.

What else do we need?

Experience shows that those patients, who receive competent *social support*, do much better in a rehabilitation program. When the going gets tough, encouragement keeps patients going.

It's easy to imagine how Irene's partner plays a role in her rehabilitation. If he wants to party and drink a lot and persuades her to join him, then her comeback is in grave danger. If he is truly supportive, he'll drive her to the rehab center, encourage her to do her homework assignments and take over some household duties.

Even when support is available, some migraineurs struggle with their own perceived unworthiness and therefore don't ask for aid and succor. The *putting-others-first syndrome* is a frequent occurrence in migraineurs and needs to be addressed. People, who fail to look after themselves and excuse that with explanations like "I don't want to be a burden", can actually become a very *heavy* burden for their family (see chapter 2).

Sadly, some patients simply don't have the *resources* (money, knowledge, abilities, social support etc.) to do what needs to be done and so they are stuck with their migraine. On the other hand, there is a lot that patients can do for themselves.

Don't try everything!

"I'VE TRIED EVERYTHING, BUT NOTHING HAS HELPED" is a frequent complaint in migraine land. Typically this sentence is followed by a list of a) *abortive* medications, b) *passive medical* treatments and c) *passive alternative* treatments. Not always, but often.

'Trying' can lead to *practicing failure*. Although it is a good thing not to give up and resign, a series of aimless attempts to find the 'magic bullet', the passive treatment that solves all problems, can easily lead to frustration and hopelessness. Before trying the next treatment, patients should ask themselves: "What is the rationale for this treatment? What is the reason for doing this? What do I expect from this? How is this going to help me? How am I going to track my progress?"

If the answer is nebulous like: "Yubyub-therapy smooths your rough nano-structure and balances subtle energies" or "I hope this will cure my migraine" then you might want to think twice.

The successful rehabilitation of migraine—by learning, practicing, training and applying new skills, knowledge and abilities—is not a new concept and not unique to our migraine revolution. Behavioral therapies have been helpful for decades, but in our drug-obsessed societies it seems to become ever more difficult to inform patients that there are ways out of their misery.

Once patients are severely disabled by chronic migraine and medication-overuse headache (MOH) they might eventually get a recommendation to try e.g. thermal biofeedback ("hand-warming"). This is a well established method to improve the regulation of arousal and the balance of the autonomic nervous system. In simple and easy cases thermal biofeedback alone can sometimes be sufficient to stop migraine attacks altogether.

However, in *severe* cases (chronic migraine, MOH) hand-warming biofeedback alone is probably *not enough* to save a patient from sinking deeper into the soft ground of chronification; especially not, when it's wrongly used like an abortive drug.

The hope must be that the innovative methods of applied neuroscience, backed by tons of scientific research, have a stronger impact and receive more attention than the true-and-tested older methods of behavioral therapy—but that is up to the patients.

The solution for migraineurs is to increase their own resilience and resistance to *all* the factors that drive their brain into migraine.

Reaching for the stars

The goal of the migraine revolution is to end the migraine tyranny. That means we're aiming for:

- no more migraine attacks (or at least a *drastic* reduction)
- prevention of comorbidities (e.g. stroke, depression etc.)
- decrease of draining and bothersome symptoms like reactivity, defensiveness, neuroticism, bad thinking habits, alexithymia etc.
- in extreme cases: at least prevention of further deterioration

Treatments *during* an attack may still be necessary for a while in order to alleviate the misery, but these treatments have no future: The migraine revolution doesn't want to make the suffering more comfortable, but put an end to it; once and for all.

The principles of the migraine revolution

In order to achieve these ambitious goals, most will need a comprehensive, individually tailored rehabilitation program which addresses *all the factors* in body, mind and brain that contribute to the generation of migraine attacks:

- 'weakness' of the prefrontal cortex?
- over-activity of the limbic system (e.g. amygdala)?
- lack of electrical stability in the cortex?
- traumatic brain injury?
- emotional trauma history?
- high reactivity?
- food allergies and intolerances (e.g. gluten)?
- toxins and detoxification? nutritional deficiencies?
- immature coping strategies (e.g. fearful-avoidant)?
- bad thinking habits, victim attitude, hopelessness etc.?

Of course, it would be awesome if there were appropriate rehab centers for migraine patients in every city; but since that is not the case, patients themselves need to step up to the plate, rise to the challenge, pull out all the stops and lift their game. They need to become their own *rehabilitation manager*, who makes sure that they get the help they need on every level.

Also, it could be prudent to ask a trusted and competent person 1.) to read this book and 2.) to become *assistant manager*; because many struggle to look after themselves (e.g. Erica).

Are you ready for battle?

Here are 15 pairs of statements. Please pick from every pair the statement which you consider true (or more true than the other one):

When things are bad, I prefer trying to tackle the problem if I can.	O	O	When things are bad, I prefer being emotional and to wait until it's over.
Migraine is a progressive *disorder* of body, mind and brain.	O	O	Migraine is a neurological *disease*.
I need more stability in body, mind & brain to resist the migraine tyranny.	O	O	Migraine is not psychological.
The attack is a slow seizure ('nerve storm') in the brainstem.	O	O	The attack is blood vessel swelling, inflammation or pinched nerves.
There are fabulous therapies available that can help migraineurs a lot.	O	O	There is no migraine cure; or it would be on the title of every newspaper.
I'm excited that I'll be able do something about my migraine.	O	O	There isn't much that I can do about my migraine.
Sadly I have the genetic 'talent' for it, but I can still be free of migraine.	O	O	Migraine is genetic and therefore pre-programmed into my life.
My migraine and my 'revolution' are my responsibility.	O	O	My migraine is my doctor's problem, because it's a medical disease.
I need and I really want to solve or reduce my migraine problem.	O	O	I ask myself: Why can't someone resolve my migraine problem.
I'm going to confront any issue, even unpleasant/scary/painful ones.	O	O	I don't have any 'issues' whatsoever apart from my migraine disease.
I'm willing to do what needs to be done to get rid of my migraine.	O	O	I'll wait for the day they'll come up with a magical medical migraine cure.
Difficulties along the way will only strengthen my determination.	O	O	I've tried once to get rid of my migraine and the result was hell.
I'm actually quite confident that I can improve my migraine situation.	O	O	Nothing will ever help, because my migraine can't be cured.
I would be grateful if I could reduce the number of attacks by 75%.	O	O	Nothing will help me, because there is no miracle cure that helps everyone.
I have people in my life who support and encourage me in this endeavor.	O	O	Nobody in my life would support these false hopes anyway.
If you have picked mainly from this white side, then you are ready for the battle against the migraine tyranny.		sums	If you have picked mainly from this gray side, you might want to re-read the chapters 5 to 8 of this book.

Part III:

Weapons for the Revolution

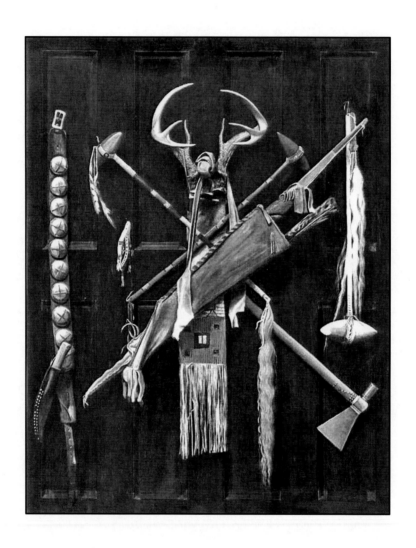

Chapter 10

Choose Your Weapons!

"We are twice armed if we fight with faith."
Plato

Learning from Jenny

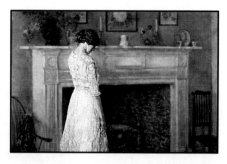

Jenny has inherited a valuable old heritage-listed house. It's not in perfect condition, but who is? The walls seem pretty solid and so she moves in; besides, she had to leave her former place anyway. One day she notices flecks of mold on the walls of her living room. Knowing that mold is toxic she buys some anti-mold spray at the drugstore and starts treating the unpleasant fungal spots. The next day they're gone thanks to the power of 4-KO-dihydroxi-trichlori-pcbtphtnyltnolyloline.

Several weeks later the moldy flecks are back, Jenny squirts her spray and it 'kinda' works again. Yet shortly thereafter she needs to repeat that treatment again, and again and again. "Enough is enough" she says and calls in a wall-fungus professional. He's got a more powerful mold spray, which gets rid of the ugly spots in no time. Jenny is happy as a clam.

Unfortunately, although the professional's mold spray keeps 'kinda' working okay, she notices that the mold is spreading, since it's now in her bedroom too. Jenny starts worrying and begins collecting advice from books and websites like wallmold.com:

> "Mold is caused by stagnant air and humidity. Avoid taking showers in your house and air all your rooms regularly. Other than that, there are these brands of freely available mold sprays (lists 10 brands) and these professional fungicides (lists 20 products). Good luck!"

Of course, Jenny stops taking showers, ventilates vigorously and sees a few more mold experts for further advice in chemical fungus warfare. After some time the mold has become a chronic problem, which makes her sick and severely interferes with her life.

Imagine for a moment that you are an architect and builder, specialized in the renovation and restoration of old houses. We don't know how Jenny got your number, perhaps she read your famous book ("The Mold Renovation") and now wants your help.

At least, that is what she says: "I really need your help here, please?" You pack your camera and a couple of funky building inspector tools and drive over to Jenny's house for an examination.

It doesn't take you too long to identify the old building's weak spots: When the house was built, a certain glue was hard to come by and the builders at the time had to improvise a little during the attachment of the termite protection sheets to the foundations. So it could have happened that the wind pulled those sheets off a smidge, before the foundations could harden up enough. That gave termites the opportunity to get into the walls of the house during the building phase and make their way up to the roof.

Over the years the termites damaged the rafters, at least enough that the roof ended up a little crooked. As a consequence the gutters don't drain the rain very well and leaf debris periodically blocks the drainage pipes, leaving the gutters full of rainwater, which then dribbles through cracks into the walls of the house, eventually supplying sufficient moisture for the mold to spread into all the rooms.

So you think to yourself: "Wow, Jenny will be so relieved that she can fix her precious home at last: Dig up the protective sheets around the foundation and re-attach them, drain the walls, renew the gutters, gas the termites, restore the rafters, re-tile the roof and give all the walls in the house a coat of fungicide paint. That'll do."

So you go ahead and start your explanation, but halfway through your lecture you notice that she isn't listening anymore: "Jenny, what is it?" She umms and ahhhs, but finally summons her courage to say: "*I was hoping that you would have a better mold spray and could simply make the flecks go away.*"

What's your reply to that?

I would tell Jenny ...

_____

_____

_____

Considering R-words

Once again, the drug *treatment* of migraine symptoms is warranted during an attack; but, no matter how well that works for different people, it doesn't lead to freedom from migraine.

Medical *treatments* for attack prevention are not very effective and even when they are, they barely ever lead to freedom from migraine *and* drugs. In a catchy phrase: Drugs don't end the tyranny.

Since the beginning of this Rebellion I've been talking about the need for *Rehabilitation* to gain freedom from symptoms on all levels of body, mind and brain, without further treatments.

Rehabilitations and Renovations follow the same principle: Fix everything that's wonky, decrepit or kaput. Once it's back in working order, look after it to keep it in good condition. That's a fairly *simple* principle, but does it mean it's *easy*?

There are people who enjoy buying a run-down ancient castle, chateau, lighthouse or farm and renovating it far beyond its former glory, including under-floor heating, double-glazed windows, fully integrated multimedia system and automatic roller-shutters. That is awesome if you have a lot of something else with R: *Resources* (money, knowledge, abilities, social support etc.). We've already mentioned in chapter 5 that there is a *snowballing* effect for personal Resources called 'cumulative advantage', which means that people with a lot of Resources have access to even more Resources, while people with poor Resources are struggling to keep afloat.

As an example, people who are born into a prosperous, highly educated family will probably end up starting the next wealthy, academic family, because they have the means to increase their Resources even further (= cumulative advantage). People who are born into a penniless, underprivileged family barely have a chance to become rich and highly educated, no matter how much effort they put in. The majority will end up without a degree and just as broke because of their *cumulative disadvantage*: They don't even have the means to protect their already meager Resources.

Migraineurs, on average, tend to have a cumulative disadvantage even if they are born into a wealthy, educated family. For example, they typically *seek* and *receive* less social support.[1]

---

[1] Rutberg S et al "Migraine – more than a headache: Women's experiences of living with migraine" Disabil Rehabil 2012;34(4):329–336

The Rebellion in chapter 6 failed, because the proletarian army led by the schoolteacher didn't have the gumption to overcome the pathetic difficulty of a single unarmed guard. Bertrand paid a bitter price for starting a revolution with a bunch of lethargic morons who abandoned their mission after exhausting themselves with spiteful slogans. Too much excitement can be draining, it seems.

The right Resources could have helped them to pursue their goal to bring down the despot, to terminate the tyrant's terror and gain their freedom at last: Levelheaded comrades who remind them of their common vision, who demand discipline during the mission, who help them to separate the emotions from the actions in order to save energy for the battle. Or shorter: social support.

Any endeavor needs appropriate Resources. Social support, level-headedness and energy are only some of the Resources one needs to overcome a vicious tyrant like migraine and the current regime. What else do we need to consider? Here is the list I've come up with; I've left one cell empty for *your* idea:

awareness	courage	constructive coping
creativity	determination	discipline
energy	helpful knowledge	levelheadedness
money	motivation/inspiration	skills and abilities
social support	strategy	thoughtfulness
time	winner's attitude	

Just in case anyone believes that Resources are *overrated* and you just need to go ahead and do what needs to be done, I've made a second list with words expressing roughly the opposite:

IGNORANCE	HELPLESSNESS	EMOTIONAL COPING
NARROW-MINDEDNESS	WORRY/OBEDIENCE	HYSTERIA
LETHARGY	MISLEADING MYTHS	FOOLISHNESS
AUSTERITY	INDIFFERENCE	INCOMPETENCE
ISOLATION	AIMLESSNESS	STUPIDITY
HASTE	VICTIM ATTITUDE	

Those who still opine that discussing Resources is *nonsense* may please step forward and explain to me how Hillary and Tenzing (page 131) would have successfully conquered Mt Everest with only a single 'un-Resource' from the negative list.

What do you reckon? Is *securing Resources* a good idea?

All the listed Resources are necessary to some degree and I'm sure there are other ones of which I have no *awareness*. One of them can make up for slight deficits in many others and that is *social support*. Hardly anybody is so Resourceful that they don't need any support whatsoever. Sure, there are a few who have heaps of money and can afford to travel around the world to consult with extraordinary therapists. They will now get the job done in no time.

Call me a dreamer, but I believe that highly privileged people who are lucky enough to have the *financial Resources* to simply pay their way out of the tyranny have an obligation to share at least their experiences and findings with others. What do you think?

Money is perhaps the most tricky Resource of all. People often behave as if money was scarce and the next thing they tell you is how unhappy they were on that five-star cruise to Bora Bora due to frequent migraine attacks. It is everybody's personal decision what their priorities are in life and what it's worth to them to become migraine-free (or at least drastically improved). Nobody wants a lesson about that. My only advice would be to undergo a Reality check and calculate *the costs of being a migraineur,* including drugs, doctor visits, complementary treatments and lost time.

Time is the only Resource that is definitely limited and every day lost to migraine or to migraine management is gone forever. You can recover lost money, but you can never recover *lost time*.

I hope this book contains enough helpful *knowledge* and here and there a little bit of *inspiration*. Yet, a book can't replace the direct contact with other people who are in a similar position. *Social support* is an amazing resource, perhaps the most essential one.

Humans are social animals and need Recognition, Respect, Reminding Remarks, Reassurance, Recommendations, Refinement of skills as well as Regular contact to Rebels like you. It all starts with a *vision*, for instance "to end the migraine tyranny", then you decide to make it your *mission*. This is the Right moment to turn the mission into a *team effort*. Therefore I urge everybody who finds this book even remotely helpful to take action to combine their *Resources* and *support* one another by creating a *strong community* and by initiating *a worldwide movement;* to unleash their wrath to liberate not only themselves, but *every migraineur in the world*. In short: Join the Migraine **R**evolution!

The empire strikes back

One of the many astounding abilities of the human prefrontal cortex (PFC) is making predictions about the future. Patients with damage to a certain area of the PFC lose that ability, leading to absurd flaws in decision-making[1] and a lack of consideration of the consequences of their actions in the future.[2]

For the preparation and the strategic planning of a revolution it is crucial to foresee potential difficulties and predict backlashes. I don't believe that Hillary and Tenzing expected escalators and balmy weather conditions on Mt Everest. They were certainly fully aware that they had to overcome steep icy passages, fierce weather conditions and their own desire for a hot shower, a take-away pizza and a cozy couch in front of a fireplace.

We can easily predict that the current regime will not be too supportive of our attempt to inform the migraine world how to end the tyranny. Luckily, the pharma industry and medical organizations are way too aloof to dignify our revolution with attention.

The truly dangerous opposition are the *soldiers* of the regime; the *obedient* patients who are scared they might lose their access to *drugs*; the *fearful* ones who believe it is up to others to decide their fate; the notoriously *helpless* ones who find their fulfillment in *complaining*; the *dismissive* pessimists who want to *prove* that the future is grim and their destructive *negativity* completely justified; the migraine bloggers whose *identity* is in danger, if they get better; the patient advocates whose mission it is to guide others down the same medical path that led *them* into *chronification*; the bitter ones whose expressive suffering is meant to be a public *accusation* of abuse; the resentful *persecutors* who create situations of *failure* to take *revenge;* or the snippy know-it-alls who enjoy a feeling of superiority from the position of a *deflating sniper* rather than risking an enriching contribution that would expose *them* to possible criticism.

Additionally there will be stuff-ups and errors, misfortunes and disappointments, fraudsters and morons, parasites and fools; in short: the usual difficulties of every successful revolution. That's why the most powerful weapon of our revolution is the *revolution*.

---

[1] Bechara A et al "Characterization of the decision-making deficit of patients with vm prefrontal cortex lesions" Brain 2000;123(Pt11):2189-202
[2] Bechara A et al "Insensitivity to future consequences following damage to human prefrontal cortex" Cognition 1994;50(1-3):7-15

Section One:
Weapons for the Body

"I think of my body as a side effect of my mind."
Carrie Fisher

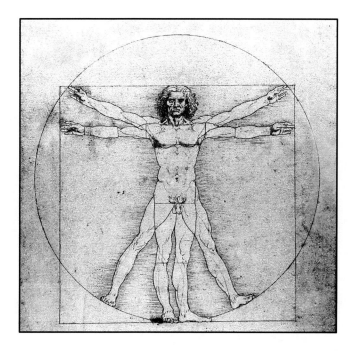

Body, mind and brain[1]

With the exception of academics, people have an intuitive understanding of the words body, mind and brain: '*Body*' stands for physical and biochemical qualities, including breathing, digestion and metabolism; '*mind*' represents thoughts, beliefs, values and conscious behaviors; and '*brain*' is the mysterious clump in the head that we don't know much about.

Let's keep things that simple and only clarify that the brain is part of our body and the mind is one of the functions of our brain, dead easy. Sophisticated questions like "What is consciousness?" can be left to unemployed neuroscientists with a second major in philosophy or theology, okay?

---

[1] Leonardo daVinci "Vitruvian Man" adapted from a photo by Luc Viatour www.lucnix.be

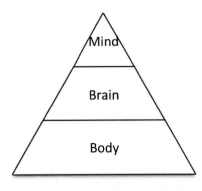

This also makes clear that body, mind and brain are not three distinctly separate categories, that they're not mutually exclusive and certainly not independent from one another: Whilst being a *mind-less body* can be a pleasurable experience every now and then, a *body-less brain* can't even switch the telly[1] on.

Even 'feelings' (body), 'emotions' (brain+mind) and 'subconscious mind' (right half of the brain+body) can be tidied up with this model until some academics come along, insist on accuracy and stuff up our clarity and simplicity.

Migraine and 'body'

During a migraine attack our mind's attention is drawn to the 'body' symptoms like neck-ache, nausea and especially head pain.

And although it is always and exclusively *brain and mind* who *experience* neck-ache, nausea and head pain, we tend to focus on the body as the *venue of remedy*, by swallowing medication, undergoing PFO closure procedures or by having Botox® injections. We've thoroughly discussed the lack of logic of some of these treatments, for instance the amputation of allegedly nerve-pinching muscles without any explanation as to how that fits with the story of SWELLING AND INFLAMMATION OF BLOOD VESSELS AROUND YOUR HEAD.

Here let's talk about the habit in migraine therapy to degrade the body's role to being the receptacle for the drugs. Listening in on the exchanges between the most '*advanced*' severe and 'difficult' complex migraine sufferers (as opposed to *completely normal* severe, complex and 'difficult' migraine patients) one can't help it but admire the vast and detailed knowledge about *medication* and other *medical migraine treatments* they've accrued. At the same time there seems to be a huge lack of knowledge and understanding, not only of mind and brain therapies, but even of *non-drug body therapies*.

This part of the book is intended to explore the many options there are to (at least) decrease migraine attack frequency and intensity; to start the revolution off with better *weapons for the body*.

---

[1] British and Australian English for a television set

Chapter 11

Let's get physical

> "Exercise relieves stress. Nothing relieves exercise."
>
> T. Ikkaku, A. Hosaka and T. Kawabata

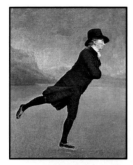

If sport did nothing for migraine, it still would have to be part of a decent rehabilitation program, because regular exercise reduces the risk of stroke, heart attack and many other ailments.[1] Migraineurs are at a higher risk for these anyway (see chapter 1) and tend to be less physically active than controls;[2] so a little bit of encouragement to workout seems appropriate.

But wait, there is more! One study compared the effect of

- a moderate, aerobic training program (= 40 min indoor cycling, 3 x/week) to
- relaxation exercises (=1x/week tuition and daily home practice) and
- the daily intake of Topiramate® (= anti-epilepsy medication).[3]

All three groups had roughly the same reduction of migraine attack-rate after three months: Aerobic endurance sport or regular relaxation practice were *just as effective* as a frequently prescribed anti-epilepsy drug with its well-known bad side effects.[4]

That is quite remarkable given that the participants were completely untrained 30-50 year old adults. In this age group the adaptation to training takes way longer than in young ones and we can safely say that the potential which regular physical exercise could have has not been exhausted in this study.

And here lies the problem; medical studies are mostly funded by drug companies and, naturally, none of them is particularly eager to prove that sport and exercise are overall better than drugs. Thus the analysis of this topic rests on a few small studies, which can easily be criticized and discredited, if one wishes to do so.[5,6]

---

[1] Thompson PD et al "Exercise and physical activity in the prevention and treatment of atherosclerotic cardiovascular disease: a statement from the Council on Clinical Cardiology and the Council on Nutrition, Physical Activity, and Metabolism" Circulation 2003;107(24):3109–3116
[2] Varkey E et al "Physical activity and headache: results from the Nord-Trøndelag Health Study (HUNT)" Cephalalgia 2008;28(12):1292-7
[3] Varkey E et al "Exercise as migraine prophylaxis: a randomized study using relaxation and topiramate as controls" Cephalalgia 2011;31(14):1428-38
[4] Coppola F et al "Language disturbances as a side effect of prophylactic treatment of migraine" Headache 2008;48(1):86-94
[5] Darling M "Exercise and migraine. A critical review" J Sports Med Phys Fitness 1991;31(2):294-302
[6] Busch V et al "Exercise in migraine therapy--is there any evidence for efficacy? A critical review" Headache 2008;48(6):890-9

Interestingly, even the most critical medical commentators recognize and acknowledge the potential of sport and exercise as a therapeutic option for migraine and demand further trials.[1] Good idea, but show me the money!

A popular tactic of medical experts to protect their turf and turnover against more benign therapeutic alternatives is to publicly criticize the quality-standard of scientific studies supporting their drug-free opponents. That is clever, because laypeople often falsely assume that all 'medical' therapies were supported by sound scientific evidence and that any therapy alternative is quackery unless proven otherwise by a double-blinded, placebo-controlled, randomized multi-center study with thousands of participants.

These, however, are the requirements for *drug trials* and neither valid nor helpful for sport, exercise or any other behavioral therapy, because the underlying question is completely different.

For the approval of a drug the pharma company has to prove that their new chemical concoction actually creates a benefit large enough to justify the inevitable risks and side effects. To isolate the drug effect from psychological influences (e.g. the placebo effect), randomization, blinding and placebo-control are required.

In contrast, behavioral therapies (including sport or exercise) require motivation and voluntary participation and *are meant* to elicit psychological effects, e.g. increased self-efficacy, self-confidence and self-regulation. They are supposed to *empower* patients and make them feel good about themselves. Logically, simple outcome studies are completely sufficient to answer the underlying question: *How much* do patients benefit from taking part in that behavioral therapy? That's all you need to find out since risks and side effects (permanent and temporary damage) are typically known and negligible (here: sore muscles).

But the propaganda of the 'drug lords' is effective: A study on back pain patients showed that many would seriously dismiss the findings of a study with "only" 50 subjects, but are willing to try a therapy, which worked for their neighbor (1 subject).[2] This is a good example that human behavior is not always driven by logic.

---

[1] Busch V et al "Exercise in migraine treatment. Review and discussion of clinical trials and implications for further trials" Schmerz 2008;22(2):137-47

[2] Glenton C et al "Lay perceptions of evidence-based information--a qualitative evaluation of a website for back pain sufferers" BMC Health Serv Res 2006;6:34

Is it worth the effort?

The beneficial effect of regular sport and exercise on overall health and disease-risk is largely known by the general public. The positive effect of physical training on the structure and the many functions of the brain is less well-known, but just as amazing.[1,2,3,4,5]

Especially the prefrontal cortex benefits from getting off the couch with more gray matter volume, white matter connections, blood perfusion and neuronal activity, which results in better cognitive function.[6] In simple words: Sport makes you fitter, healthier *and* smarter. Not too shabby, ey?

It would be interesting to find out, if regular aerobic exercise is capable of compensating for the cognitive impairment,[7] which comes as a frequent side effect with some migraine drugs.[8] As an added bonus, sport also reduces anxiety, depression[9] and even neuroticism,[10,11] and also protects against osteoporosis;[12] a relevant detail for migraineurs, who often end up with brittle bones from migraine medication.[13,14]

The increase in aerobic fitness is reflected in the reduction of the migraine attack *intensity and frequency*.[15] And it doesn't seem to take much to see a substantial effect when sport is combined with relaxation: One study could prove significant benefits after only twelve workouts in six weeks; 45 min gymnastics with music and 15 min of relaxation exercises.[16] That doesn't sound too hard.

---

[1] Cotman CW et al "Exercise: a behavioral intervention to enhance brain health and plasticity" Trends Neurosci 2002;25(6):295-301
[2] Hillman CH et al "Be smart, exercise your heart: exercise effects on brain and cognition" Nat Rev Neurosci 2008;9(1):58-65
[3] Gondoh Y van Praag H "Exercise and the brain: something to chew on" Trends Neurosci 2009;32(5):283-90
[4] Erickson KI et al "Exercise training increases size of hippocampus and improves memory" Proc Natl Acad Sci USA 2011;108(7):3017-22
[5] Gondoh Y et al "Effects of aerobic exercise training on brain structure and psychological well-being in young adults" J Sports Med Phys Fitness 2009;49(2):129-35
[6] Erickson KI et al "Aerobic exercise effects on cognitive and neural plasticity in older adults" Br J Sports Med 2009;43(1):22-4
[7] Baker LD et al "Effects of aerobic exercise on mild cognitive impairment: a controlled trial" Arch Neurol 2010;67(1):71-9
[8] Bendtsen L et al "Reference programme: Diagnosis and treatment of headache disorders and facial pain. Danish Headache Society, 2nd Edition" J Headache Pain. 2012;13(Suppl 1):1–29
[9] Carek PJ et al "Exercise for the treatment of depression and anxiety" Int J Psychiatry Med 2011;41(1):15-28
[10] De Moor MH et al "Regular exercise, anxiety, depression and personality: a population-based study" Prev Med 2006;42(4):273-9
[11] Potgieter JR et al "Relationship between adherence to exercise and scores on extraversion and neuroticism" Percept Mot Skills 1995;81(2):520-2
[12] Czarkowska-Paczek B et al "Physical exercise prevents osteoporosis" Przegl Lek 2011;68(2):103-6
[13] Pack AM et al "Adverse effects of antiepileptic drugs on bone structure: epidemiology, mechanisms and therapeutic implications" CNS Drugs 2001;15(8):633-42
[14] Pack AM et al "Bone disease associated with antiepileptic drugs" Cleve Clin J Med 2004;71 Suppl 2:S42-8
[15] Darabaneanu S et al "Aerobic exercise as a therapy option for migraine: a pilot study" Int J Sports Med 2011;32(6):455-60
[16] Dittrich SM et al "Aerobic exercise with relaxation: influence on pain and psychological well-being in female migraine patients" Clin J Sport Med 2008;18(4):363-5

Exercise-induced migraine

A small minority of migraineurs can initiate a migraine attack with exercise. This is a difficulty to be dealt with, but not an excuse. It rather shows that the overall resistance is so low that even normal activities can result in another migraine episode or at least in exertion-induced headaches. That can understandably lead to fear of physical activity, which is completely unacceptable.

During the supervised training of an outcome study, exercise-induced migraine did not happen once.[1] The plausible suspicion is that other factors (e.g. dehydration, low blood sugar, no warm-up etc.) are the real culprits. My advice for those who fear exercise-induced migraine: Drink enough plain water, eat regularly, warm up thoroughly and increase the level of exertion slowly.[2] If needed, ask your doctor about a temporary drug solution. One dose of Aspirin or Ibuprofen before the training might do the trick.

General recommendations

- *Check your heart first*: Adults over 40 should ask their doctor before rushing to the gym; a stress EKG to complete exhaustion can be advisable, depending on existing risk factors.
- *Suitable activities*: Aerobic endurance exercises are walking, running, swimming, cycling, rowing and the like, but also ball sports or workouts like 'Spinning', 'Aerobics', 'Circuit', 'Zumba' or whatever takes your fancy and makes you pant and sweat. The aim is to raise your heart rate moderately, depending on your age and fitness level. If it feels too hard, then it is too much; "a bit strenuous", but not "very", is just right.
- *Choose wisely*: Not everybody has the motivation to set the alarm and go for a long run in the morning. Pick the type of workout that you'll actually do, even when the weather is bad.
- *Begin slowly*: Untrained adults are often very unfit. Brisk walking for 5 to 10 min may well be an appropriate start.
- *Regular is the key*: A daily workout would be ideal; two to three times a week 30-60 min is an effective compromise to strive for.
- *My own solution*: Daily 45-90 min walking (up to 15% uphill) with earphones on a treadmill in front of a TV with a TiVo®.

---

[1] Varkey E et al "A study to evaluate the feasibility of an aerobic exercise program in patients with migraine" Headache 2009;49(4):563-70
[2] Lambert RW Jr et al "Prevention of exercise induced migraine by quantitative warm-up" Headache 1985;25(6):317-9

Chapter 12

Passing Gas

"As we free our breath, we relax our emotions and let go our body tensions."

Gay Hendricks

Abdominal breathing

When people are distressed or otherwise aroused, they breathe faster and deeper without actually using up more oxygen. This acute *hyperventilation* (= over-breathing), for instance during a panic attack, can cause even more aggravation, confusion, tingling, dizziness, muscle twitching and fainting.[1]

It also works the other way round: When people breathe too much, their stress level goes up.[2] Especially *thoracic breathing* (= into

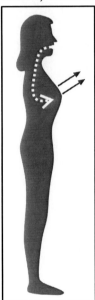

the chest; left pic) has an activating or 'distressing' effect.[3] Even without hyperventilation or overbreathing, the dysfunctional thoracic breathing pattern is suspiciously common in the so-called medically unexplained, or functional syndromes.[4]

On the contrary, *diaphragmatic breathing* (= into the belly; right pic) has a calming effect on the nervous system[5] and is therefore a highly endorsed, universal stress reduction technique,[6] because it elicits a relaxation response,[7] which is the exact opposite to the stress reaction.

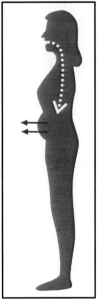

---

[1] Cowley DS et al "Hyperventilation and panic disorder" Am J Med 1987;83(5):929-37
[2] DeBeck LD et al "Heart rate variability and muscle sympathetic nerve activity response to acute stress: the effect of breathing" Am J Physiol Regul Integr Comp Physiol 2010;299(1):R80-91
[3] Fried R. "The Psychology and Physiology of Breathing" Springer - New York 1993
[4] Courtney R et al "Medically unexplained dyspnea: partly moderated by dysfunctional (thoracic dominant) breathing pattern" J Asthma 2011;48(3):259-65
[5] Bacon M et al "A behavioral analysis of diaphragmatic breathing and its effects on peripheral temperature" J Behav Ther Exp Psychiatry 1985;16(1):15-21
[6] Conrad A et al "Psychophysiological effects of breathing instructions for stress management" Appl Psychophysiol Biofeedback 2007;32(2):89-98
[7] Benson H et al "The relaxation response: psychophysiologic aspects and clinical applications" Int J Psychiatry Med 1975;6(1-2):87-98

A study on migraineurs compared the effect of biofeedback-assisted diaphragmatic breathing-retraining with a beta-blocker medication and found a drastic reduction of frequency, severity and duration of attacks, as well as number of vomiting episodes. One year later, more than 50% of the medication responders had relapsed, but less than 10% of the belly-breathing group.[1]

Can you believe that? A breathing exercise is significantly better than the most popular prophylactic migraine drug. And when you combine the behavioral therapies with a beta-blocker, results get even better.[2] The idea to combine several effective therapies to a multi-modal rehab-program is not unique to our revolution.[3] Anyway, one crucial step for migraine rebels is to *change the habitual breathing pattern* from thoracic to abdominal.

The gas whose absence causes seizures

We breathe, in order to get oxygen into the body. Everybody knows that. The oxygen uptake is not a problem for migraine sufferers. But there is a second gas that we should watch and that is CO_2, carbon dioxide, because that is a biggie for migraineurs.

Carbon dioxide is a gas that humans release with every breath. When people hyperventilate, e.g. during a panic attack, they lose too much CO_2, which causes the symptoms mentioned earlier.

In addition, a lack of CO_2 (called *hypocapnia*) also causes a sharp increase in excitability of the cortex.[4,5] The effect is so strong that hyperventilation (leading to hypocapnia) reliably triggers seizures in patients with epilepsy. Neurologists use this mechanism to initiate seizures for diagnostic purposes.[6,7,8]

Given that it is a form of slow seizure in the brainstem, could a migraine attack be promoted by too much breathing?

---

[1] Kaushik R et al " Biofeedback assisted diaphragmatic breathing and systematic relaxation versus propranolol in long term prophylaxis of migraine" Complement Ther Med 2005;13(3):165-74

[2] Holroyd KA et al "Effect of preventive (beta blocker) treatment, behavioural migraine management, or their combination on outcomes of optimised acute treatment in frequent migraine: randomised controlled trial" BMJ 2010;341:c4871

[3] Gunreben-Stempfle B et al "Effectiveness of an intensive multidisciplinary headache treatment program" Headache 2009;49(7):990-1000

[4] Tomita-Gotoh S et al "Scalp-recorded direct current potential shifts induced by hypocapnia and hypercapnia in humans" Electroencephalogr Clin Neurophysiol 1996;99(1):90-7

[5] Leistner S et al "Combined MEG and EEG methodology for non-invasive recording of infraslow activity in the human cortex" Clin Neurophysiol 2007;118(12):2774-80

[6] Guaranha MS et al "Hyperventilation revisited: physiological effects and efficacy on focal seizure activation in the era of video-EEG monitoring" Epilepsia 2005;46(1):69-75

[7] Sawayama E et al "Moderate hyperventilation prolongs electroencephalogram seizure duration of the first electroconvulsive therapy" J ECT 2008;24(3):195-8

[8] Arain AM et al "Utility of daily supervised hyperventilation during long-term video-EEG monitoring" J Clin Neurophysiol 2009;26(1):17-20

Does overbreathing promote migraine attacks?

Don't ask me why, but there are no *direct* scientific studies about this question. Nevertheless, the circumstantial evidence would be more than sufficient in a court case.

- Hypocapnia (lack of CO_2) does indeed activate brainstem cells,[1] which subsequently release the neuropeptide CGRP, a known villain in the biochemistry of migraine.
- Carbon dioxide nasal spray does inhibit overexcited brainstem neurons.[2]
- CO_2 nasal spray has also been tested as abortive migraine medication and showed substantial symptom relief in the majority of participants.[3]
- Some migraineurs can abort oncoming migraine attacks by breathing into a bag, so that they rebreathe their own CO_2.[4,5]
- Carbon dioxide inhalations and baths are moderately effective treatments for migraine prevention in some European countries.[6]
- In physiology studies migraineurs appear to be hypocapnic.[7,8]
- Overbreathing/hypocapnia wreaks havoc in the bowel[9] and is a frequent finding in patients with IBS (irritable bowel syndrome).[10] Many severe migraineurs have either IBS or other digestive irregularities.
- Overbreathing/hypocapnia sabotages the production of serotonin.[11] Migraine patients do have low levels of serotonin.[12] – (I could go all day.)

Let's stop the arguing and simply say: Migraineurs who overbreathe are probably in more trouble. Patients with epileptic seizures can cut their episodes with calm abdominal breathing;[13] overbreathing migraineurs should consider practicing the same.

There are instructions for abdominal breathing exercises available for free on the internet. In case I find an outstanding program, I'll put it up on www.TheMigraineRevolution.com.

---

[1] Vause C et al "Effect of carbon dioxide on calcitonin gene-related peptide secretion from trigeminal neurons" Headache 2007;47(10):1385-97
[2] Tzabazis AZ et al "Trigeminal antihyperalgesic effect of intranasal carbon dioxide" Life Sci 2010;87(1-2):36-41
[3] Spierings LH et al "Abortive treatment of migraine headache with intranasal, non-inhaled carbon dioxide: a randomized, double-blind, placebo-controlled, parrallel-group study" Headache 2005;45(6):809
[4] Dexter SL "Rebreathing aborts migraine attacks" Br Med J (Clin Res Ed)1982;284(6312):312
[5] Pradalier A et al "Trial treatment of migraine attack by rebreathing of expired air" Presse Med 1984;13(31):1901
[6] Brockow T et al "Clinical evidence of subcutaneous CO2 insufflations: a systematic review" J Altern Complement Med 2000;6(5):391-403
[7] Kastrup A et al "Cerebral blood flow and CO2 reactivity in interictal migraineurs: a transcranial Doppler study" Headache 1998;38(8):608-13
[8] Liboni W et al "Spectral changes of near-infrared spectroscopy signals in migraineurs with aura reveal an impaired carbon dioxide-regulatory mechanism" Neurol Sci 2009;30 Suppl 1:S105-7
[9] Bharucha AE et al "Hyperventilation alters colonic motor and sensory function: effects and mechanisms in humans" Gastroenterology 1996;111(2):368-77
[10] Chambers JB et al "Hyperventilation and irritable bowel syndrome" Lancet 1986;1(8474):221
[11] Hoes MJ "Pharmacotherapy of the hyperventilation syndrome" Ann Med Psychol (Paris) 1983;141(8):859-74
[12] Ferrari MD et al "Serotonin metabolism in migraine" Neurology 1989;39(9):1239-42
[13] Fried R et al "Effect of diaphragmatic respiration with end-tidal CO2 biofeedback on respiration, EEG, and seizure frequency in idiopathic epilepsy" Ann N Y Acad Sci 1990;602:67-96

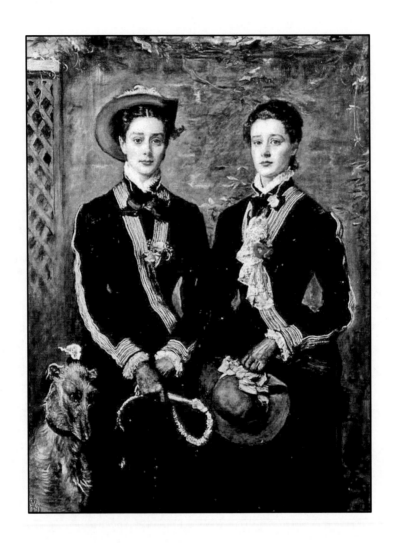

Chapter 13

Making a Difference

> "Some think it's holding on that makes one strong;
> sometimes it's letting go."
>
> Sylvia Robinson

Progressive muscle relaxation

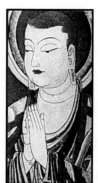

If we were all capable of meditating deeply for hours like a Buddhist monk, we wouldn't need trivial relaxation exercises, biofeedback or autogenic training. We would also be less distressed[1] and I daresay we would have fewer migraine attacks, if any at all.[2] Alas, not everybody is blessed with a life of deliberate poverty, dependence on alms, complete celibacy and hours of daily meditation.

And so we need to find other solutions in our quest to prevent our troubled mind from pushing our already agitated brain over the cliff into the next migraine abyss. Perhaps the body can lend us a helping hand? Pretty please?

When people are emotionally tense, their muscles typically aren't very relaxed either. In the 1920s the American physician Edmund Jacobson had the idea to reduce emotional tension by practicing muscular relaxation.[3] It did work.

Progressive muscle relaxation (PMR) is a two-step process. First you tense a muscle group; for instance you make a fist. Then you direct your *feeling awareness* to those muscles in your forearm that are still holding your fist clenched. After about ten seconds of tension—the muscles might even start burning a wee bit—you let your fist go and consciously sense how the muscles soften and how the uncomfortable tightness in your forearm dissipates.

The PMR procedure is normally applied to all major muscle groups in sequence with the objective to increase the awareness for the distinction between tension and relaxation.

---

[1] Verma G et al "The effect of meditation on psychological distress among Buddhist Monks and Nuns" Int J Psychiatry Med 2010;40(4):461-8
[2] Carter OL et al "Meditation alters perceptual rivalry in Tibetan Buddhist monks" Curr Biol 2005;15(11):R412-3
[3] Jacobson E "Progressive Relaxation: A Physiological & Clinical Investigation of Muscular States & Their Significance in Psychology & Medical Practice" Univ of Chicago Pr; 3 Revised edition 1974

This is made easy by the stark difference between the *feelings of tense discomfort* versus the *sensations of relaxation* within each muscle group. That's why PMR is such an ideal learning tool for those clients whose restless minds won't allow for spiritual growth during pure meditation in an attitude of loving kindness:

"Gosh, this is boring—What a waste of my precious time—I could get some work done—I'm not good at this ~~crap~~ stuff—Are we done soon?"

Highly-strung and reactive people are often surprisingly insensitive *of* themselves. That means they often miss their own body's subtle clues and don't feel the beginning of a state shift, only its end. Migraineurs with alexithymia (see chapter 5) often can't recognize when they're *becoming* tired or hungry, until they're completely spent or starved; or run into a hunger headache.

Therefore it makes a lot of sense for these migraineurs to increase their acumen and sensitivity for superfluous inner tension by practicing PMR and applying their increased awareness in life.

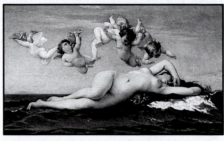

It normally doesn't take too long before clients can completely relax their entire body and don't even need to tense their muscles first. Once the body is calm and cozy, mind and brain will follow and adopt poise and equanimity.

Meanwhile Dr. Jacobson's progressive muscle relaxation has become the psychotherapeutic 'workhorse' in the complementary treatment of chronic pain,[1] cancer,[2] multiple sclerosis,[3] asthma[4] and high blood pressure[5], as well as for almost any mind disorder[6] including schizophrenia,[7] stress[8] and anxiety.[9]

---

[1] Carroll D et al "Relaxation for the relief of chronic pain: a systematic review" J Adv Nurs 1998;27(3):476-87

[2] Baider L et al "Progressive muscle relaxation and guided imagery in cancer patients" Gen Hosp Psychiatry 1994;16(5):340-7

[3] Ghafari S et al "Effectiveness of applying progressive muscle relaxation technique on quality of life of patients with multiple sclerosis" J Clin Nurs 2009;18(15):2171-9

[4] Nickel C et al "Effect of progressive muscle relaxation in adolescent female bronchial asthma patients: a randomized, double-blind, controlled study" J Psychosom Res 2005;59(6):393-8

[5] Sheu S et al "Effects of progressive muscle relaxation on blood pressure and psychosocial status for clients with essential hypertension in Taiwan" Holist Nurs Pract 2003;17(1):41-7

[6] Chen WC et al "Efficacy of progressive muscle relaxation training in reducing anxiety in patients with acute schizophrenia" J Clin Nurs 2009;18(15):2187-96

[7] Golombek U "Progressive muscle relaxation (PMR) according to Jacobson in a department of psychiatry and psychotherapy - empirical results" Psychiatr Prax 2001;28(8):402-4

[8] Khanna A et al "A study to compare the effectiveness of GSR biofeedback training and progressive muscle relaxation training in reducing blood pressure and respiratory rate among highly stressed individuals" Indian J Physiol Pharmacol 2007;51(3):296-300

[9] Canter A et al "A comparison of EMG feedback and progressive muscle relaxation training in anxiety neurosis" Br J Psychiatry 1975;127:470-7

The mere performance of PMR is not quite enough to limit migraine attacks; just like mortar alone is not enough to build a stable brick wall. The decisive step is the transfer of emotional aplomb into real life, to acquire the habit of remaining soft during daily hassles and to replace rigid reactivity with sensible flexibility. Newly learnt capabilities need to be applied to come to fruition or for country folks: Growing without harvesting won't fill the silo.

I recommend learning and practicing PMR *after* mastering calm abdominal breathing and *before* attempting autogenic training. Any one of these techniques has the potential to facilitate sufficient change to produce a considerable reduction in migraine frequency or even—not rarely—result in the cessation of attacks.

However, none of these nor other relaxation methods target migraine attacks directly; so the complaint

> "I've tried PMR exercises, but they failed to stop my migraine attacks."

indicates a severe and widespread error and that is to mistake a behavioral therapy as comparable to drugs or surgery. A relaxation routine can indeed 'fail', but only fail to induce relaxation:

> "The music on that sleep CD makes me wanna dance all night."

And utter inner tranquility, once achieved, may still not be enough:

> "Although I have become a different person—all my friends call me 'The Levitator'—I still have migraine attacks before my period."

But relaxation exercises cannot 'fail' to stop migraine, because that's neither their intention nor their purpose. They also don't stop global warming and so cannot 'fail' at that either. Roger?

Although reviews in medical journals typically attest that PMR and other relaxation methods have a *statistically significant* and *moderately large positive* effect on migraine,[1] progressive muscle relaxation alone is probably not sufficient to turn a life-long, severe, complex and difficult migraine patient into an ex-migraineur.

On the other hand, as part of a comprehensive rehabilitation program, a daily relaxation ritual can definitely make the difference between eternal migraine tyranny and triumphant victory. Instructions for PMR can be found for free on the internet and for money everywhere else. Ommm.

---

[1] Campbell K et al "Evidence-Based Guidelines For Migraine Headache: Behavioral and Physical Treatments" US Headache Consortium, available from the American Academy of Neurology, 2000; accessed April 9, 2012

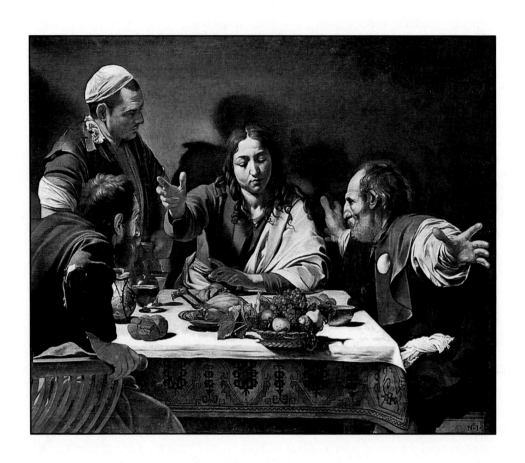

Chapter 14

Thought for Food

> "Eating is always a decision,
> nobody forces your hand to pick up food and put it into your mouth."
>
> Albert Ellis

There is not much talk in migraine land about nutritional therapy as a way of increasing stability and resistance; nor are food sensitivities, malnutrition or metabolic syndrome much of a topic. The public discussion revolves around the alarming powers of 'trigger' foods.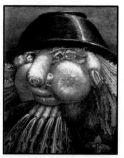

Does food pull the trigger?

We've talked about it at length in chapters 4 and 8, but since the misinformation is so persistent and omnipresent, we need to say it again: There is no such thing as a 'trigger food': No food has the power to trigger migraine attacks in the majority of migraineurs.

In a placebo-controlled British study[1], out of 88 patients, who believed chocolate to be a 'trigger' for them, 25 were selected for their alleged high reactivity to "even small amounts of chocolate". Those 25 received separate samples of real and fake chocolate, ate it and reported their chocolate-induced migraine headaches.

11 had no headache after either sample, 8 reported attacks after real chocolate only, 5 after the fake sample only and 1 subject after either. 15 of the 25 went into a second study with a different supplier for the samples. Again, 5 reacted to neither sample, 5 to the real chocolate only, 3 to the fake sample only and 1 to either.

Only 5 subjects reported the same response in both rounds of which only 2 out of 15 showed a consistent reaction to the real chocolate, but not to the fake sample.

The law of probability would explain one person reporting headaches after real chocolate only, based on pure chance. But let's say that *both* these British 'responders' were *sensitized* to chocolate and that the results were *representative* for all chocolate-victims.

---

[1] Moffett AM et al "Effect of chocolate in migraine: a double-blind study" J Neurol Neurosurg Psychiatry 1974;37(4):445-8

This means: Up to 25% of sufferers believe that their migraine can be triggered by chocolate, but in only 3% of all cases may that actually be true. 97% of migraineurs *do not react* to chocolate, 22% erroneously *believe* they do. Unhelpful beliefs obviously are a more common problem in migraine land than sensitization to food.

Is migraine a form of food allergy?

Instead of banning certain foods based on rumors and superstition, what about finding out which foods actually trigger allergic or otherwise untoward reactions?

In a proper *allergy* one would expect elevated levels of IgE (immunoglobulin E), which is one of the immune systems weapons (antibodies) against an intruder. One study measured IgE levels in migraine patients with and without a known allergic condition, of course in comparison to a healthy control group:[1]

Test	healthy controls:	migraine, no allergy	migraine and allergy
serum histamine	48 ng/ml	105 ng/ml	159 ng/ml
serum IgE	38 IU/ml	79 IU/ml	303 IU/ml

The allergy markers were significantly elevated even in unallergic migraine patients. Is migraine half an allergy? Other studies found that "an IgE mechanism seems to be unimportant in the process of food-induced migraine".[2] This is so confusing.

In 2001 a review of 45 studies[3] came to the conclusion, that

- migraineurs *only* show elevated IgE levels, when they also have an 'atopic' disorder (e.g. eczema, hay fever, allergic asthma)
- histamine levels are usually elevated in migraine sufferers
- there are signs of immune suppression due to chronic stress

What does this all mean? Whilst migraine is a common symptom in food allergies[4], IgE-mediated allergic mechanisms do not explain the idea of "dietary migraine" or "food triggers".

That is so weird. Everywhere you look you find migraineurs discussing trigger foods and doctors prescribing elimination diets. Is that nothing but mass hysteria?

---

[1] Gazerani P et al "A correlation between migraine, histamine and immunoglobulin e" Scand J Immunol 2003;57(3):286-90
[2] Pradalier A et al "Immunological aspects of migraine" Biomed Pharmacother 1996;50(2):64-70
[3] Kemper RH et al "Migraine and function of the immune system: a meta-analysis of clinical literature published between 1966 and 1999" Cephalalgia 2001;21(5):549-57
[4] Lingam S et al "Neurological features of children with food allergies" Clin Transl Allergy 2011;1(Suppl 1):P85

Migraine and food sensitivity

Welcome to the wonderfully weird world of food 'sensitivities' and 'intolerances'. The underlying idea here is that there might be patients out there, who—although not IgE-allergic to certain foods—wither away, when they eat those, and flourish, when they don't. In other words, is there a second form of food intolerance? And does this have an impact on migraine?

One possible approach is testing for a different antibody: IgG, the immunoglobulin G. A study in 2007 ran IgG tests on therapy-resistant migraine patients to identify offending foods; interestingly they had more 'IgG-reactions' (6-30 foods) than the healthy controls (0-4). As one would expect, the patients had to eliminate those foods from their diet, to which they were proven 'sensitive'. After one month on an individualized IgG-based elimination diet, 43 out of 65 participants (=66%) were migraine-free, after six months 76% were migraine-free.[1] Have we found the miracle cure here?

A similar study tested the same concept in a double blind, randomized, crossover design.[2] After IgG-testing migraineurs were put for six weeks on an individualized nutrition plan, based on their individual test results: either an *elimination* diet without 'offending foods' or a *provocation* diet with lots of those IgG-positive foods. In a second six-week phase they received the other food-plan, so that every participant had six weeks on IgG-based food *elimination* and six weeks on IgG-based food *provocation*. The difference was significant with an average of 10.5 headache days during the provocation phase and 7.5 during the elimination phase.

A third study with initially 167 probands comparing a true IgG-based elimination diet with a sham diet showed a significant reduction of migraine-like headaches after four weeks, but not after twelve weeks. The authors suspected that many participants, in the knowledge of the study design with a sham diet, did not follow the diet instructions, but simply waited for their real IgG-test results.[3]

The failure of this study confirms that sham control doesn't make sense in trials of behavioral therapies (here: diet changes).

---

[1] Arroyave Hernández CM et al "Food allergy mediated by IgG antibodies associated with migraine in adults" Rev Alerg Mex 2007;54(5):162-8

[2] Alpay K et al "Diet restriction in migraine, based on IgG against foods: a clinical double-blind, randomised, cross-over trial" Cephalalgia 2010;30(7):829-37

[3] Mitchell N et al "Randomised controlled trial of food elimination diet based on IgG antibodies for the prevention of migraine like headaches" Nutr J 2011 Aug;10:85

Studies of IgG-based food elimination diets yielded positive results in patients with IBS (irritable bowel syndrome),[1,2] one of migraine's sister disorders. When patients strictly followed their true diet, they were 26% better off than on a sham or placebo diet.[3]

Nevertheless, other 'experts' dismiss IgG testing as unreliable and ruthless money making[4] — without offering better alternatives: "The mechanisms of IgG-mediated food allergy have not been fully elucidated."[5]

One study found that IgG antibodies to foods are associated with *systemic* inflammation in obese adolescents;[6] another one showed that there was no correlation between symptom severity and IgG findings.[7]

Where does this leave the patients? Well, they have the choice to engage in this fascinating discussion and wait until further studies reveal the 'truth' about IgG antibodies, chronic systemic inflammation and symptoms of IBS or migraine. Alternatively, they could accept that there will always be a number of unanswered questions and a variety of opinions. Then they could simply look at the *usefulness* of a test or a therapy, instead of waiting for a 'truth', which might never be discovered. Fact is that many patients seem to benefit greatly from not eating foods, to which their IgG test showed a positive reaction.[8] Isn't that what counts?

These findings also mirror the relative success of the *oligoantigenic* diet in children with migraine or epilepsy:[9,10] no individualized testing, only those few foods are allowed, to which hardly anyone is allergic or sensitive; therefore very restrictive.

Those unwilling to adjust their diet, need not bother with an IgG test. For those, who want to make a change, diet modification based on IgG testing appears to be a promising weapon.

---

[1] Zar S et al "Food-specific IgG4 antibody-guided exclusion diet improves symptoms and rectal compliance in irritable bowel syndrome" Scand J Gastroenterol 2005;40(7):800-7

[2] Yang CM et al "The therapeutic effects of eliminating allergic foods according to food-specific IgG antibodies in irritable bowel syndrome" Zhonghua Nei Ke Za Zhi 2007;46(8):641-3

[3] Atkinson W et al "Food elimination based on IgG antibodies in irritable bowel syndrome: a randomised controlled trial" Gut 2004;53(10):1459-64

[4] Wüthrich B " Unproven techniques in allergy diagnosis" J Invest Allergol Clin Immunol 2005;15(2):86-90

[5] Pascual J et al "IgG-mediated allergy: a new mechanism for migraine attacks?" Cephalalgia 2010;30(7):777-9

[6] Wilders-Truschnig M et al "IgG antibodies against food antigens are correlated with inflammation and intima media thickness in obese juveniles" Exp Clin Endocrinol Diabetes 2008;116:241–245

[7] Zuo XL et al "Alterations of food antigen-specific serum immunoglobulins G and E antibodies in patients with irritable bowel syndrome and functional dyspepsia" Clin Exp Allergy 2007;37(6):823-30

[8] Mullin GE et al "Testing for food reactions: the good, the bad, and the ugly" Nutr Clin Pract 2010;25(2):192-8

[9] Egger J et al "Is migraine food allergy? A double-blind controlled trial of oligoantigenic diet treatment" Lancet 1983;2(8355):865-9

[10] Egger J et al "Oligoantigenic diet treatment of children with epilepsy and migraine" J Pediatr 1989;114(1):51-8

Migraine and gluten

If you think that the last topic was complicated and confusing, wait until you've read this bit about migraine and gluten!

Gluten is a protein in wheat, rye, barley and many processed foods. It is composed of gliadin and glutenin, which doesn't make things easier. Celiac disease is a severe intolerance to the gliadin part of the gluten with various gastro-intestinal symptoms and eventually leads to serious decay of the intestinal tissue.

The diagnosis of celiac disease is straightforward as long as patients have the classical symptoms and expected test results, e.g. certain markers in the blood and a ruined gut lining. Here too, experts argue about the best tests, but the ultimate proof for celiac disease is the damage in the bowel wall.[1] Nasty as this may be, it affects less than 1% of the population.

28% of patients with celiac disease also have migraine,[2] 35% have 'neurologic' problems (like movement disorders, sensory loss) or 'psycho' symptoms (like depression, personality changes, even psychosis). Finally it is accepted that classic celiac disease with gut symptoms is only *one* of many presentations of gluten intolerance.[3] Some scientific articles suspected that 'neurologic' symptoms like migraine might be the *result* of a gluten intolerance,[4,5] sparking the idea to screen healthy people for it as early detection/prevention.[6]

71% of celiac patients have abnormalities in the blood supply to the prefrontal cortex.[7] What a coincidence, just like migraineurs![8] And that supports new conclusions that gluten intolerance, irritable bowel syndrome and migraine have one common *cause*: an edgy nervous system[9] with a shaky prefrontal cortex[10] affecting the gut's nervous regulation and inflammatory immune responses.[11]

---

[1] Scanlon SA et al "Update on celiac disease – etiology, differential diagnosis, drug targets, and management advances" Clin Exp Gastroenterol 2011;4:297–311
[2] Bürk K et al "Neurological symptoms in patients with biopsy proven celiac disease" Mov Disord 2009;24(16):2358-62
[3] Hadjivassiliou M et al "Gluten sensitivity: from gut to brain" Lancet Neurol 2010;9(3):318-30
[4] Hernandez-Lahoz C et al "Neurological disorders associated with gluten sensitivity" Rev Neurol 2011;53(5):287-300
[5] Jackson JR et al "Neurologic and psychiatric manifestations of celiac disease and gluten sensitivity" Psychiatr Q 2012 Mar;83(1):91-102
[6] Aggarwal S et al "Screening for celiac disease in average-risk and high-risk populations" Therap Adv Gastroenterol 2012;5(1):37-47
[7] Usai P et al "Frontal cortical perfusion abnormalities related to gluten intake and associated autoimmune disease in adult coeliac disease: 99mTc-ECD brain SPECT study" Dig Liver Dis 2004;36(8):513-8
[8] Cavestri R et al "Interictal abnormalities of regional cerebral blood flow in migraine with and without aura" Minerva Med 1995;86(6):257-64
[9] Cady RK et al "The bowel and migraine: update on celiac disease and irritable bowel syndrome" Curr Pain Headache Rep 2012;16(3):278-86
[10] Piché M, et al "Decreased pain inhibition in irritable bowel syndrome depends on altered descending modulation and higher-order brain processes" Neuroscience 2011;195:166-75
[11] Kalafatakis K et "Contribution of neurotensin in the immune and neuroendocrine modulation of normal and abnormal enteric function" Regul Pept 2011;170(1-3):7-17

Now, what does all that mean, particularly for migraineurs? First, we need to address the popular idea that gluten intolerance *causes* migraine; or—to be more precise—the theory that the gut's immune reaction to gluten *causes* migraine: If that were true, then patients with celiac disease who follow a strictly gluten-free diet wouldn't have migraine attacks anymore. That, however, is not the case: Even without eating any gluten whatsoever, celiac patients do still have migraine attacks.[1] There goes a charming theory.

It is currently very popular to emphasize the newly found connections from the enteric nervous system (= the 'second brain' in the gut)[2] to the brain in the head,[3] to the extent of ideas to treat neuropsychiatric disorders with diet.[4] Is that a good idea?

The unambiguous answer is "yes and no". Whilst it is sensible to stop provoking the gut's agitated immune response, it would be foolish to conclude that *the gut rules the brain* and blindly follow catchy phrases like "you are what you eat".[5] Unfortunately, things are not that simple and neither are human beings.

For celiac disease, the most severe form of gluten intolerance, but also for irritable bowel syndrome, it is clear that psycho-social factors (e.g. attachment, abuse, early life stress, anxiety, depression, health beliefs, coping style etc.) play *the dominant role* in the progression and prognosis,[6,7] similar to what we've already found for migraine. Nevertheless, let's get back to gluten.

Since gluten-free nutrition doesn't even liberate celiac patients with migraine from attacks, why would any patient without celiac disease even think about the drag of a gluten-free diet?

Although the gut's reaction to gluten is neither *the origin* of migraine nor of the reduced blood supply to the prefrontal cortex, those gluten-reactive migraineurs who strictly avoid gluten, have a better blood flow to the PFC[8] and so *fewer* migraine attacks.[1]

---

[1] Gabrielli M et al "Association between migraine and Celiac disease: results from a preliminary case-control and therapeutic study" Am J Gastroenterol 2003;98(3):625-9
[2] Gershon MD "The enteric nervous system: a second brain" Hosp Pract (Minneap) 1999;34(7):31-42
[3] Remes-Troche JM et al "A bi-directional assessment of the human brain-anorectal axis" Neurogastroenterol Motil 2011;23(3):240-8
[4] Fetissov SO et al "The new link between gut-brain axis and neuropsychiatric disorders" Curr Opin Clin Nutr Metab Care 2011;14(5):477-82
[5] Cizza G et al "Was Feuerbach right: are we what we eat?" J Clin Invest 2011;121(8):2969-71
[6] Dorn SD et al "Psychosocial factors are more important than disease activity in determining gastrointestinal symptoms and health status in adults at a celiac disease referral center" Dig Dis Sci 2010;55(11):3154-6
[7] Surdea-Blaga T et al "Psychosocial determinants of irritable bowel syndrome" World J Gastroenterol 2012;18(7):616-26
[8] Usai P et al "Frontal cortical perfusion abnormalities related to gluten intake and associated autoimmune disease in adult coeliac disease: 99mTc-ECD brain SPECT study" Dig Liver Dis 2004;36(8):513-8

The logical conclusions from our investigation are as follows: Migraine sufferers who also happen to be diagnosed with *celiac disease* are on a strictly gluten-free diet anyway. They might have learnt from this chapter that the label "gluten *allergy*" does not mean: "It has nothing to do with me, my history or my personality. It's 'medical', because it's an allergy." Sorry, but it doesn't work that way; mind and brain rule the immune system,[1] like it or not.

Migraine patients, who don't have celiac disease, but a *positive IgG test* to gluten, should seriously consider adopting a gluten-free lifestyle. The expectation of a reduction in migraine symptoms is justified, but not of a complete cessation. That would be a bonus.

Those migraineurs, who neither have celiac disease nor a positive IgG test to gluten, but *irritable bowel syndrome* or some other autoimmune trouble, need to think about how difficult it would be for them to give a gluten-free diet a shot. There is a fair chance that it leads to worthwhile improvements, but complete freedom from migraine attacks should not be the benchmark.

All the celiac-free migraine sufferers who show no reaction to gluten in the IgG test and who have neither autoimmune nor bowel issues are certainly allowed to try their luck with a gluten-free diet, but in *difficult and complex* cases I'm concerned, that the vague chance of improvements won't outweigh the likely disappointment of "YET ANOTHER FAILURE" in countless attempts to find the magic cure.

More thoughts about food and migraine

Migraineurs tend to have higher blood sugar and insulin levels than healthy controls,[2,3,4] which is consistent with a relative insulin resistance [5] and metabolic syndrome.[6] Obesity—not an unlikely consequence of metabolic syndrome—is a risk factor for migraine chronification[7] and migraine itself is a risk factor for stroke and heart attack.[8] It's a bit of a trap, ey?

---

[1] Forsythe P "The Nervous System as a Critical Regulator of Immune Responses Underlying Allergy" Curr Pharm Des 2012;18(16):2290-304
[2] Hamed SA et al "Vascular risk factors, endothelial function, and carotid thickness in patients with migraine: relationship to atherosclerosis" J Stroke Cerebrovasc Dis 2010;19(2):92-103
[3] Cavestro C et al "Insulin metabolism is altered in migraineurs: a new pathogenic mechanism for migraine?" Headache 2007;47(10):1436-42
[4] Kokavec A et al "Sugar alters the level of serum insulin and plasma glucose and the serum cortisol:DHEAS ratio in female migraine sufferers" Appetite 2010;55(3):582-8
[5] Rainero I et al "Insulin sensitivity is impaired in patients with migraine" Cephalalgia 2005;25(8):593-7
[6] Bhoi SK et al "Metabolic syndrome and insulin resistance in migraine" J Headache Pain 2012;13(4):321-6
[7] Bigal ME et al "Obesity and chronic daily headache" Curr Pain Headache Rep 2012;16(1):101-9
[8] Hamed SA et al "Vascular risk factors, endothelial function, and carotid thickness in patients with migraine: relationship to atherosclerosis" J Stroke Cerebrovasc Dis 2010;19(2):92-103

Surprisingly, it might even be that *habitual overbreathing* and the resulting hypocapnia (= low CO_2 levels) play a worsening role here: Low CO_2 leads to nitric oxide stress,[1] which in turn reduces insulin sensitivity.[2] Now migraineurs have one more reason to do their abdominal breathing exercises.

The second conclusion from the aforementioned trap is, that sport and exercise become even more important for migraineurs to kick-start their metabolism[3] and manage their weight, if necessary.

A third idea could be to look into a low-insulin diet with limited intake of carbohydrates, especially refined carbs (sugar, white flour). The *ketogenic diet* (= low in carbs, high in fat; used for children with intractable severe epilepsy) has recently been mentioned as a potential treatment option for chronic migraine.[4] As *'modified Atkins diet'* a similar concept showed promising results for adult epilepsy.[5] In contradiction to that are the results of a study with a *low-fat diet*, which allegedly lead to significant reductions in frequency and severity of migraine attacks.[6]

At this point there is no substantiated concept of a migraine diet beyond the always valid advice to eat healthy food. What *that* means is subject to heated debates amongst nutrition gurus. General consensus is that fast food, high fructose corn syrup, sugar and white flour are bad, whereas unprocessed food and vegetables are good. Anything else is highly disputed.

MSG and aspartame are no-nos for migraineurs, everybody knows that. I suggest to extend that to all stimulating substances like energy drinks and caffeine-containing beverages, including cola and diet-cola, but also <u>coffee</u>![7]   (Okay, but only one small cup in the morning!)

Lastly, drink plenty of *water*! Dehydration does promote migraine attacks,[8] possibly due to a parched prefrontal cortex.[9,10]

---

[1] Fathi AR et al "Carbon dioxide influence on nitric oxide production in endothelial cells and astrocytes: cellular mechanisms" Brain Res 2011;1386:50-7

[2] Gruber HJ et al "Hyperinsulinaemia in migraineurs is associated with nitric oxide stress" Cephalalgia 2010;30(5):593-8

[3] Joseph LJ et al "Weight loss and low-intensity exercise for the treatment of metabolic syndrome in obese postmenopausal women" J Gerontol A Biol Sci Med Sci 2011;66(9):1022-9

[4] Maggioni F et al "Ketogenic diet in migraine treatment: a brief but ancient history" Cephalalgia 2011;31(10):1150-1

[5] Kossoff EH et al "A prospective study of the modified Atkins diet for intractable epilepsy in adults" Epilepsia 2008;49(2):316-9

[6] Bic Z et al "The influence of a low-fat diet on incidence and severity of migraine headaches" J Womens Health Gend Based Med 1999;8(5):623-30

[7] Smith JE et al "Storm in a coffee cup: caffeine modifies brain activation to social signals of threat" Soc Cogn Affect Neurosci 2011 Nov 16 [Epub ahead of print]

[8] Blau JN et al "Water-deprivation headache: a new headache with two variants" Headache 2004;44(1):79-83

[9] Shirreffs SM et al "The effects of fluid restriction on hydration status and subjective feelings in man" Br J Nutr 2004;91(6):951-8

[10] Farrell MJ et al "Effect of aging on regional cerebral blood flow responses associated with osmotic thirst and its satiation by water drinking: a PET study" Proc Natl Acad Sci U S A 2008;105(1):382-7

Chapter 15

Doping for Migraine

> "Friendship is like vitamins,
> we supplement each other's minimum daily requirements"
> Unknown

Herbs and supplements

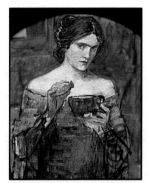

Don't we all love swallowing something potent in order to get better? Medication for everything 'medical', diet pills to lose body fat, vitamins for vigor and vitality and herbal remedies for a bit of nature's magic. Rather than facing the roots of a problem, we prefer fixing the symptoms by popping a pill.

It's easy to be cynical about and critical of the growing supplement industry; but what about nutritional deficiencies due to processed food, depleted soil, malabsorption or due to an increased demand thanks to the excessively draining effect of constant relentless distress?

Severe migraineurs cannot afford to be slack or aloof towards the world of nutraceuticals, nor can they possibly gulp down all the minerals, herbs and vitamins that anyone has ever recommended.

Let's have a look at what is known, at what the studies say and make up our minds as we go. Deal?

Magnesium

Magnesium (Mg) is needed for more than 300 biochemical reactions in the body. It helps maintain normal nerve and muscle function, a steady heart rhythm, a healthy immune system and strong bones.[1] A healthy adult human body contains 24g (0.85oz) of magnesium, 99% of which is stored in bones and cells.[2] That leaves only 1% for outside the cells (extracellular) and raises questions as to what to measure for the identification of a Mg *deficiency*.[3]

---

[1] Office of Dietary Supplements, NIH (National Institutes for Health, USA), http://ods.od.nih.gov/factsheets/magnesium-HealthProfessional/
[2] Wester PO "Magnesium" Am J Clin Nutr 1987;45(5 Suppl):1305-12
[3] Reinhart RA "Magnesium metabolism. A review with special reference to the relationship between intracellular content and serum levels" Arch Intern Med 1988;148(11):2415-20

Doctors often request the test for Mg in *serum* (= blood fluid) and whilst a low result does indeed indicate a severe Mg shortage,[1] normal serum levels can also be found in patients with magnesium deficiency *in other body tissues*.[2] Tricky, isn't it?

To make matters worse, an abnormally low serum Mg level is called "hypomagnesemia", which sounds a lot like magnesium 'deficiency' to the average medic; and so it can easily happen that doctors misinterpret a normal *serum* magnesium level as evidence against Mg deficiency in the *tissues* and logically advise against magnesium supplementation although clinical signs speak for it.

Measuring the magnesium content of *red blood cells* (erythrocytes) yields different results,[3] which do not correlate with serum levels.[4] And still, that doesn't mean they represent Mg levels inside other body tissues very well.

Luckily, there are heaps more magnesium tests, some are even available outside research projects; for instance the EXA test, which is done on a sample of cells scraped out from under the tongue (for details see www.exatest.com).[5] Real experts opine that only a 'magnesium loading' test[6] with a 24-hour urine collection can identify Mg deficiency;[7] yet other real experts dispute that too.[8]

All this leads to two questions:

1. "How do I know if I'm deficient and therefore should be taking a Mg supplement?" and
2. "What the devil has all of that to do with migraine?"

Magnesium and migraine

During migraine attacks magnesium levels in the brain are abnormally low,[9] which could be expected, because a low level of magnesium in the brain *promotes seizure activity*.[10,11] (By the way, have I mentioned that a migraine attack is a brainstem seizure?)

---

[1] Whang R et al "Frequency of hypomagnesemia and hypermagnesemia. Requested vs routine" JAMA 1990;263(22):3063-4
[2] Rob PM et al "Magnesium deficiency after renal transplantation and cyclosporine treatment despite normal serum-magnesium detected by a modified magnesium-loading-test" Transplant Proc 1995;27(6):3442-3
[3] Millart H et al "Red blood cell magnesium concentrations: analytical problems and significance" Magnes Res 1995;8(1):65-76
[4] Ulger Z et al "Intra-erythrocyte magnesium levels and their clinical implications in geriatric outpatients" J Nutr Health Aging 2010;14(10):810-4
[5] Silver BB "Development of cellular magnesium nano-analysis in treatment of clinical magnesium deficiency" J Am Coll Nutr 2004;23(6):732S-7S
[6] Vizinová H et al "The oral magnesium loading test for detecting possible magnesium deficiency" Cas Lek Cesk 1993;132(19):587-9
[7] Huijgen HJ et al "Magnesium levels in critically ill patients. What should we measure?" Am J Clin Pathol 2000;114(5):688-95
[8] Cieslinski G et al "Magnesium excretion in urine is not a marker of magnesium deficiency. Reliability of an oral magnesium administration test" Med Klin (Munich) 1999;94(2):82-7
[9] Ramadan NM et al "Low brain magnesium in migraine" Headache 1989;29(9):590-3
[10] Morris ME "Brain and CSF magnesium concentrations during magnesium deficit in animals and humans: neurological symptoms" Magnes Res 1992;5(4):303-13
[11] Nuytten D et al "Magnesium deficiency as a cause of acute intractable seizures" J Neurol 1991;238(5):262-4

Does that mean that the low magnesium level *caused* the brainstem seizure that we call *migraine* attack? Hard to say, but an intravenous magnesium infusion is known to abort all symptoms of a migraine attack in up to 80% of patients within 15 minutes.[1,2,3] Of course, not only migraine seizures, but also epileptic seizures can be stopped with magnesium infusions.[4]

Just like patients with epileptic seizures,[5,6] migraine patients seem to have *lower than normal* magnesium levels also between attacks (= 'interictally') no matter what exactly the researchers measured: blood, saliva, brain, whatever.[7,8,9,10,11,12,13]

Given that low magnesium levels promote epileptic seizures and migraine attacks, and given that migraineurs tend to have low magnesium levels, wouldn't it be a good idea for migraineurs to take a magnesium supplement and see whether that is helpful?

Some are not convinced; have look at this expert:

> "With a good side effect profile, **magnesium** is a relatively safe **drug** with a possible beneficial effect in the prophylaxis of migraine headache, and it may have its niche in the **treatment** of migraine patients. However, the current **medical** evidence that has accumulated and the fact that there are far more effective **treatment** possibilities clearly indicate that this **drug** is definitely not to be used by every migraineur."[14]

Isn't that interesting? Magnesium is an elementary mineral in our food and body. There is a lot of it in beans, almonds, spinach and bananas.[15] This above quoted doctor is trying to turn magnesium into a "*drug*"! If we accept that, we mustn't complain, if he starts believing that he can turn water into wine.

---

[1] Mauskop A et al "Intravenous magnesium sulfate rapidly alleviates headaches of various types" Headache 1996;36(3):154-60
[2] Bigal ME et al "Intravenous magnesium sulphate in the acute treatment of migraine without aura and migraine with aura. A randomized, double-blind, placebo-controlled study" Cephalalgia 2002;22(5):345-53
[3] Demirkaya S et al "Efficacy of intravenous magnesium sulfate in the treatment of acute migraine attacks" Headache 2001;41(2):171-7
[4] Stewart CE "Anticonvulsant medications" Emerg Med Serv 2001;30(7):56-66
[5] Benga I et al "Plasma and cerebrospinal fluid concentrations of magnesium in epileptic children" J Neurol Sci 1985;67(1):29-34
[6] Oladipo OO et al "Plasma magnesium in adult Nigerian patients with epilepsy" Niger Postgrad Med J 2003;10(4):234-7
[7] Sarchielli P et al "Serum and salivary magnesium levels in migraine and tension-type headache. Results in a group of adult patients" Cephalalgia 1992;12(1):21-7
[8] Gallai V et al "Serum and salivary magnesium levels in migraine. Results in a group of juvenile patients" Headache 1992;32(3):132-5
[9] Gallai V et al "Red blood cell magnesium levels in migraine patients" Cephalalgia 1993;13(2):94-81
[10] Thomas J et al "Free and total magnesium in lymphocytes of migraine patients - effect of magnesium-rich mineral water intake" Clin Chim Acta 2000;295(1-2):63-75
[11] Talebi M et al "Relation between serum magnesium level and migraine attacks" Neurosciences (Riyadh) 2011;16(4):320-3
[12] Qujeq D et al "Evaluation of intracellular magnesium and calcium concentration in patients with migraine" Neurosciences 2012;17(1):85-6
[13] Samaie A et al "Blood Magnesium levels in migraineurs within and between the headache attacks: a case control study" Pan Afr Med J 2012;11:46
[14] Pardutz A et al "Should magnesium be given to every migraineur? No" J Neural Transm 2012;119(5):581-5
[15] http://magnesiumrichfoods.com

Here is the problem: When you want to find out, if a *drug* is any good, you first give it to a bunch of sick rats and if that goes well, you try it out on patients with a promising ailment. If the drug heals more patients than it damages, then it's a good one and everybody is happy: patients, doctors and the pharma company.

Magnesium is *not a drug* and magnesium supplementation can only help those migraineurs, who are deficient in magnesium. As an abortive infusion, magnesium is particularly helpful in those migraineurs with *low* levels of magnesium, the lower, the better![1,2]

If magnesium infusions work like a charm as an abortive treatment for Mg deficient migraineurs, it begs the question, if magnesium supplementation could be helpful to prevent migraine attacks, doesn't it?

Several studies have investigated this burning question and the results have been found to be *inconsistent*:

> Study 1 found a 42% reduction in attack rate with 600mg *magnesium citrate* compared to 16% with placebo after 12 weeks and concluded: High-dose oral magnesium appears to be effective in migraine prophylaxis.[3]
>
> Study 2, oddly designed, aimed at a more than 50% reduction in migraine attacks and 30% of both the *Mg injection* group and the placebo injection group reached that goal: "With regard to the number of migraine days or attacks there was no benefit with magnesium compared to placebo."[4]
>
> Study 3 tested the effect of daily 600mg *magnesium citrate* and found not only significant improvements in migraine symptoms, but also renormalizations of a few funky brain measurements.[5]
>
> Study 4 tested *magnesium oxide* versus placebo on children for 16 weeks, found a slight decrease in headache frequency, but not in severity, and concluded: "Larger trials of this safe, appealing complementary therapy are needed."[6]

Since the results apparently are so *inconsistent*, treatment guidelines *do not recommend* magnesium supplementation for the preventive treatment of migraine, despite the successful studies with magnesium citrate. Is that weird or what?

---

[1] Mauskop A et al "Intravenous magnesium sulphate relieves migraine attacks in patients with low serum ionized magnesium levels: a pilot study" Clin Sci (Lond) 1995;89(6):633-6
[2] Mauskop A et al "Intravenous magnesium sulfate rapidly alleviates headaches of various types" Headache 1996;36(3):154-60
[3] Peikert A et al "Prophylaxis of migraine with oral magnesium: results from a prospective, multi-center, placebo-controlled and double-blind randomized study" Cephalalgia 1996;16(4):257-63
[4] Pfaffenrath V et al "Magnesium in the prophylaxis of migraine--a double-blind placebo-controlled study" Cephalalgia 1996;16(6):436-40
[5] Köseoglu E et al "The effects of magnesium prophylaxis in migraine without aura" Magnes Res 2008;21(2):101-8
[6] Wang F et al "Oral magnesium oxide prophylaxis of frequent migrainous headache in children: a randomized, double-blind, placebo-controlled trial" Headache 2003;43(6):601-10

> "What is going on here? And why are we wasting so much time and paper on a such an insignificant topic like magnesium, which doesn't seem to cut it, according to all those 'inconsistent' studies?"

What studies? Have they managed to trick you too? Yes, those medical researchers are pretty clever and sneaky. Pay careful attention: As I said earlier, magnesium is not a medical drug and it is *not a medication* for migraine. The objective of magnesium supplementation is to make up for a lack of magnesium in food or for a higher Mg demand, both of which can lead to low magnesium levels in the body's tissues, called deficiency.

It would be interesting to measure the impact of magnesium supplementation on magnesium tissue levels and to find out which magnesium compound is best absorbed by the body.

And once you have an idea how supplements can or cannot compensate for the effect of *fluoride in drinking water*, which seems to interfere with magnesium metabolism a fair bit,[1,2] then it would be informative to measure how much magnesium-deficient migraineurs benefit from effective magnesium supplementation.

A study that investigates magnesium in migraine patients, *without testing* magnesium levels before and after, doesn't tell us much: Did study 2 (see previous page) fail, because it was done in Vienna, where they have *no water fluoridation* and therefore perhaps no magnesium deficiency? Who knows?

And did study 4 produce a lame result, because they used *magnesium oxide*, which is famous amongst nutritionists for its low bioavailability (= can't get used well by the body)?[3] Why would you even bother doing a study with magnesium oxide, when you know about its pathetic 4% absorption rate?[4]

Magnesium supplementation

As frustrating as all of this may be, Mg is a *crucial* topic for all migraineurs.[5] Remember that there is a very decent chance that this innocuous element alone may significantly reduce attack rate and severity; and it might even prolong your life![6]

---

[1] Machoy-Mokrzynska A "Fluoride-Magnesium Interaction" J Int Soc Fluor Res 1995;28(4):175-177
[2] Marier JR "Observations and implications of the (Mg F) interrelations in biosystems" J Int Soc Fluor Res 1981;14:142
[3] Lindberg JS et al "Magnesium bioavailability from magnesium citrate and magnesium oxide" J Am Coll Nutr 1990;9(1):48-55
[4] Firoz M et al "Bioavailability of US commercial magnesium preparations" Magnes Res 2001;14(4):257-62
[5] Mauskop A et al "Why all migraine patients should be treated with magnesium" J Neural Transm 2012;119(5):575-9
[6] Rowe WJ "Correcting magnesium deficiencies may prolong life" Clin Interv Aging 2012;7:51-4

It depends on the individual situation, but the assumption that every patient with migraine has *lower than optimal* tissue Mg levels is not far-fetched; and so every migraineur might want to presume being magnesium-deficient until proven otherwise.

Processed food, fluoride in water and our frantic lifestyle are sufficient reasons why that may be true for the vast majority of the population anyway, many experts say. — So, what do we do now?

First, some form of magnesium level *laboratory test* would be helpful; if not reliable for the identification of a deficiency, then at least in order to track and monitor the effect of an increased intake. Since the ionized Mg test—the gold standard in research—is not readily available, the EXA test could be the next best choice (see www.exatest.com), followed by measuring magnesium in red blood cells (RBC); forget 'normal' and consider it a starting point.

Second, *magnesium citrate* is an inexpensive supplement, which is seen as a safe and solid choice[1] in the jungle of nutraceuticals. Additionally the use of *transdermal magnesium oil*, which is a magnesium chloride solution, might help to compensate for the suspected shortage within weeks instead of months. Mg oil can tickle, tingle or slightly burn on sensitive skin; a test on the outside of one leg is advisable. In contrast to most oral supplements, magnesium oil does *not* have a laxative effect and is thought to 'refill' the tissues much faster than any ingested Mg concoction.

Thirdly, *magnesium-rich food* and a restriction of excessive calcium intake may be worth considering; all of it, of course, after consulting your doctor or an expert (e.g. nutritionist or naturopath).

Fourthly, a *repetition* of the first test for Mg levels after three months might aid in finding a connection between symptom improvement and supplementation and help adjust the dose.

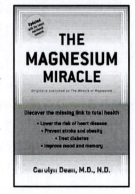

For even more details and further study of this unfortunately very important topic I wholeheartedly recommend the book "The Magnesium Miracle" by Carolyn Dean, who is not only a medical and naturopathic doctor, but also a well-informed expert in all things 'magnesic'.

---

[1] Walker AF et al "Mg citrate found more bioavailable than other Mg preparations in a randomised, double-blind study" Magnes Res 2003;16(3):183-91

Vitamin B2 (Riboflavin)

B vitamins play an important role in cell energy metabolism, which is generally impaired in patients with migraine attacks[1,2] or other seizures.[3] This diminished energy production can partly be explained with reduced tissue levels of carbon dioxide[4,5] due to habitual *overbreathing* (see chapter 12).

So it makes sense to look into natural substances which could lift the cell's energy metabolism enough to have an impact on migraine symptoms. Riboflavin (vitamin B2) is such a substance and well-controlled studies have shown its impressive efficacy as a safe preventive at high doses of *400mg daily* in adults.[6,7,8,9] Up to 60% of the studied migraineurs at least halved their attack rate.

Studies with vitamin B2 for children with migraine weren't quite as consistent, because the strong placebo effect in all migraine patients—made possible by their 'wobbly' prefrontal cortex (see chapter 8)—stuffed up the statistical analysis of one study a bit.[10] A second trial with kids, however, was successful.[11]

Even at these high doses, riboflavin doesn't seem to cause any *serious* side effects, but a funny one: It tints the wee neon-yellow.

A genetic study has given hints that riboflavin may be particularly effective as migraine preventive in populations of *non-European* ethnicity,[12] which is amazing, given that several of these already very successful vitamin B2 trials took place in Europe.

Despite its good effect in migraine attack reduction, vitamin B2 (riboflavin) is <u>not</u> a drug, but a *cell energy metabolism booster*[13] and it may well take a few months until the full effect kicks in.

---

[1] Lodi R et al "Energy metabolism in migraine" Neurol Sci 2006;27 Suppl 2:S82-5
[2] Sparaco M et al "Mitochondrial dysfunction and migraine: evidence and hypotheses" Cephalalgia 2006;26(4):361-72
[3] Folbergrová J et sl "Mitochondrial dysfunction in epilepsy" Mitochondrion 2012 Jan;12(1):35-40
[4] MacMillan V et al "The effect of combined hypocapnia and hypoxemia upon the energy metabolism of the brain" Can J Physiol Pharmacol 1974;52(6):1136-46
[5] Fritz KI et al "Effect of moderate hypocapnic ventilation on nuclear DNA fragmentation and energy metabolism in the cerebral cortex of newborn piglets" Pediatr Res 2001;50(5):586-9
[6] Schoenen J et al "High-dose riboflavin as a prophylactic treatment of migraine: results of an open pilot study" Cephalalgia 1994;14(5):328-9
[7] Schoenen J et al "Effectiveness of high-dose riboflavin in migraine prophylaxis. A randomized controlled trial" Neurology 1998;50(2):466-70
[8] Yee AJ et al "Effectiveness of high-dose riboflavin in migraine prophylaxis" Neurology 1999;52(2):431-2
[9] Boehnke C et al "High-dose riboflavin treatment is efficacious in migraine prophylaxis: an open study in a tertiary care centre" Eur J Neurol 2004;11(7):475-7
[10] MacLennan SC et al "High-dose riboflavin for migraine prophylaxis in children: a double-blind, randomized, placebo-controlled trial" J Child Neurol 2008;23(11):1300-4
[11] Condò M et al "Riboflavin prophylaxis in pediatric and adolescent migraine" J Headache Pain 2009 Oct;10(5):361-5
[12] Di Lorenzo C et al "Mitochondrial DNA haplogroups influence the therapeutic response to riboflavin in migraineurs" Neurology 2009;72(18):1588-94
[13] Henriques BJ et al "Emerging roles for riboflavin in functional rescue of mitochondrial flavoenzymes" Curr Med Chem 2010;17(32):3842-54

Coenzyme Q10 (CoQ10)

The coenzyme Q10 too is involved in a cell's energy production and frequently mentioned as a potential 'doping' substance for migraineurs. Though the evidence base is not quite as impressive as for magnesium citrate and vitamin B2:

- A pilot study without placebo control ("open label") showed promising results of 150mg of CoQ10 per day: 61% of Q10-swallowing sufferers at least halved their days with migraine per month.[1]
- A randomized, placebo-controlled trial found that CoQ10 significantly decreased attack frequency, headache days, and days with nausea; roughly 50% of the patients at least halved their attack rate with 3x100mg CoQ10 per day vs. 15% in the placebo group. No serious side effects were reported.[2]
- Measurements in a headache center on more than 1,500 children and adolescents with frequent headaches discovered that one third of the brats had abnormally low CoQ10 levels. Supplementation doubled their levels within 100 days into the reference range; their headache frequency went down by only a third, but their headache disability by a decent 50%.[3]
- A way cooler study with all the bells and whistles in the same headache center tested CoQ10 as an addition to a comprehensive rehabilitation program. They found that the kids with the CoQ10 did better in the first four weeks, than their buddies on placebo. In the end all the kids got so much better in that rehabilitation program, that CoQ10 didn't leave a lasting impression.[4]

Here is what I think: All these studies are trying to tell us, whether CoQ10 is any *good for migraine*. That is nonsense. CoQ10 supplementation can only be *good for CoQ10 deficiency* and in some cases—so it seems—correcting low levels of that enzyme has lead to clinical improvements in several patients. That's awesome.

Now there are two options: 1. Either you start by measuring CoQ10 levels and in case of a low result ('deficiency') begin taking a supplement, or 2. you begin taking it and document the effect. If there is one, you can conclude that you've *'corrected'* the deficit.

---

[1] Rozen TD et al "Open label trial of coenzyme Q10 as a migraine preventive" Cephalalgia 2002;22(2):137-41
[2] Sándor PS et al "Efficacy of coenzyme Q10 in migraine prophylaxis: a randomized controlled trial" Neurology 2005;64(4):713-5
[3] Hershey AD et al "Coenzyme Q10 deficiency and response to supplementation in pediatric and adolescent migraine" Headache 2007;47(1):73-80
[4] Slater SK et al "A randomized, double-blinded, placebo-controlled, crossover, add-on study of CoEnzyme Q10 in the prevention of pediatric and adolescent migraine" Cephalalgia 2011;31(8):897-905

Butterbur (petasites hybridus)

Plant extracts as *herbal medicines* are very different from nutritional supplements. Supplemental vitamins and minerals are thought to make up for the shortcomings of our modern diet; they are basically a form of food. Risks and serious side effects are not likely unless the dosage is extremely off (Just like too many dried apricots can have an 'explosive' effect; still not serious though).

Since nobody suffers from migraine due to a 'butterbur deficiency', herbal remedies have to be considered as a form of *medication* and there is no logic behind the assumption that plant-based products are always harmless, only because they are 'natural'. That's not necessarily true; take cigarettes as an example.

Butterbur is not tobacco, but the plant contains pyrrolizidine alkaloids (PA), which are liver-toxic and promote cancer. It might be a good idea to make sure that a butterbur product is "PA-free".

Another tricky detail with herbal remedies is the question, how much of the active ingredient is actually in every capsule? In the case of butterbur the beneficial substance is petasin, which is available and well tested in a patented, standardized form with the name Petadolex®:

- A first randomized, placebo-controlled study found an average reduction from 3.4 to 1.8 migraine attacks per month on 2x50mg Petadolex® daily vs no significant change in the placebo group. 45% of the patients had at least halved the number of their migraine episodes. The stuff was well tolerated.[1]
- A larger study with 245 human guinea pigs compared 2x75mg to 2x50mg Petadolex® and 2x placebo daily. After 4 months the attack rate was reduced by 48% on the higher dose, by 36% on the lower dose and by 26% on placebo. Of those migraineurs on 2x75mg, 68% had at least halved their attack rate;[2] best effect was reached after 3 months. As side effect, burping was reported.
- An open study tested Petadolex® on children and adolescents with migraine. After four months on an age-dependent dose ranging from 50-150mg daily 77% of the kids reported at least a 50% reduction in attack rate. The average attack frequency went down by 63%. Seven percent burped.[3]

---

[1] Diener HC et al "The first placebo-controlled trial of a special butterbur root extract for the prevention of migraine: reanalysis of efficacy criteria" Eur Neurol 2004;51(2):89-97

[2] Lipton RB et al "Petasites hybridus root (butterbur) is an effective preventive treatment for migraine" Neurology 2004;63(12):2240-4

[3] Pothmann R et al "Migraine prevention in children and adolescents: results of an open study with a special butterbur root extract" Headache 2005;45(3):196-203

- The last study—on migraine kids in primary school—compared Petadolex® to 'music therapy' (psychotherapy and relaxation exercises) in addition to standard care (headache education). With more than 50% responders, both were significantly better than placebo; 'music therapy' had the advantage.[1]

Like other herbs, Petadolex® butterbur extract is not recommended for *pregnant women*, because there are no studies which tell us anything about how it affects a fetus.[2] Also, patients with a confirmed liver disease shouldn't take it. Cautious doctors recommend running liver function tests after starting migraine prevention with Petadolex®.[2] This shouldn't frighten migraineurs with a healthy liver; it's a safe,[3] well-tolerated and apparently pretty effective herbal medicine, that could help reduce migraine a fair bit (and perhaps make you burp a little).

Other butterbur extracts may also be safe and effective, but only Petadolex® can be recommended based on evidence.

Feverfew (tanacetum parthenium)

A second herb that is frequently mentioned in migraine land for *attack prevention* is feverfew. Possibly due to different preparations and variations of the strength of the (suspected) active substance, a bunch of studies came to inconsistent results.[4,5,6,7] A Cochrane review in 2004 found *insufficient evidence* from the existing randomized controlled trials.[8]

Interestingly, two favorable studies tested a *powdered* plant extract, whereas two unsuccessful trials used an *alcoholic* extract. Forest Gump pointed out the problem with unstandardized herbs: "My mama said, you never know what you're gonna get."

- MIG-99, a much 'better' feverfew extract with CO_2 was tested on 147 patients; only those patients with more than four attacks per month had a benefit from 3x6.25mg compared to placebo.[9]

---

[1] Oelkers-Ax R et al "Butterbur root extract and music therapy in the prevention of childhood migraine" Eur J Pain 2008;12(3):301-13
[2] Evers S. "Pestwurz in der Behandlung der Migräne" Nervenheilkunde 2009;28:548-552
[3] Danesch U et al "Safety of a patented special butterbur root extract for migraine prevention" Headache 2003;43(1):76–78
[4] Johnson ES et al "Efficacy of feverfew as prophylactic treatment of migraine" Br Med J 1985;291:569-573
[5] Murphy JJ et al "Randomised double-blind placebo-controlled trial of feverfew in migraine prevention" Lancet 1988;2:189-192
[6] De Weerdt CJ et al "Herbal medicines in migraine prevention: Randomized double-blind placebo-controlled crossover trial of feverfew preparation" Phytomedicine 1996;3:225-230
[7] Palevitch D et al "Feverfew (Tanacetum parthenium) as a prophylactic treatment for migraine: A placebo- controlled double-blind study" Phytother Res 1997;11:508-51
[8] Pittler MH et al "Feverfew for preventing migraine" Cochrane Database Syst Rev 2004;(1):CD002286
[9] Pfaffenrath V et al "The efficacy and safety of Tanacetum parthenium (feverfew) in migraine prophylaxis--a double-blind, multicentre, randomized placebo-controlled dose-response study" Cephalalgia 2002;22(7):523-32

Allegedly about one third of the study participants reported adverse effects, to the same degree on placebo and feverfew.

- Yet another study with 3x6.25 MIG-99 feverfew extract daily for migraine prevention finally was successful. The average migraine frequency of 4.8 per month went down by 1.9 on the real herb and by 1.3 on placebo. Only 30% on MIG-99 at least halved their attack rate. Side effects were reported by about 10% of either group.[1]

Despite many *good* studies, feverfew is not overly impressive for attack prevention on average. On the other hand, for individual patients, especially those with frequent attacks, it may do the trick.

To me, it makes more sense to first identify individual deficits in the body's biochemistry by screening and testing than trying to hit unknown targets with shots in the dark. It appears that so many migraineurs are deficient in magnesium and vitamin B2 that even aimless supplementation leads to positive *group results*.

That, however, can cause a lot of frustration for the individual patient, who now tries one substance after the other, herb after herb, anxiously hoping that the next one might be the '*magic*' bullet.

With that being said, there may be an important role for feverfew. Mixed with ginger it has been tested as an attack abortive:

- An open-label study tried GelStat Migraine® on 29 patients at the beginning of the headache phase of a migraine attack; 48% were pain-free after two hours and 34% ended up with mild headaches only. 60% of the study participants were satisfied with this comparably harmless product.[2]
- A second trial with GelStat Migraine®, this time randomized and placebo-controlled, wasn't published in a medical journal, but presented during a conference. 65% of the treatment group reported headache relief vs 36% in the placebo group. Almost 20% became pain-free after two hours.[3]
- Under the brand name LipigesicM® the same combination of feverfew and ginger was tested by 45 migraineurs on 151 attacks;[4] 32% became pain-free (16% on placebo) and 63% had pain relief (39% on placebo) after two hours.

---

[1] Diener HC et al "Efficacy and safety of 6.25 mg t.i.d. feverfew CO2-extract (MIG-99) in migraine prevention--a randomized, double-blind, multicentre, placebo-controlled study" Cephalalgia 2005;25(11):1031-41
[2] Cady RK et al "Gelstat Migraine (sublingually administered feverfew and ginger compound) for acute treatment of migraine when administered during the mild pain phase" Med Sci Monit 2005;11(9):PI65-9
[3] Aurora SK et al "GelStat is effective relieving migraine pain in a double-blind, placebo-controlled study" 58th Annual Meeting of the American Academy of Neurology, 2006 San Diego, CA
[4] Cady RK et al "A double-blind placebo-controlled pilot study of sublingual feverfew and ginger (LipiGesic™ M) in the treatment of migraine" Headache 2011;51(7):1078-86

Omega-3 fatty acids

Even in skinny people the human brain consists of 60% fat.[1] Several sources of information suggest that the human brain developed on a diet, which had a 1:1-ratio of omega-6 to omega-3 fatty acids.[2] In contrast, Western diets have a ratio between 10:1 and 25:1, indicating a deficiency in Ω (oops) omega-3 fatty acids (FA).

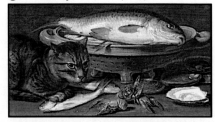

These nutrients are *essential*, because, like all mammals, humans don't have the necessary enzyme to produce'em themselves.[3] They are *important*, because more and more studies find a connection between omega-3 FA (= fatty acids) deficiency and a heap of health issues over the lifespan:[4] from developmental disorders in childhood, to depression, aggression, and schizophrenia in adulthood, and cognitive decline, dementia and Alzheimer's disease in late life; as well as cancer, inflammation, heart and autoimmune diseases.[5]

It would be interesting to find out, if migraine too is negatively affected by an omega-3 FA deficiency. For that, one would have to measure the omega-3 concentration of migraine brains in comparison to healthy brains. Nobody seems to have done that yet, but there is a clue from patients with depression, the number one comorbidity for migraineurs:

DHA (= docosahexaenoic acid, one of the omega-3 fatty acids) was missing in parts of the *prefrontal cortex* of patients with major depression compared to normals, especially in women (-32%).[6]

Neuronal membranes (= the walls of nerve cells) contain up to 50% DHA,[7] which *lowers* the brain's excitability.[8] As outlined in chapter 8, migraine brains tend to be a bit too excitable.[9]

---

[1] Chang CY "Essential fatty acids and human brain" Acta Neurol Taiwan 2009 Dec;18(4):231-41
[2] Simopoulos AP "Evolutionary aspects of diet: the omega-6/omega-3 ratio and the brain" Mol Neurobiol 2011;44(2):203-15
[3] Simopoulos AP et al "The importance of the omega-6/omega-3 fatty acid ratio in cardiovascular disease and other chronic diseases" Exp Biol Med (Maywood) 2008;233(6):674-88
[4] Sinn N et al "Oiling the brain: a review of randomized controlled trials of omega-3 fatty acids in psychopathology across the lifespan" Nutrients 2010;2(2):128-70
[5] Swanson D et al "Omega-3 fatty acids EPA and DHA: health benefits throughout life" Adv Nutr 2012 Jan;3(1):1-7
[6] McNamara RK et al "Selective deficits in the omega-3 fatty acid docosahexaenoic acid in the postmortem orbitofrontal cortex of patients with major depressive disorder" Biol Psychiatry 2007;62(1):17-24
[7] Singh M "Essential fatty acids, DHA and human brain" Indian J Pediatr 2005;72(3):239-42
[8] Saugstad LF "A "new-old" way of thinking about brain disorder, cerebral excitability--the fundamental property of nervous tissue" Med Hypotheses 2005;64(1):142-50
[9] Gunaydin S et al "Motor and occipital cortex excitability in migraine patients" Can J Neurol Sci 2006;33(1):63-7

Supplementation with omega-3 FA has been shown to reduce uncontrolled epileptic seizures[1] and to increase activation in the prefrontal cortex.[2] It looks as if this would be exactly the stuff that migraine patients could benefit from. Has anyone tried?

- A first uncontrolled pilot study in Sweden over 3 months with 41 participants resulted in significant reductions of attack frequency and intensity by about 30%. Yet, in the subgroup of migraineurs with more than one attack per week, 67% were significantly improved. Side effects were fishy burps.[3]
- A second uncontrolled trial in Denmark with the same product and dosage also came to promising findings; 57% of those with frequent attacks and 43% of the others experienced fewer attacks; 87% in total answered that the fish-oil capsules had improved their migraine condition. Eight burped fishily.[4]
- Time for 'real' science: A randomized, double-blind, placebo-controlled study with 196 participants over 16 weeks including 4-week placebo run-in and run-out periods made the French researchers scratch their heads: With fish oil the participants experienced a 55% reduction, with placebo a 45% reduction in migraine attacks, which they interpreted as *failure of omega-3 FA* in the prevention of migraine as the study title forcefully expressed.[5]

As you can see, omega-3 FA supplementation for migraineurs is not justified by studies and can't be recommended, right?

What do you think about that? Did the third study set the record straight? Were the promising results in Sweden and Denmark based on placebo? What happened here that makes the 87% happy customers in Denmark look like idiots now?

First of all, *absence of proof* is not *proof of absence*. If a trial fails to prove a benefit, that does not mean that there is none. Secondly, they've tested fish oil like a drug. Fatty acids are natural substances in food, bodies and brains, *not migraine drugs*. If those researchers can't be bothered to measure the FA levels in their subjects, how do they know they were deficient and the supplement changed that? (If the attack rate does go down, one can simply conclude that.)

---

[1] Taha AY et al "Assessing the link between omega-3 fatty acids, cardiac arrest, and sudden unexpected death in epilepsy" Epilepsy Behav 2009;14(1):27-31

[2] McNamara RK et al "Docosahexaenoic acid supplementation increases prefrontal cortex activation during sustained attention in healthy boys: a placebo-controlled, dose-ranging, functional magnetic resonance imaging study" Am J Clin Nutr 2010;91(4):1060-7

[3] Hansen K "Kan migræne påvirkes av fiskeolje? Et åbent studie" Migrænenyt 1990;5:20-22

[4] Lejnemark NO "Fiskolja hjälp mot migrän?" Migränbladet 1995;20:9

[5] Pradalier A et al "Failure of omega-3 polyunsaturated fatty acids in prevention of migraine: a double-blind study versus placebo" Cephalalgia 2001 Oct;21(8):818-22

Thirdly, what makes anybody assume that 16 weeks of real omega-3 FA supplementation is a time frame in which a noticeable result should be expected? Fourthly, why did the French do a study on *patients with very rare migraine attacks* — about 0.4 per week — although they already knew from the Scandinavian trials that infrequent migraineurs are unlikely to show a big response.

Fifthly, given the gigantic placebo response in that study, it is actually very impressive that the fish oil still managed to generate a *statistically significant difference* to the placebo group in the *number of attacks* (7 vs 6 within the 16 weeks). It was the difference in duration and the intensity of the remaining attacks that didn't reach the level of statistical significance. Did this study really show a "failure of omega-3 fatty acids for migraine prevention"? I can't help it, but something smells fishy here.

And lastly, even if omega-3 fatty acid supplementation had no effect whatsoever for attack prevention, *especially migraineurs* might also want to benefit from the (relative) protective effect against depression, aggression, Alzheimer's, as well as inflammatory, auto-immune and cardiovascular diseases. Don't you think?

You won't believe it, but it gets even better:

- A trial in the US set out to investigate whether supplementation with fish oil rich in omega-3 FA might reduce frequency and severity of migraine attacks in adolescents in a randomized, double-blind, cross-over design; after two months on either placebo or the real stuff, they paused for a month (= 'wash-out' period) and then restarted taking capsules, but now the groups were swapped for placebo or real fish oil. In the end they found massive, reductions of about 80% in headache frequency, duration and severity on fish oil, and about 70% on the placebo capsule. 90% of the patients would recommend either one to friends and relatives! [1]
Amazing, but how could the placebo too cause such a humungous effect? The placebo capsules contained olive oil, which also has omega-3 fatty acids!

The scientists understood the outcome as a clue that olive oil might be beneficial too. That is not completely new: olive oil seems to lower the omega-6 FA and so improve the "Ω-6 to Ω-3" ratio. [2]

---

[1] Harel Z et al "Supplementation with omega-3 polyunsaturated fatty acids in the management of recurrent migraines in adolescents" J Adolesc Health 2002;31(2):154-61

[2] Haban P et al "Dietary supplementation with olive oil leads to improved lipoprotein spectrum and lower n-6 PUFAs in elderly subjects" Med Sci Monit 2004;10(4):PI49-54

I hope that they don't repeat the study with linseed or borage oil in their 'ineffective' placebo capsule. Linseed oil is rich in ALA (alpha linolenic acid, an Ω-3 FA) and borage oil is a source of GLA (gamma linolenic acid, an anti-inflammatory Ω-6 FA).

- After 6 months of supplementation with ALA and GLA, 86% of 129 patients experienced a reduction in frequency, severity and duration of their migraine attacks, 22% became migraine-free, 90% had reduced nausea and vomiting[1]

Some people would argue that this could have been the result of a placebo effect and that there is not enough evidence to support omega-3 FA supplementation. *On the other hand*, how much scientific evidence is typically required and reasonable, when it comes to food and nutritional supplements?

Since an increase of omega-3 intake is recommended anyway, all these studies merely serve as motivating and encouraging 'infotainment': Don't be too surprised, when you notice the impact of fish oil capsules on your migraine!

In principle, humans can convert ALA to EPA[2] and DHA,[3] but this production line might be a bit unreliable or inefficient.[4] The preferred ratio of EPA to DHA in supplements is still under investigation and it may well turn out to depend on the intended purpose: more DHA seems good for a healthy body[5] and more EPA fosters health of mind and brain.[6,7]

Just for the average migraineur's orientation and education: In the Scandinavian fish oil studies they used an omega-3 FA dose of 2,000mg daily with a ratio of 3:2 between EPA and DHA.

Difficult, complex severe migraineurs with frequent attacks might consider taking up to 3,000mg per day for a while and/or trying out, whether they like a higher ratio of EPA to DHA better.

The fatty acid profile in the body can be tested; in red blood cells it reflects the dietary intake during the last 120 days.

---

[1] Wagner W et al "Prophylactic treatment of migraine with gamma-linolenic and alpha-linolenic acids" Cephalalgia 1997;17(2):127-30
[2] EPA = eicosapentaenoic acid, another famous omega-3 PUFA (polyunsaturated fatty acids)
[3] Burdge GC et al "Conversion of a-linolenic acid to longer-chain polyunsaturated fatty acids in human adults" Reprod Nutr Dev 2005;45:581-597
[4] Hussein N et al "Long-chain conversion of [13C]linoleic acid and alpha-linolenic acid in response to marked changes in their dietary intake in men" J Lipid Res 2005;46(2):269-80
[5] Vemuri M et al "Docosahexaenoic Acid (DHA) But Not Eicosapentaenoic Acid (EPA) Prevents Trans-10, Cis-12 Conjugated Linoleic Acid (CLA)-Induced Insulin Resistance in Mice" Metab Syndr Relat Disord 2007;5(4):315-22
[6] Martins JG et al "EPA but not DHA appears to be responsible for the efficacy of omega-3 long chain polyunsaturated fatty acid supplementation in depression: evidence from a meta-analysis of randomized controlled trials" J Am Coll Nutr 2009 Oct;28(5):525-42
[7] Kidd PM et al "Omega-3 DHA and EPA for cognition, behavior, and mood: clinical findings and structural-functional synergies with cell membrane phospholipids" Altern Med Rev 2007;12(3):207-27

Vitamin D (cholecalciferol)

Vitamins are substances that we need to take in, because our bodies can't make them. With the help of a bit of sunshine our skin can actually produce the so-called 'vitamin' D. Nevertheless, due to limited sun exposure, vitamin D deficiency is a common problem.

With growing distance from the equator, Vitamin D levels strongly decrease and the prevalence of headaches and migraine increases.[1] Data also show more headaches and migraine attacks in autumn and winter. Is that a coincidence?

Tests in a Norwegian clinic on patients with chronic pain, chronic fatigue or a headache disorder discovered that 60% of them had low vitamin D levels; the average of the headache patients was the worst amongst the three groups.

There are two articles with case reports about successful migraine treatment with vitamin D supplementation[2,3] and neurologists report their findings on the internet, but that's about it.

Let's simply say that migraineurs are probably better off when they don't add a vitamin D deficiency to their plight. Doctors can request a blood test, the *25-hydroxyvitamin D* (calcidiol) is the right one; the 1,25-OH is the wrong one.[4] Ideally, the level should be 60-80ng/ml (USA) or 150-200nmol/L (SI units).

Typical dosage for vitamin D_3 (cholecalciferol) supplementation is 10,000 IU in winter and 5,000 IU in summer, according to neurologist Dr. Stasha Gominak (www.drgominak.com). She recommends up to 20,000 IU for up to 3 weeks, if the test results are below 50 ng/ml and a re-check after 4-6 weeks.

Lowering homocysteine in some with aura

There is a connection between migraine with aura and higher levels of *homocysteine*[5] (not in Portugal though[6]), which can be treated with supplementation of 2mg of folic acid, 25mg vitamin B6 and 400mcg vitamin B12, a study found.[7] So, why not check for it?

---

[1] Prakash S et al "The prevalence of headache may be related with the latitude: a possible role of Vitamin D insufficiency?" J Headache Pain 2010;11(4):301-7

[2] Thys-Jacobs S "Alleviation of migraines with therapeutic vitamin D and calcium" Headache 1994;34(10):590-2

[3] Thys-Jacobs S "Vitamin D and calcium in menstrual migraine" Headache 1994;34(9):544-6

[4] http://www.vitamindcouncil.org

[5] Oterino A et al "The relationship between homocysteine and genes of folate-related enzymes in migraine patients" Headache 2010;50(1):99-168

[6] Ferro A et al "The C677T polymorphism in MTHFR is not associated with migraine in Portugal" Source Dis Markers 2008;25(2):107-13

[7] Lea R et al "The effects of vitamin supplementation and MTHFR (C677T) genotype on homocysteine-lowering and migraine disability" Pharmacogenet Genomics 2009;19(6):422-8

On the soapbox

As we've seen in this chapter, herbs and supplements can have quite an impact on migraine-attack frequency, duration and severity, when used correctly and with the right understanding. However, I see certain pitfalls and up here on my soapbox I feel confident enough to address them.

Medical doctors may or may not know about magnesium citrate, vitamin B2, Petadolex, coenzyme Q10, omega-3 fatty acids, vitamin D and feverfew, but doctors are typically not aware that, on average, these benign substances are *just as effective* as prescription drugs for attack prevention.[1] Let's talk about their advantages:

- Serious risks and side effects practically don't exist.
- You can combine as many as you need.
- They have multiple effects in the body, think of omega-3 FA!
- Patients can buy'em themselves, adjust the dosage themselves.
- They can still be combined with prescription drugs, if need be.

Problems arise, when patients mistake them for drugs and expect immediate and absolute protection against attacks. On internet forums I frequently find posts like "I'VE TRIED (NAME OF THE STUFF), BUT IT DIDN'T DO MUCH FOR ME." That's discouraging for others, isn't it?

How do you know that it didn't do much for you? Have you measured the levels before supplementation and after? What were the attack frequency, duration and severity before and after supplementation? "DIDN'T DO MUCH" is not informative, but the expression of hurt and disappointment: Hurt by what? Disappointed by whom?

Taking supplements against nutritional deficiencies is not in all cases enough to stop migraine attacks, perhaps not even enough to reduce anything in some cases; but it's a constructive step.

In most difficult and complex cases *one* productive step is probably not sufficient; many more are necessary. Some patients typically experience '*insurmountable*' *difficulties* at every single step, like Erica: "I'VE TRIED IT ONCE, AND THE RESULT WAS HELL."

In the world of supplements this sentence translates to: "I'VE TRIED TAKING MAGNESIUM, BUT IT GAVE ME HORRIBLE DIARRHEA." Okay, but why are you telling me that? How is this helpful for you or me?

---

[1] Diener HC et al "Effectiveness of chemical, herbal and dietetic migraine prophylactis. An overview of randomized controlled double-blind studies" MMW Fortschr Med 2009;151(24):42-5

Reactive migraineurs are well advised to slowly slowly slowly ease into taking magnesium. Starting with 600mg magnesium *oxide* daily is possibly not the best idea, but even after learning that lesson, there is no reason to give up: shit happens!

Patients respond differently to the various magnesium products and sometimes one needs to swap from one to the other. As transdermal 'oil', magnesium chloride normally has no accelerating effect on the digestion, but we need to be prepared that some reactive migraine patients may prove us wrong.

Skin reactions are also likely in some and it might take some hefty diluting with water before *hyperreactive* migraineurs can tolerate magnesium oil.

The example of Erica (see chapter 6) demonstrates that some 'difficult' and complex migraineurs don't have the skills to protect themselves against their own reactivity by taking sensible baby steps. It seems as if the "WORLD IS HOSTILE", particularly towards *them* and anything can potentially attack and hurt them ("ANYTHING CAN BE A MIGRAINE TRIGGER"). Supplements can easily end up in the role of the *assassin* and the reactive migraineur as the *victim* in this drama.

Psychodynamic psychologists would possibly interpret these scenarios as "re-enactment of abuses", which many difficult patients have suffered, as studies show (see chapter 5). We *mustn't reward* them with our sympathy and thereby make matters worse. Instead, we must teach them what *reasonable* steps to take and how to protect oneself by increasing resistance and stability.

There are many more vitamins, minerals and herbs that are discussed in migraine forums and websites, almost always in their potential role as drug replacement, as protective agent, as savior. Whilst some simple and easy migraineurs (think of Clare in chapter 5) will tolerate everything and thrive on anything, 'difficult' and complex cases like Erica or Daisy are urgently advised to take a way more scientific approach: Testing levels at every corner may be cumbersome, but it reduces the guesswork and the emotional load.

Testing versus trying

In severe, 'difficult' and complex cases it can be a smart move to put a bit more effort in to guarantee that the body's biochemistry is in good balance and no potential poison is forgotten.

There are several useful tests available that allow a detailed view into the body's biochemistry, for instance:

Hair mineral analysis (HMA or HTMA = hair trace mineral analysis) is a relatively cost-effective way to screen for mineral 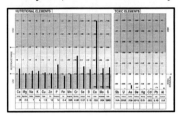 deficiencies and heavy metal poisoning. There is no shortage of passionate reviews in medical journals, condemning the use of HMA,[1] based on a few dodgy labs. If performed by a lab that doesn't wash the hair sample with chemicals, HMA is a reliable[2,3] screening tool and used in research.[4,5] Confirmatory tests with other body tissues for critical parameters are always a good idea. Recommended by experts (drlwilson.com) are these labs: Analytical Research Labs in Arizona (arltma.com), Trace Elements Inc. in Texas (traceelements.com) and InterClinical Laboratories in NSW, Australia (interclinical.com.au).

An *Organix Comprehensive Profile* informs about energy production, detoxification, neurotransmitter breakdown and intestinal microbial activity. Naturopaths, nutritionists and other practitioners of Functional Medicine, who professionally test and tweak the body's biochemistry with diet and nutraceuticals, typically use tests like these.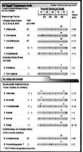

A case in point

A 7 year-old boy started having terrible migraine attacks. His parents took him to the family doctor, who referred them on to a neurologist. The expert doctor ordered an MRI brain scan (see chapter 7) to rule out tumors and demons. Neither one were found and so the neurologist shrugged his shoulders.

Unhappy with the lack of therapeutic progress, the concerned parents took their suffering offspring to a naturopathic doctor.

---

[1] Seidel S et al "Assessment of commercial laboratories performing hair mineral analysis" JAMA 2001;285(1):67-72
[2] Shamberger RJ "Validity of hair mineral testing" Biol Trace Elem Res 2002;87(1-3):1-28
[3] Miekeley N et al "Elemental Anomalies in Hair as Indicators of Endocrinologic Pathologies and Deficiencies in Calcium and Bone Metabolism" J Trace Elem Med Biol 2001;15(1):46-55
[4] Kim YS et al "Women with fibromyalgia have lower levels of calcium, magnesium, iron and manganese in hair mineral analysis" J Korean Med Sci 2011;26(10):1253-7
[5] Rahman A et al "Zinc, manganese, calcium, copper, and cadmium level in scalp hair samples of schizophrenic patients" Biol Trace Elem Res 2009;127(2):102-8

Dr. Sharrie Hanley,[1] the naturopath, suggested a hair mineral analysis (HMA) to get an overview of the status of 35 nutrient and toxic minerals (As we already know, that is a "money-making quack test" that no serious mainstream doctor would ever consider). Anyway, the desperate parents followed the naturopath's idea and sent a lock, freshly cut off the boy's scalp, to the laboratory.

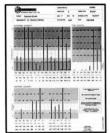

← The report exposed an excessively elevated copper level (700%) and a severe deficiency in zinc. Hereupon it turned out that the father did copper flashings on roofs for a living and stored the leftovers in the yard. Guess who played with it?

Zinc and copper need to be in balance, since zinc is required for copper metabolism.[2] Brains are clearly better off without *copper toxicity*, a suspected risk factor for Alzheimer's disease[3] and migraine.[4]

Long story short: "Copper-boy" was given a zinc supplement, daddy cleared the yard of scrap metal and voilà, the terrible migraine attacks ceased. The second HMA shows copper levels coming down, even without *liposomal glutathione* and vitamin C, which is the present remedy for excess copper.[5] The moral of this story: A bit of *detective work* can pay off big time.

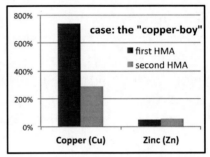

My favorite supplier for any type of supplement is iherb.com with good prices and fast delivery. My esteemed readers can save $5 at iHerb with *discount code* "ICA553".

The many placebo-controlled studies that we've reviewed so far remind us of a greater power: Study subjects know that they only have a *50%-chance* of getting just a test substance of *uncertain efficacy* and still up to 45% had noticeably fewer migraine attacks on placebo. This shows the unparalleled potency of one of the most mighty supplements in migraine therapy: a glimmer of hope.

---

[1] Dr. Sharrie Hanley, Rutland,Vermont/USA; www.drsharrie.com (Thanks for the case example, Sharrie)
[2] Harris ED "Zinc and Copper: Evidence for Interdependence, Not Antagonism" Nutrition 2001;17:734–742
[3] Brewer GJ "Copper excess, zinc deficiency, and cognition loss in Alzheimer's disease" Biofactors 2012;38(2):107-13
[4] Harrison DP "Copper as a factor in the dietary precipitation of migraine" Headache 1986;26(5):248-50
[5] Hatori Y et al "Functional partnership of the copper export machinery and glutathione balance in human cells" J Biol Chem 2012;287(32):26678-87

Chapter 16

Being Watched by Angels

"When I woke up this morning my girlfriend asked me, 'Did you sleep good?'
I said, 'No, I made a few mistakes.'"

Steven Wright

Migraine and sleep

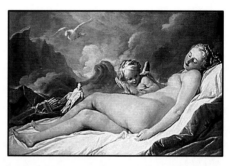

According to a study, 50% of migraineurs indicate that their migraine attacks are 'triggered' by "poor" sleep.[1] Another one found that sleep quality and duration were reduced in nights before an attack.[2] For many migraineurs the majority of their episodes start at night or in the early morning.[3] But also between attacks patients report a diminished quality[4] and duration[1] of sleep; most wake up with headaches.[1] *Bad sleepers* typically have more severe attacks.[1]

Further down the track, chronic migraineurs apparently display *poor sleeping habits* and suffer from non-restorative sleep. No wonder that 84% wake up tired[5] and two thirds of them meet the criteria for *chronic fatigue syndrome*.[6] Squashed into a catchy slogan we could summarize: Episodic migraine plus insomnia equals chronic migraine with 'cream' (e.g. fatigue, depression[7]).

Sleeping correctly

It doesn't take much effort to apply a few simple principles for improved sleep "hygiene", which can be found in many books and all over the internet. They do indeed increase sleep duration and reduce migraine attack rates in children as well as in adults.[8]

---

[1] Kelman L et al "Headache and sleep: examination of sleep patterns and complaints in a large clinical sample of migraineurs" Headache 2005;45(7):904-10
[2] Niederberger U et al "Sleeping behavior and migraine. An evaluation by daily self-reports" Schmerz 1998;12(6):389-95
[3] Gori S et al "Sleep quality, chronotypes and preferential timing of attacks in migraine without aura" J Headache Pain 2005;6(4):258-60
[4] Seidel S et al "Quality of sleep, fatigue and daytime sleepiness in migraine - a controlled study" Cephalalgia 2009;29(6):662-9
[5] Calhoun AH et al "The prevalence and spectrum of sleep problems in women with transformed migraine" Headache 2006;46(4):604-10
[6] Peres MF et al "Fatigue in chronic migraine patients" Cephalalgia 2002;22(9):720-4
[7] Fava M et al "Daytime sleepiness and insomnia as correlates of depression" J Clin Psychiatry 2004;65 Suppl 16:27-32
[8] Bruni O et al "Sleep hygiene and migraine in children and adolescents" Cephalalgia 1999;19 Suppl 25:57-9

Moreover, adopting good sleeping habits helped almost 50% of the chronic migraineurs in one study to revert back to episodic migraine.[1] That is remarkable, but why weren't they taught earlier?

Hygienic slumber advice can be found on many websites, for example at "www.sleepoz.org.au" under "Fact Sheets". Sleep well!

When warm milk doesn't work

As we've seen, insomnia in addition to migraine can be a real complication. So let's put our thinking caps on and leave the beaten path to find sincere solutions for those serious cases with severe migraine and persistent sleep issues.

We've learnt that the more severe, complex and difficult migraineurs don't sleep all that well anyway. Could it be that they would revert back to simple and easy cases, if only they slept well?

What happens to healthy people, when their sleep is badly sabotaged, e.g. by a baby? After a couple of bad nights they ...

... can't concentrate at work[2]	... struggle remembering stuff[3]
... are tense and distressed[4]	... are grumpy and irritable: tetchy[5]
... become a bit clumsy[6]	... are nervous and upset[7]
... start complaining about headaches[8] and other pains.[9]	

Now listen carefully, because I have a question for you: When 1. you look at this list and 2. consider everything I've taught you about the functions of the *prefrontal cortex* — e.g. in chapter 8 — which prefrontal area of the brain seems to pay the price, when good sleep is in short supply?

        a) area 51   O

        b) the *prefrontal cortex*   O ← !!!

        c) where the hair is longest   O

Well done, I knew you wouldn't disappoint me.

---

[1] Calhoun AH et al "Behavioral sleep modification may revert transformed migraine to episodic migraine" Headache 2007;47(8):1178-83
[2] Alhola P et al "Sleep deprivation: Impact on cognitive performance" Neuropsychiatr Dis Treat 2007;3(5):553–567
[3] Boonstra TW et al "Effects of sleep deprivation on neural functioning: an integrative review" Cell Mol Life Sci 2007;64(7-8):934–946
[4] Kato M et al "Effects of sleep deprivation on neural circulatory control" Hypertension 2000;35(5):1173-5
[5] Babson KA et al "A test of the effects of acute sleep deprivation on general and specific self-reported anxiety and depressive symptoms: an experimental extension" J Behav Ther Exp Psychiatry 2010;41(3):297-303
[6] Ayalon RD et al "The effect of sleep deprivation on fine motor coordination in obstetrics and gynecology residents" Am J Obstet Gynecol 2008;199(5):576.e1-5
[7] Kahn-Greene ET et al "The effects of sleep deprivation on symptoms of psychopathology in healthy adults" Sleep Med 2007;8(3):215-21
[8] Blau JN "Sleep deprivation headache" Cephalalgia 1990;10(4):157-60
[9] Pieh C et al "Sleep and pain: a bi-directional relation?" Psychiatr Prax 2011;38(4):166-70

Exactly, it's the prefrontal cortex (PFC) which is particularly vulnerable to sleep disturbances.[1,2,3,4,5,6] When the PFC doesn't get its beauty sleep, things can get ugly pretty quickly. The 'animal' parts of the brain take over (see page 186 about the triune brain) and our behavior becomes more emotional and instinctive. Since the PFC is too tired to keep the 'beasts' in their cages, we tend to be a bit stupid,[7] anxious and depressed,[8] as well as a little more crazy[9] and aggressive[10] than we would like to be.

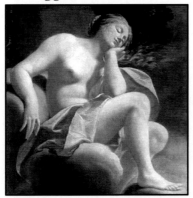

Lack of good sleep also promotes more seizure activity in the cortex,[11,12] a fact that neurologists use to provoke epileptic activity in patients' brains for diagnostic purposes.[13] They know that a tired prefrontal cortex can't constrain the brain's neuronal 'tension', and so the cortex ends up highly excitable and ready to seize.[14] In migraine it's the brainstem that ends up in a seizure, but the migraineur's hyperexcitable cortex[15] seems to intensify the reported sleep problems. Especially the visual cortex was found to be hyperexcitable,[16] thereby probably increasing the sensitivity to light,[17] which in turn is thought to interfere with the release of the 'sleep hormone' melatonin.[18] In short:

poor sleep → lame PFC → bad arousal control → hyperexcitable cortex → increased light sensitivity → reduced melatonin release → poor sleep ...

[1] Harrison Y et al "Sleep loss impairs short and novel language tasks having a prefrontal focus" J Sleep Res 1998;7(2):95-100
[2] Harrison Y et al "Prefrontal neuropsychological effects of sleep deprivation in young adults" Sleep 2000;23(8):1067-73
[3] Muzur A et al "The prefrontal cortex in sleep" Trends Cogn Sci 2002;6(11):475-481
[4] Schwartz J et al "Neurophysiology of Sleep and Wakefulness: Basic Science and Clinical Implications" Curr Neuropharmacol 2008;6(4):367–37
[5] Altena E et al "Prefrontal Hypoactivation and Recovery in Insomnia" Sleep 2008;31(9):1271–1276
[6] Tucker AM et al "The prefrontal model revisited: double dissociations between young sleep deprived and elderly subjects on cognitive components of performance" Sleep 2011;34(8):1039-50
[7] Curcio G et "Sleep loss, learning capacity and academic performance" Sleep Med Rev 2006;10(5):323-37
[8] Terauchi M et al "Associations between anxiety, depression and insomnia in peri- and post-menopausal women" Maturitas 2012;72(1):61-5
[9] Brand S et al "Sleep and its importance in adolescence and in common adolescent somatic and psychiatric conditions" Int J Gen Med 2011;4:425–442
[10] Kamphuis J et al "Poor sleep as a potential causal factor in aggression and violence" Sleep Med 2012;13(4):327-34
[11] Méndez M et al "Interactions between sleep and epilepsy" J Clin Neurophysiol 2001;18(2):106-27
[12] Kwan SY "Sleep in patients with epilepsy" Acta Neurol Taiwan 2011;20(4):229-131
[13] Wassmer E et al "The acceptability of sleep-deprived electroencephalograms" Seizure 1999;8(7):434-5
[14] Scalise A et al "Increasing cortical excitability: a possible explanation for the proconvulsant role of sleep deprivation" Sleep 2006;29(12):1595-8
[15] Mulleners WM et al "Visual cortex excitability in migraine with and without aura" Headache 2001;41(6):565-72
[16] Gunaydin S et al "Motor and occipital cortex excitability in migraine patients" Can J Neurol Sci 2006;33(1):63-7
[17] Claustrat B et al "Melatonin secretion is supersensitive to light in migraine" Cephalalgia 2004;24(2):128-33
[18] Claustrat B et al "Nocturnal plasma melatonin levels in migraine: a preliminary report" Headache 1989;29(4):242-5

Slumber doping

Melatonin can be supplemented and, according to the studies, it might even be a good idea for those migraineurs who have serious difficulties with sleep and who are getting worse.

Study 1: Children with migraine and tension-type headaches were given 3mg of melatonin for three months. 66% reported at least a halving of their headache attacks, 20% became headache-free. One kid had to stop taking the melatonin, because of excessive daytime sleepiness[1] (I would have tried a lower dose first).

Study 2: 80% of adults who were taking 3mg melatonin at night had fewer headaches.[2] Sounds promising, doesn't it?

Study 3, however, wrecked it: In a double blind, randomized, placebo-controlled cross-over study a dose of only 2mg of melatonin daily reduced the average number of migraine attacks from 4.2 to 2.8 per month, just like the placebo pill.[3]

Melatonin is not a dangerous drug; it's a hormone that gets released from the pineal gland. As a supplement, it's not overly expensive. I can't think of a compelling reason why migraineurs with sleep issues shouldn't give melatonin a try until the real insomnia therapies are in place—despite conflicting study results. A meta-analysis did find melatonin effective in the treatment of 'delayed sleep phase disorder' (e.g. jet lag, shift workers).[4]

An alternative to swallowing additional melatonin could be to protect the body's own production. Especially the blue part of the light spectrum, present in artificial light and emitted from TVs and computer monitors, interferes with natural melatonin release.[5,6]

Amber tinted glasses that block out blue light have been found quite effective in boosting melatonin levels[7] and thereby as sleep enhancing aid.[8] They also help shift workers sleep well.[9] Thumbs up for sleep thanks to amber, low-blue-light glasses in the evening!

---

[1] Miano S et al "Melatonin to prevent migraine or tension-type headache in children" Neurol Sci 2008;29(4):285-7
[2] Peres MF et al "Melatonin, 3 mg, is effective for migraine prevention" Neurology 2004;63(4):757
[3] Alstadhaug KB et al "Prophylaxis of migraine with melatonin: a randomized controlled trial" Neurology 2010;75(17):1527-32
[4] van Geijlswijk IM et al "The use of exogenous melatonin in delayed sleep phase disorder: a meta-analysis" Sleep 2010;33(12):1605-14
[5] Gooley JJ et al "Exposure to room light before bedtime suppresses melatonin onset and shortens melatonin duration in humans" J Clin Endocrinol Metab 2011;96(3):E463-72
[6] Figueiro MG et al "The impact of light from computer monitors on melatonin levels in college students" Neuro Endocrin Lett 2011;32(2):158-63
[7] Sasseville A et al "Blue blocker glasses impede the capacity of bright light to suppress melatonin production" J Pineal Res 2006;41(1):73-8
[8] Burkhart K et al "Amber lenses to block blue light and improve sleep: a randomized trial" Chronobiol Int 2009;26(8):1602-12
[9] Sasseville A et al "Wearing blue-blockers in the morning could improve sleep of workers on a permanent night schedule: a pilot study" Chronobiol Int 2009;26(5):913-25

Killing three birds with one stone

Insomnia is the result of difficulties with the regulation of brain arousal. When the balance between the prefrontal cortex, the limbic system and the brainstem is out of whack, all sorts of problems arise — for instance poor sleep, mood issues or migraine attacks in predisposed patients — as an expression of the underlying problem of uncontrolled *hyperarousal*.[1,2,3,4,5]

Instead of taking drugs for the headaches, drugs for anxiety, drugs for depression and sleeping pills as 'dessert', wouldn't it be a smart move to improve the ability to regulate one's brain's arousal?

In the case of migraine and poor sleep, the appropriate therapies for the *underlying* problem (right brain hyperarousal) are:

- PFC infrared neurofeedback training[6]
- symptom-based neurofeedback training[7]
- infra-low frequency neurofeedback training[8]
- Z-score neurofeedback training[9]
- QEEG-guided neurofeedback training[10]
- LoRETA neurofeedback training
- low energy neurofeedback (LENS)[11]
- EMG biofeedback, progressive muscle relaxation[12]
- autogenic training[13]
- mind therapies/psychological coaching[14]
- moderate aerobic exercise[15]

---

[1] Bastien CH et al "Chronic psychophysiological insomnia: hyperarousal and/or inhibition deficits? An ERPs investigation" Sleep 2008;31(6):887-98

[2] Bonnet MH et al "Hyperarousal and insomnia: state of the science" Sleep Med Rev 2010;14(1):9-15

[3] Riemann D et al "The hyperarousal model of insomnia: a review of the concept and its evidence" Sleep Med Rev 2010;14(1):19-31

[4] Terzano MG et al "Neurological perspectives in insomnia and hyperarousal syndromes" Handb Clin Neurol 2011;99:697-721

[5] Fernández-Mendoza J et al "Cognitive-emotional hyperarousal as a premorbid characteristic of individuals vulnerable to insomnia" Psychosom Med 2010;72(4):397-403

[6] Carmen JA "Passive infrared hemoencephalography: Four years and 100 migraines" Journal of Neurotherapy 2004;8(3),23-51

[7] Hoedlmoser K et al "Instrumental conditioning of human sensorimotor rhythm (12-15 Hz) and its impact on sleep as well as declarative learning" Sleep 2008;31(10):1401-8

[8] Massimini M et al "EEG slow (approximately 1 Hz) waves are associated with nonstationarity of thalamo-cortical sensory processing in the sleeping human" J Neurophysiol 2003;89(3):1205-13

[9] Hammer BU et al "Neurofeedback for insomnia: a pilot study of Z-score SMR and individualized protocols" Appl Psychophysiol Biofeedback 2011;36(4):251-64

[10] Walker JE "QEEG-guided neurofeedback for recurrent migraine headaches" Clin EEG Neurosci 2011;42(1):59-61

[11] Larsen S et al "The LENS (Low Energy Neurofeedback System): A Clinical Outcomes Study on One Hundred Patients at Stone Mountain Center" Journal of Neurotherapy 2006;10:2-3,69-78

[12] Morin CM et al "Nonpharmacologic treatment of chronic insomnia. An American Academy of Sleep Medicine review" Sleep 1999;22(8):1134-56

[13] Bowden A et al "Autogenic Training as a behavioural approach to insomnia: a prospective cohort study" Prim Health Care Res Dev 2012;13(2):175-85

[14] Wang MY et al "Cognitive behavioural therapy for primary insomnia: a systematic review" J Adv Nurs 2005;50(5):553-64

[15] Passos GS et al "Effects of moderate aerobic exercise training on chronic primary insomnia" Sleep Med 2011;12(10):1018-27

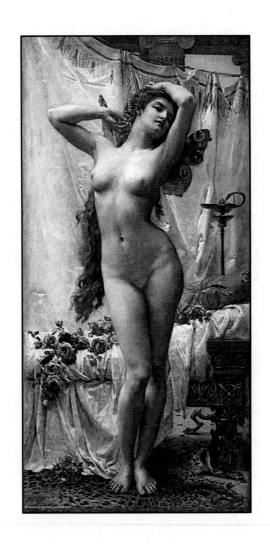

Chapter 17

Balancing Your Urges

> "Hormones, like a family, function together
> – and they dysfunction together."
> Janet Lang

Hormones

The word 'hormone' allegedly comes from the Greek word for urge, impulse or impetus. More than 50 different hormones act as messenger substances in body and brain, not dissimilar to neurotransmitters (see page 160) since they also dock onto specific receptors on the cell's surface.

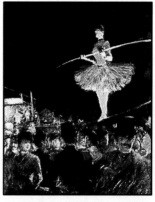

Unfortunate limits

This may well be a disappointing chapter, because I'm going to point out problems without offering a perfect solution. Prescribing bio-identical hormone supplementation is a task reserved for medical doctors. Therefore, all I can do is inform you and keep my fingers crossed that you can find a doc who is up to that task.

A second limitation is the fact that this book is about migraine, which by itself is a gigantic topic and it is simply not possible to squeeze another huge subject like *migraine and the 50 hormones* into a chapter; it would take a separate book.

For some readers, the revelation that migraine is more than a very bad headache—caused by cheese, red wine and chocolate—might be too challenging already, but many others will (hopefully) appreciate gaining at least some insight into the involvement of the hormone system in the multi-faceted body-mind-&-brain disorder that is migraine.

What about Estrogens?

Strictly speaking, there are three hormones in the group called *estrogens*: estradiol (E2), estriol and estrone. Articles for laypeople often refer to the most abundant of the three, estradiol (E2), when they say "estrogen". I'll also use 'estrogen' or 'estradiol' for 'E2'.

In childhood the occurrence of migraine is roughly the same amongst boys and girls (4%). As soon as puberty strikes, the distribution of migraine shifts in dubious favor of the women (18%) versus men (6%).[1] Is there something else that changes at that time?

During puberty, estradiol levels rise in girls *and* boys, but in girls to *five times* the boys' levels, which leads to the widely known and obvious consequences: Little girls turn into young women and some of them start having migraine attacks. Why is that?

Estrogen (E2) does not only have various effects on the body, but also acts as a neuromodulator in the brain: E2 increases excitability and *promotes seizure activity*.[2,3] Logically, those girls who are predisposed—due to genetic 'talent', early life stress, imperfect attachment experiences, overbreathing, 'wobbly' PFC, low magnesium or omega-3 FA levels etc.—develop the episodic brainstem seizures that we know as migraine attacks: the higher the estrogen levels, the more encouragement for seizure activity.[4,5] That's old hat in epileptology (= seizure knowledge).

Are we drowning in estrogen?

Let's keep this short. It is common knowledge and rather obvious that the age at which girls start developing bosoms, is dropping.[6] Boobies are the work of estrogen and even boys, ambitious bodybuilders and men beyond their prime grow boobs when estradiol levels are too high.

Surprisingly, studies don't find elevated *natural* hormone levels in prematurely buxom maidens.[7] This supports horror stories and conspiracy theories that are popular amongst environmentalists and other new-age party poopers: Allegedly—but who would ever believe such nonsense—our environment, drinking water and food supply is heavily polluted with chemicals that act like estrogen in the human body: xenoestrogens.[8]

---

[1] Silberstein SD et al "Sex hormones and headache" Rev Neurol (Paris) 2000;156 Suppl 4:4S30-41
[2] Scharfman HE et al "The Influence of Gonadal Hormones on Neuronal Excitability, Seizures, and Epilepsy in the Female" Epilepsia 2006;47(9):1423–1440
[3] Frye CA "Hormonal influences on seizures: basic neurobiology" Int Rev Neurobiol 2008;83:27-77
[4] Herzog AG et al "A comparison of anastrozole and testosterone versus placebo and testosterone for treatment of sexual dysfunction in men with epilepsy and hypogonadism" Epilepsy Behav 2010;17(2):264-71
[5] Velíšková J et al "Sex and hormonal influences on seizures and epilepsy" Horm Behav 2012 Apr [Epub ahead of print]
[6] Parent AS et al "The Timing of Normal Puberty and the Age Limits of Sexual Precocity: Variations around the World, Secular Trends, and Changes after Migration" Endocr Rev 2003;24(5):668-93
[7] Aksglaede L et al "Recent decline in age at breast development: the Copenhagen Puberty Study" Pediatrics 2009;123(5):e932-9
[8] Watanabe H et al "Tissue-specific estrogenic and non-estrogenic effects of a xenoestrogen, nonylphenol" J Mol Endocrinol 2004;33(1):243-52

"Xeno" (from the Greek word 'xenos') means 'foreign' and so xenoestrogens are foreign compounds with estrogenic consequences in body and brain (e.g. more seizure activity, soft chest tissue growth etc.). They are only one group in the opulent world of EDCs (= endocrine disrupting chemicals). "Endocrine" refers to the hormone system and EDCs—allegedly—wreak havoc there.

According to a statement paper issued by the Endocrine Society (USA) there is strong and mounting evidence that EDCs play a role in infertility, breast and prostate cancer, malformations, thyroid problems, obesity and diabetes, to mention just a few growing concerns in the industrialized world. Since they only list 485 scientific references, I think we can dismiss that society's statement with one convincing argument: "If our environment were full of xenoestrogens and other EDCs, *they* would have told us on TV and IT WOULD HAVE BEEN ON THE FRONT PAGE OF EVERY NEWSPAPER!"

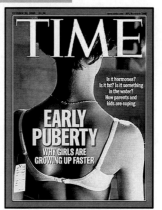

Instead it was the cover story of only one, little known, regional magazine of debatable reputation in October 2000 named CLOCK or something like that.

Also, xenoestrogens can be found in mother's milk.[1] So *they* can't be feminizing the hormone system: 8-year-old girls who enter puberty have normally been *weaned* several years prior. How about that?

What about menstrual migraine?

The final argument against the ridiculous idea that estradiol and xenoestrogens promote migraine attacks is the connection between menstruation and migraine. Most women—but especially those with menstrual/menstrually related migraine—know that near the beginning of the period migraine attacks are more likely and more severe. That proves impressively that *falling* estrogen levels promote attacks, everybody knows that and everybody says that, therefore it must be true. For that reason, *estrogen* replacement therapy is frequently used in the treatment of menstrual migraine and is *extraordinarily successful*.

Okay, that is not entirely correct. In fact, that is **not true** at all.

---

[1] Massart F et al "Human breast milk and xenoestrogen exposure: a possible impact on human health" J Perinatol 2005;25(4):282-8

Strangely, estrogen replacement therapy was repeatedly found to provoke and *promote* migraine attacks in women.[1,2,3] This is so weird. How can falling estrogen levels be a migraine 'trigger', but avoiding that 'trigger' with estrogen replacement doesn't work?

What a pity!

If migraine attacks were seizures—for instance in the brainstem—then we could ask eliptologists (seizure doctors) about what they know about seizures and the menstrual cycle. They would say that we should also look at *progesterone*, because *progesterone reduces seizure activity*. Consequently, the ratio between estradiol and progesterone relates well to seizure propensity.[4,5]

Seizure doctors also know that it's not the falling *estrogen levels* that promote seizure activity, but the dropping *progesterone levels* before the period. It's old hat![6] To be more precise, it's not the progesterone itself, but the *allopregnenolone*, a metabolite of progesterone, that inhibits seizure activity directly.[7]

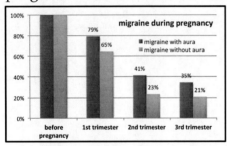 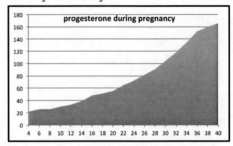

⬆ With a "bun in the oven" most migraine women lose their attacks; the effect *increases* during baking time,[8] *just like progesterone levels*. Or is that just a coincidence?

Women with menstrually related epilepsy (called catamenial) get successfully treated with natural progesterone replacement therapy.[9] *What a pity* that migraine attacks are not a form of seizure in the brainstem; at least not in the eyes of most doctors. Not yet.

What do you reckon, is it time for a migraine revolution?

---

[1] Silberstein SD "Sex hormones and headache" Rev Neurol (Paris) 2000;156 Suppl 4:4S30-41
[2] Brandes JL "The influence of estrogen on migraine: a systematic review" JAMA 2006;295(15):1824-30
[3] Loder E et al "Hormonal management of migraine associated with menses and the menopause: a clinical review" Headache 2007 Feb;47(2):329-40
[4] Bonuccelli U et al "Unbalanced progesterone and estradiol secretion in catamenial epilepsy" Epilepsy Res 1989;3(2):100-6
[5] Herzog AG "Reproductive endocrine considerations and hormonal therapy for women with epilepsy" Epilepsia 1991;32 Suppl 6:S27-33
[6] Cogen PH et al "Ovarian steroid hormones and cerebral function" Adv Neurol 1979;26:123-33
[7] Reddy DS, et al "Neurosteroid replacement therapy for catamenial epilepsy" Neurotherapeutics 2009;6(2):392-401
[8] Serva WA et al "Course of migraine during pregnancy among migraine sufferers before pregnancy" Arq Neuropsiquiatr 2011;69(4):613-9
[9] Stevens SJ et al "Hormonal therapy for epilepsy" Curr Neurol Neurosci Rep 2011;11(4):435-42

Well, it looks as if estrogen is quite ghastly and progesterone is very kind and friendly, am I right?

And yet another twist!

On the other hand, estradiol replacement is popular for women during and after menopause to prevent hot flushes, vaginal dryness, osteoporosis and heart disease, but also to avert *mood swings*, *insomnia* and *memory problems*.[1] Does that ring a bell?

Ladies, what have I taught you? Which prefrontal area of the brain is responsible for preventing the *mood* from swinging? What's behind the forehead that can appease the arousal control in the brainstem, so that we can sleep and not suffer from *insomnia*? Who, if not the prefrontal cortex, might show its weakness as a lack of concentration and *memory* problems?[2]

And, ladies, while we're at it: Has anyone ever told you that you're not quite as gorgeous and lovable as normal in the days leading up to your period? Well, now is the time.

Estradiol has an overall activating effect on the brain; we've talked about that, right? Now think hard about this extremely difficult question: Which prefrontal area of the brain's cortex behind the forehead *also loses activation* when estrogen levels plummet before the monthly 'crimson tide'?[3] (Okay, I'll give you a hint: it is often wonky, shaky or wobbly in migraine patients)

a) PVC O   b) KFC O   c) PFC (prefrontal cortex) O

Exactly, when estradiol runs out, the prefrontal cortex so sadly misses estrogen's encouragement that it can't be bothered to do a good job anymore. That's why some chicks are a bit cranky[4] before 'Eva's curse' and other dames have a really tough time with PMS (= premenstrual syndrome) or even PMDD (= premenstrual dysphoric disorder),[5,6,7,8] which actually is not funny.

---

[1] U.S. Department of Health & Human Services "Facts about Menopausal Hormone Therapy" /women/pht_facts.pdf 2012 Apr 25
[2] Resnick SM et al "Effects of estrogen replacement therapy on PET cerebral blood flow and neuropsychological performance" Horm Behav 1998;34(2):171-82
[3] Shansky RM et al "Estrogen prevents norepinephrine alpha-2a receptor reversal of stress-induced working memory impairment" Stress 2009;12(5):457–463
[4] Ossewaarde L et al "Neural mechanisms underlying changes in stress-sensitivity across the menstrual cycle" Psychoneuroendocrinology 2010;35(1)
[5] Baehr E et al "Premenstrual dysphoric disorder and changes in frontal alpha asymmetry" Int J Psychophysiol 2004;52(2):159-67
[6] Accortt EE et al "Frontal EEG asymmetry and premenstrual dysphoric symptomatology" J Abnorm Psychol 2006;115(1):179-84
[7] Batra NA et al "Proton magnetic resonance spectroscopy measurement of brain glutamate levels in premenstrual dysphoric disorder" Biol Psychiatry 2008;63(12):1178-84
[8] Accortt EE et al "Prefrontal brain asymmetry and pre-menstrual dysphoric disorder symptomatology" J Affect Disord 2011;128(1-2):178-83

"That is so interesting, but what the (beep) does all that have to do with migraine?"

We've learnt in chapter eight that the PFC has to maintain control over the limbic system and the brainstem, not unlike a lion tamer in a circus: If he is not up to the task, the beasts get out of control. Same thing for the PFC: If the PFC is weakened by the drop in estrogen, it can't control the *limbic system*, which makes women cranky before 'code red'; and it can't control the *brainstem*, which allows for a migraine attack. In a way it's quite simple.

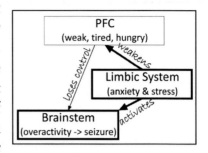

"How do I know that you're telling the truth? All the other books and websites say ..."

That is a good question and completely justified. As we've already learnt in chapter 8, the PAG in the brainstem has the task to stop body signals from activating the pain network, not too dissimilar to a bouncer in front of a nightclub who only works well when the boss keeps an eye on him. As soon as the PFC (boss) loses control over the PAG (bouncer) in the brainstem, body signals can activate the pain matrix more easily. That's what happens when estrogen in the prefrontal cortex drops before Aunt Flow's visit.

I suggest that every female reader who is still struggling with this concept, picks up the telephone, rings her favorite cosmetic parlor to make an appointment for a long and thorough *bikini wax* session late in her next premenstrual week. That should bring clarity about the connection between estradiol and the PFC on one side and the brainstem and pain on the other.

Estrogen and progesterone have *massive* effects on the brain and — when out of balance — on migraine attacks. When estradiol is not sufficiently *balanced* by progesterone (= "estrogen dominance") it can have lots of negative consequences; breast cancer is one nasty example,[1,2] epileptic and migraine seizures are two more.

Estradiol and progesterone are neither *'migraine triggers'*, nor are they *'migraine medication'*. If you ladies don't understand that, let me know and I'll change your booking to a full 'Brazilian'.

---

[1] Cowan LD et al "Breast cancer incidence in women with a history of progesterone deficiency" Am J Epidemiol 1981;114(2):209-17
[2] Lyytinen H et al "Breast cancer risk in postmenopausal women using estrogen-only therapy" Obstet Gynecol 2006;108(6):1354-60

How do you balance hormones?

In a perfect world, every patient with diminished wellbeing or health issues, especially those with a *disorder*, would first undergo an examination of the main *regulatory* systems: brain/nervous system, hormone and immune system. And while you're at it, you would have all the major biochemical pathways checked for roadblocks and the mind for unhelpful, unbalanced beliefs.

That is different in the real world, because conventional medicine is caught in the lopsided model of disease and looks for promising targets for drugs and surgery. The concept of symptoms as an expression of an '*out of whack*' system is completely foreign, perhaps even repulsive to the medical establishment. (A small but growing number of thoughtful doctors are aware of that and have begun to practice a more 'holistic' or 'integrative' approach.)

You would think that, in order to check and correct hormone imbalances, you simply see an *endocrinologist* (hormone doctor); he measures all your levels, compares them to optimal values and then tweaks everything into a perfectly healthy equilibrium with comparably harmless bio-identical hormone supplements, right? Not in this world, you dreamer!

Hormones are natural substances, invented by God, refined by evolution and produced by the body itself. Pharmaceutical companies can't get patents on natural hormones and so they're forced to invent *non-natural* products in order to make endocrinology profitable; hence many doctors diligently prescribe "conjugated estrogen" and "progestins" under the banner 'hormone therapy'.

Conjugated equine estrogens (CEE) are mainly estrone sulphate, not estradiol, and won from horse wee. The brand name Premarin® reminds you of the 'natural' source: **pre**gnant **ma**re **uri**ne. CEE (conjugated equine estrogens) don't get cleared well by the liver[1,2] and increase the stroke risk in women after menopause:

"CEE should <u>not</u> be recommended for prevention in postmenopausal women."[3]

---

[1] Schindler AE et al "Comparative pharmacokinetics of oestradiol, oestrone, oestrone sulfate and "conjugated oestrogens" after oral administration" Arzneimittelforschung 1982;32(7):787-91

[2] Shifren JL et al et al "A comparison of the short-term effects of oral conjugated equine estrogens versus transdermal estradiol on C-reactive protein, other serum markers of inflammation, and other hepatic proteins in naturally menopausal women" J Clin Endocrinol Metab 2008;93(5):1702-10

[3] Anderson GL et al "Effects of conjugated equine estrogen in postmenopausal women with hysterectomy: the Women's Health Initiative randomized controlled trial" JAMA 2004;291(14):1701-12

Synthetic progestins are the drug companies' interpretation of progesterone. A trial, investigating the health effects of 'hormone replacement therapy' (HRT) with a combination of synthetic progestins and conjugated equine estrogens, had to be *stopped*, because the incoming data flagged more strokes, more heart disease, more blood clots in the lungs and more invasive breast cancer in women who were taking the 'hormone-imposter' drugs.[1] A later study even found an increased mortality in these women.[2]

Many doctors still prescribe these substances and call it *'hormone replacement therapy'* (HRT), perhaps in the understanding that they are indeed *replacing* missing hormones—with drugs!

Other docs have read the studies and are now *opposed to hormones*. Into this atmosphere of 'pro-versus-con' HRT amongst conservative doctors comes the very different concept of balancing and supplementing hormone levels with bio-identical products, as proposed by naturopathic, integrative, holistic, anti-aging and other 'non-mainstream' doctors.

Unfortunately they haven't come up with a better name than *bio-identical hormone replacement therapy* although it's actually about supplementing and restoring hormones to healthy and youthful levels for optimal verve and vitality. Perhaps their rationale is that, in cases of severe estrogen dominance, they *replace* the urgent need for Xanax®, Zoloft®, Ambien® and especially for a divorce lawyer, *with* a bio-identical progesterone cream.

Some savvy doctors advertise bio-identical hormones like a *fountain of youth* and so it has become fashionable in selected circles of women past a certain age to get the hormone-pellet bum-implant in one session with cosmetic Botox®, laser hair removal and collagen lip upholstery. This alienates the vast majority of mainstream doctors even further from 'hormones' and leaves unbalanced patients between a rock and a hard place.

As a result, migraineurs with hormonal imbalances have two options. Either they find an 'alternative' doctor, who practices bio-identical HRT or they start studying the subject themselves by reading books and websites and by joining like-minded groups.

---

[1] Rossouw JE et al "Risks and benefits of estrogen plus progestin in healthy postmenopausal women: principal results From the Women's Health Initiative randomized controlled trial" JAMA 2002;288(3):321-33

[2] Heiss G et al "Health risks and benefits 3 years after stopping randomized treatment with estrogen and progestin" JAMA 2008;299(9):1036-45

Apart from the usual suspects like Google, yahoo, yellow pages and other local directories, an inquiry at the nearest *compounding pharmacy* might help to track down a BHRT doctor, since they typically fill the hormone masters' prescriptions.

In Australia you need a script for any hormone supplement, whereas in the U.S. and the U.K. a few products are freely available.

Measuring hormone levels

By now it should be crystal clear that any bio-identical hormone supplementation only makes sense to make up for an imbalance due to a deficiency. For that you need to know your hormone levels in *blood* and compare them to the ideal values of young healthy people. Professional hormone jugglers often insist on measuring hormone metabolite excretion in a 24-hour urine collection in addition to blood test results. The reliability of *saliva* tests is in question[1,2] with the exception of the assessment of relative changes over time; e.g. a profile of cortisol during the day or estrogen and progesterone over the menstrual cycle.[3,4]

Usually the results are displayed with reference ranges and to ease the burden on the doctor, the lab report indicates when a test result is *outside* the reference range. The docs are trained to interpret that as abnormal and meaningful. Yet, for the purpose of optimizing hormonal balance, docs and patients need to ignore reference ranges and find an *ideal value* or ratio to compare against.

Every lab sets up its own reference ranges, so that 95% of their measurements fall within that range for that age group. Since perfectly healthy young people don't have hormone tests, the lab reference range merely reflects the vast majority of sick people in that region, sorted by age group. As a consequence a 35-year-old woman with suspected estrogen dominance and progesterone deficiency gets compared by the lab to 95% of all the other anxious and distractible 35-year-old estrogen volcanoes. And the 60-year-old man with suspected low testosterone gets compared to all the other ancient grumpy buggers with excessive abdominal fat, man boobs, pre-diabetes and erectile dysfunction; result: normal!

---

[1] Granger DA et akl "The 'trouble' with salivary testosterone" Psychoneuroendocrinology 2004;29(10):1229-40
[2] Gröschl M "Current status of salivary hormone analysis" Clin Chem 2008;54(11):1759-69
[3] Chiappelli F et al "Salivary biomarkers in psychobiological medicine" Bioinformation 2006;1(8):331–334
[4] Wolfram M et al "The cortisol awakening response (CAR) across the female menstrual cycle" Psychoneuroendocrinology 2011;36(6):905-12

For that reason a test result is labeled "normal", when it is within the *majority range of results for old and sick locals*. That does not say whether a level is *just sufficient* or *good* or *ideal* or *inside the target range* for young and healthy people.

I suggest to either forget lab reference ranges completely or at least to keep in mind what they express: 95% of the results from people in the area, who had that same test probably for a reason.

Blood test results should always be expressed *with the unit* of measurement. In the U.S. it's often in mg/dL or something like that, European and Australian labs report results in SI units like pmol/L. Conversion charts can be found on the internet and being pedantic about the correct test, measurement unit and decimal point is paramount. "My doc said that 17 is too little progesterone" can be very confusing on an international internet forum, when in fact her doc said: "Without my glasses I can't read the result for 17-OH-progesterone, it's too small."

Which hormones need testing in migraineurs?

Obviously, the levels of and the balance between estrogen and progesterone need attention in menstrual migraine, but also in all difficult and complex cases, especially when other suspicious symptoms are present, e.g. severe period pain (dysmenorrhea),[1] autoimmune[2] or so-called 'psychiatric' comorbidities.[3]

Testosterone and DHEA-S are typically part of a hormone test panel, which is useful: Testosterone has a calming effect on the brain[4] and, compared to cortisol, was found to be lower in women with chronic migraine, together with lower DHEA-S.[5]

Elevated cortisol levels have been associated with chronic migraine and doubts of normal function of migraineurs' HPA-axis (hypothalamus, pituitary and adrenal gland) warrant checking blood levels of ACTH and cortisol in the morning,[6] complemented by salivary cortisol and melatonin profiles.[7]

---

[1] Harel Z "Dysmenorrhea in adolescents and young adults: from pathophysiology to pharmacological treatments and management strategies" Expert Opin Pharmacother 2008;9(15):2661-72
[2] Walker SE "Estrogen and autoimmune disease" Clin Rev Allergy Immunol 2011;40(1):60-5
[3] Peterlin BL et al "The associations between migraine, unipolar psychiatric comorbidities, and stress-related disorders and the role of estrogen" Curr Pain Headache Rep 2009;13(5):404-12
[4] Reddy DS et al "The testosterone-derived neurosteroid androstanediol is a positive allosteric modulator of GABAA receptors" J Pharmacol Exp Ther 2010;334(3):1031-41
[5] Patacchioli FR et al "Salivary cortisol, dehydroepiandrosterone-sulphate (DHEA-S) and testosterone in women with chronic migraine" J Headache Pain 2006;7(2):90-4
[6] Peres MF et al "Hypothalamic involvement in chronic migraine" J Neurol Neurosurg Psychiatry 2001;71(6):747-51
[7] Vogler B et al "Role of melatonin in the pathophysiology of migraine: implications for treatment" CNS Drugs 2006;20(5):343-50

A complete thyroid panel is probably not a bad idea either, given that analgesics (= pain killers) and antiseizure drugs are suspected to suppress thyroid function[1,2] and low thyroid function seems to promote migraine[3,4] and headaches,[5,6] as well as seizures (at least in dogs).[7] Almost 60% of migraine patients with known thyroid dysfunction showed white matter abnormalities (= detectable alterations in the brain's internal 'telephone cables').

It is common practice to measure TSH (= thyroid stimulating hormone) and call that a 'thyroid' function test. TSH, however, is secreted by the pituitary gland and represents the brain's polite request to the thyroid gland to please produce the thyroid hormone T4 (= thyroxin). Understandably, TSH levels don't inform us about the thyroid gland's hormone production or the conversion from T4 to the active form T3. You need to measure T4 and T3 as well.

Plenty of information about thyroid hormones can be found on the web at *drrind.com* and *stopthethyroidmadness.com*.

Men and hormones

Although menstrual migraine is not common in men, most men have hormones too. In fact, they have the same hormones as women and estrogen dominance in men can result from too much conversion of testosterone into estradiol by too much body fat. The conversion enzyme ("aromatase") can be blocked with medication to decrease seizure susceptibility.[8]

Recommended reading

Dr. Thierry Hertoghe, president of the International Hormone Society, has published great books, one for normal people ("solution") and one for experts ("handbook").

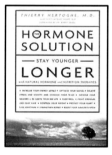
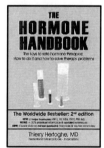

---

[1] Rainero I et al "Endocrine function is altered in chronic migraine patients with medication-overuse" Headache 2006;46(4):597-603
[2] Lossius MI et al "Reversible effects of antiepileptic drugs on thyroid hormones in men and women with epilepsy: a prospective randomized double-blind withdrawal study" Epilepsy Behav 2009;16(1):64-8
[3] Singh SK "Prevalence of migraine in hypothyroidism" J Assoc Physicians India 2002;50:1455-6
[4] Shestakov VV et al "Clinical features of migraine and parameters of trigeminal somatosensory evoked potentials in patients with different levels of thyroid-stimulating hormone" Zh Nevrol Psikhiatr Im S S Korsakova 2010;110(12):77-81
[5] Moreau T et al "Headache in hypothyroidism. Prevalence and outcome under thyroid hormone therapy" Cephalalgia 1998;18(10):687-9
[6] Hagen K et al " Low headache prevalence amongst women with high TSH values" Eur J Neurol 2001;8(6):693-9
[7] on Klopmann T et al "Euthyroid sick syndrome in dogs with idiopathic epilepsy before treatment with anticonvulsant drugs" J Vet Intern Med 2006;20(3):516-22
[8] Harden C et al "Aromatase inhibitors as add-on treatment for men with epilepsy" Expert Rev Neurother 2005;5(1):123-7

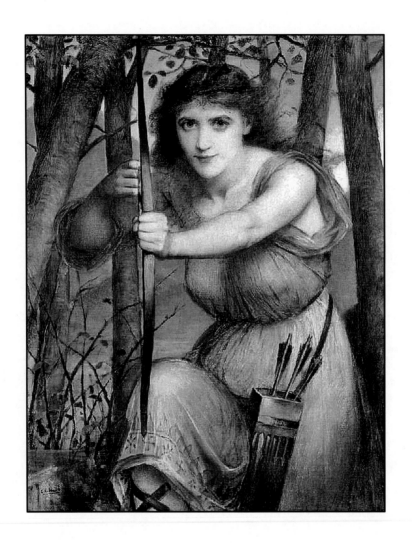

Chapter 18

Points of Pain

> "An arrow may fly through the air and leave no trace;
> but an ill thought leaves a trail like a serpent."
>
> Charles Mackay

Trigger point treatment

If all is good and dandy, muscles can take a lot of pressure without hurting. Spots that are a bit tender are called *tender points*; excellent choice of name! Spots that exhibit spontaneous electrical activity and thereby trigger the experience of pain via sensitized pathways are called *trigger points*.[1] Although they are located in muscle tissue, trigger points belong to the nervous system.

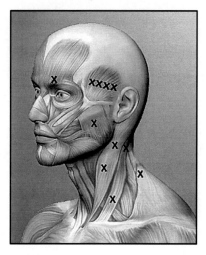

What makes trigger points a bit freaky is the fact that the area which is felt as painful is often somewhere else and that phenomenon is called *referred pain*. One study found active trigger points in 94% of migraine patients in head and neck muscles. The number of active trigger points correlated with attack frequency and the duration of the disorder. In almost a third of the migraineurs, the palpation (= medical word for fumbling) provoked a migraine attack, oooops.[2]

The sensitized pathway from the trigger point to the brain leads into the brainstem, more precisely to the PAG[3] ("the bouncer", page 175) and so the accidental provocation of migraine attacks by poking "myofascial"[4] trigger points is not too surprising for the attentive readers of this book. It would be tough to explain how digging into muscles causes **SWELLING AND INFLAMMATION OF BLOOD VESSELS**.

---

[1] Ge HY et al "Myofascial trigger points: spontaneous electrical activity and its consequences for pain induction and propagation" Chin Med 201125;6:13

[2] Calandre EP et al "Trigger point evaluation in migraine patients: an indication of peripheral sensitization linked to migraine predisposition?" Eur J Neurol 2006;13(3):244-9

[3] Niddam DM et al "Central modulation of pain evoked from myofascial trigger point" Clin J Pain 2007;23(5):440-8

[4] "myo" is Latin for muscle, "fascia" is a form of connective tissue, myofascial means "in muscles or tendons"

Instead of wasting time on the *micro-anatomy* of trigger points, let's simply say, they are the muscle's 'intercom' for listening and talking to the nervous system (brain).

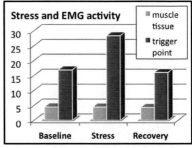

Researchers have measured the electrical activity in trigger points and in adjacent muscle tissue with needle EMG. Then their subjects had to perform a stressful task. The distress showed up as an increase of the signal in the trigger point, not in the muscle.[1]

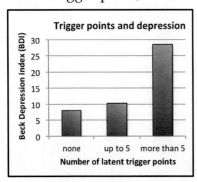

Tender points are trigger points in the making (="latent"). Their number climbs as depression levels rise.[2] These two studies already indicate who's behind the activation of trigger points: the *Lizard* and the *Horse* (see page 186), because they rule over the autonomic nervous system, which activates the points of pain.

Electrical *activation* occurs with distress, but *skyrockets* with feelings of *anger*[3] or *worry*.[4] If this wasn't such a strictly scientific book, one could characterize trigger points as "*the body's sour tears*". Autogenic Training helps to limit the stress-induced creation and activation of trigger points[5] (see chapter 24).

Popular passive trigger point treatments are dry needling, injections or transdermal patches with local anesthetics (e.g. Lidocaine),[6,7] which can reduce the intensity of migraine pain significantly, when the right spot gets found and hit.[8] Even patients with cluster headaches benefit from trigger point treatment.[9]

---

[1] McNulty WH et al "Needle electromyographic evaluation of trigger point response to a psychological stressor" Psychophysiol 1994;31(3):313-6
[2] Celik D et al "The relationship between latent trigger points and depression levels in healthy subjects" Clin Rheumatol 2012;31(6):907-11
[3] Cafaro TA et al "The exploration of trigger point and heart rate variability excitation and recovery patterns in actors performing anger inhibition and anger expression" Appl Psychophysiol Biof 2001;26:236
[4] Armm J et al "The relationship between personality characteristics and local muscle tenderness development in first year psychology graduate students: A prospective study. Applied Psychophysiol Biof 1999;24(2),125
[5] Banks S et al "Effects of autogenic relaxation training on EMG activity in myofascial trigger points" J Musculoskel Pain 1998;6,4
[6] Affaitati G et al "A randomized, controlled study comparing a lidocaine patch, a placebo patch, and anesthetic injection for treatment of trigger points in patients with myofascial pain syndrome: evaluation of pain and somatic pain thresholds" Clin Ther 2009;31(4):705-20
[7] Venancio Rde A et al "Botulinum toxin, lidocaine, and dry-needling injections in patients with myofascial pain and headaches" Cranio 2009;27(1):46-53
[8] Giamberardino MA et al "Contribution of myofascial trigger points to migraine symptoms" J Pain 2007;8(11):869-78
[9] Calandre EP et al "Myofascial trigger points in cluster headache patients: a case series" Head Face Med 2008;4:32

Here is my very biased, partial and purely personal opinion. *Finding and calming* trigger points is a very smart, highly advisable move and can help enormously with the *symptoms* of migraine.

The disadvantage of injections and dry needling are the discomfort of the treatment and the substantial soreness thereafter. I usually soothe angry trigger points with *photonic stimulation*,[1] an infrared light therapy invented by NASA.[2,3,4] In one patient with a visibly throbbing, incensed trigger point near the shoulder blade, this treatment alone aborted an acute, full-blown migraine attack, her last.

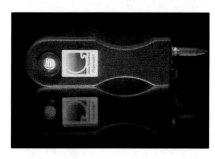

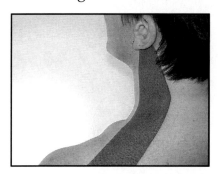

For sustained pain reduction and healing I mostly apply an elastic therapeutic sticky tape called *Meditape*,[5] which is similar to the popular Kinesiotape, but follows a different methodology. In stark conflict with my own beliefs and inexplicably, I've witnessed that the mere *color* of the tape can have a decisive impact. This surprising and admittedly weird color-effect is part of the Meditaping method. Together with the different application strategy, the choice of color may also help explain why many positive study-results with Kinesiotaping didn't quite reach the same level of success that therapists and their patients have experienced in clinical practice with Meditaping therapy.[6,7,8]

Stoked by this *risk-free symptom relief*, patients are usually very motivated to address the root causes of migraine in mind and brain.

---

[1] The device in the picture is a Photonic Stimulator (PS1) from Ochslabs Inc./CA; www.ochlabs.com
[2] see NASA press release 03-366 or 00-366 http://www.msfc.nasa.gov/news/news/releases/2000/00-336.html
[3] Eells JT et al "Mitochondrial signal transduction in accelerated wound and retinal healing by near-infrared light therapy" Mitochondr 2004;4(5-6):559-67
[4] Desmet KD et al "Clinical and experimental applications of NIR-LED photobiomodulation" Photomed Laser Surg 2006;24(2):121-8
[5] http://www.medi-tape.de/; also Sielmann D "Medi-Taping-Schmerztherapie ohne Medikamente" Bad Oldenburg 2010
[6] González-Iglesias J et al "Short-term effects of cervical kinesio taping on pain and cervical range of motion in patients with acute whiplash injury: a randomized clinical trial" J Orthop Sports Phys Ther 2009;39(7):515-21
[7] Karatas N et al "The effect of Kinesiotape application on functional performance in surgeons who have musculo-skeletal pain after performing surgery" Turk Neurosurg 2012;22(1):83-9
[8] Williams S et al "Kinesio taping in treatment and prevention of sports injuries: a meta-analysis of the evidence for its effectiveness" Sports Med 2012;42(2):153-64

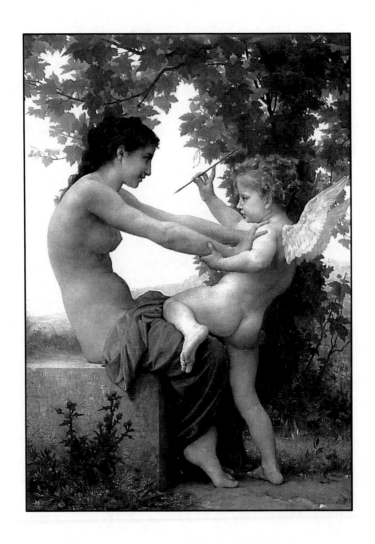

Chapter 19

Pricks with Benefits

> "Even pain pricks to livelier living."
> Amy Lowell

Acupuncture for attack prevention

Many migraineurs and many excellent therapists *swear by acupuncture* and claim good results in the treatment of migraine, be it for the prevention of attacks or even their abortion. The needle-shy author of this book neither performs acupuncture himself nor did he ever have much pleasure or success as the punctured patient.

When acupuncture gets tested like a drug, a sham treatment serves as a comparison to identify an 'unspecific' effect. Compared to a sham acupuncture (on the 'wrong' points), real acupuncture on traditional energy-meridian points was found to have *no benefits*.[1,2]

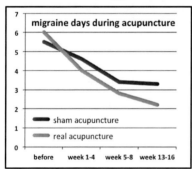

One study compared three different styles of Chinese acupuncture on 480 migraine patients against sham pricks over 16 weeks. The three varieties of real acupuncture reduced the number of migraine days by 61-65%, the fake acupuncture only by 40%. The authors found the difference "not clinically relevant".[3] Call me pedantic, but I do see a relevant difference between 2.2 or 3.3 migraine days in four weeks. On average, all groups improved a fair bit from almost 6 to 2.5 days with migraine in four weeks with nothing but a few, relatively harmless acupuncture treatments.

The danger of such studies is that some hard-core pharma friends get the opportunity to confuse laypeople with an invalid interpretation: **"ACUPUNCTURE IS A *SCAM*, BECAUSE IT'S NOT BETTER THAN *SHAM* ACUPUNCTURE."** Well, lets compare the benefit of acupuncture to the blessings that patients receive from drug treatment, shall we?

---

[1] Diener HC "Acupuncture prophylaxis of migraine no better than sham acupuncture for decreasing frequency of headaches" Evid Based Med 2012 Jun 20. [Epub ahead of print]
[2] Linde K et al "Acupuncture for migraine prophylaxis" Cochrane Database Syst Rev. 2009;(1):CD001218
[3] Li Y et al "Acupuncture for migraine prophylaxis: a randomized controlled trial" CMAJ 2012;184(4):401-10

One study comparing acupuncture to Topiramate® (an anti-seizure drug) in the treatment of chronic migraine ended with a 1:1 draw. Acupuncture took the lead with a stronger reduction in headache days, but the drug scored a late equalizer with a thrashing tenfold rate of adverse effects (66% vs 6%).[1]

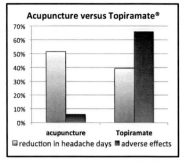

Flunarizine (Sibelium®) blocks calcium channels and so makes it harder for neurons to pass their messages on (page 161). It is used for migraine attack prevention. Common side effects are tiredness, drowsiness, weight gain, depression, muscle stiffness or shaking.[2]

Here is the design of "a single-blinded, double-dummy, randomized controlled trial" of acupuncture versus flunarizine:[3]

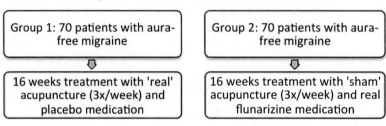

We already know that the difference between 'real' acupuncture and 'sham' acupuncture is "not relevant" and so we would expect that group 2 with the *flunarizine* plus needles has a better result than group 1 with the *placebo pill* and needles. Surprise: *Group 1* had more "responders" (= − 50% migraine days or better) and fewer migraine days than group 2. The authors concluded that "acupuncture was more effective than flunarizine", but I would find that in those migraine patients who already get treated with needles, flunarizine is worse than a placebo pill; but that's just me.

The punchline is, whether named sham or real acupuncture, needle-pricks are better than drugs for the prevention of migraine attacks, and usually have fewer side effects or adverse reactions. That's the finding of a review of 22 trials with over 4000 patients.[4]

---

[1] Yang CP et al "Acupuncture versus topiramate in chronic migraine prophylaxis: a randomized clinical trial" Cephalalgia 2011;31(15):1510-21
[2] Sibelium® manufacturer's patient information; http://home.intekom.com/pharm/janssen/sibelium.html
[3] Wang LP et al "Efficacy of acupuncture for migraine prophylaxis: a single-blinded, double-dummy, randomized controlled trial" Pain 2011;152(8):1864-71
[4] Linde K et al "Acupuncture for migraine prophylaxis" Cochrane Database Syst Rev. 2009;(1):CD001218

We can rightfully say that research hasn't come up with a reason why people should not swear by acupuncture, if they want to. And patients who aren't swearing yet, might want to give these *pricks with benefits* a try and see if it helps; especially if they're not happy with their preventive medication.

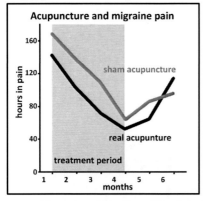

The decisive question is: "Do needles *end the migraine tyranny* and transform migraineurs into ex-migraineurs?" The answer is: "Not really." Like with preventive meds, in most cases the attacks come back when the treatment phase ends. The graph to the left is from one of the many studies and shows the total number of hours in migraine pain.[1]

By now it should also be clear that so-called 'sham' acupuncture is probably not a fake treatment, but another needle therapy.[2] One migraine patient reported on an internet forum that she tried real and *sham* acupuncture in practice, but she might have mixed it up with "dry needling", a trigger point treatment.

Acupuncture for acute attacks

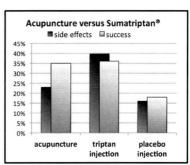

Time for a re-match. In the blue corner, the current champion in attack abortion: the injection with a triptan. In the red corner, the challenger: real acupuncture. 179 acute attacks later we have a photo finish and you will be the judge of success *and* side effects. To be fair, half of the triptan patients needed the drug twice and half of those had a benefit, but a second acupuncture didn't rescue many.[3]

Two studies found *real* acupuncture superior to *fake* needling for acute migraine attacks.[4,5] Both were done in China! Hmmm.

---

[1] Alecrim-Andrade J et al "Acupuncture in migraine prevention: a randomized sham controlled study with 6-months posttreatment follow-up" Clin J Pain 2008;24(2):98-105
[2] Moffet HH "Sham acupuncture may be as efficacious as true acupuncture: a systematic review" J Altern Complement Med 2009;15(3):213-6
[3] Melchart D et al "Acupuncture versus placebo versus sumatriptan for early treatment of migraine attacks: a randomized controlled trial" J Intern Med 2003;253(2):181-8
[4] Li Y et al "Acupuncture for treating acute attacks of migraine: a randomized controlled trial" Headache 2009;49(6):805-16
[5] Wang LP et al "Efficacy of acupuncture for acute migraine attack: a multicenter single blinded, randomized controlled trial" Pain Med 2012;13(5):623-30

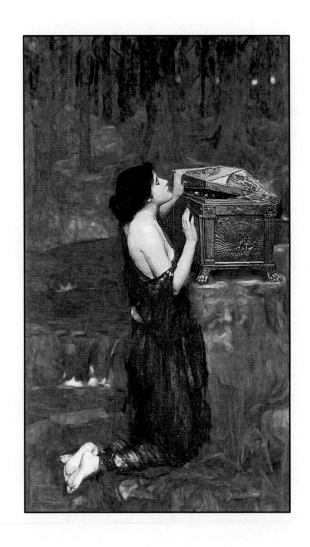

Chapter 20

Pandora's Chest of Treasures

> "Knowledge is the treasure of a wise man."
> William Penn

A plethora of non-drug migraine treatments is mentioned on websites or in books and articles. It's a piece of cake to quickly dismiss them in one fell swoop, since none of them is recognized by the medical establishment due to a lack of *accepted evidence*. However, it is my duty as a rebellious book author to scrutinize the current regime's opponents in our search for allies. We can't possibly examine every whacky idea, personal belief and odd theory out there, but it is typical for migraine that even so-called *'complete nonsense'* is sometimes helpful for someone. Let's peek into Pandora's box and see if there are any *migraine treasures* in it.

Acupressure

Pressing certain acu-points on traditional energy-meridians is known as acupressure. Some say, self-administered acupressure is helpful for the headache during an attack.[1] Since serious risks and side effects are unlikely, why not give a try? If it relieves the pain, then you know it works for you. In case acupressure does not reduce the headache, it might actually *reduce nausea*. A review of 40 trials found acupressure on wrist point Pericardium 6 (P6) as good as medication for nausea and vomiting.[2] An acupressure wrist-band was better than nothing.[3]

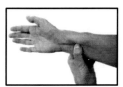

Aromatherapy

You might think I'm kidding when I say: "The number of studies about aromatherapy exceed my *reviewing capacity*", but I'm not. Admittedly, there are no studies investigating aromatherapy for migraine and if there was an essential oil that remedies migraine THAT WOULD BE ON THE TITLE PAGE OF EVERY NEWSPAPER, wouldn't it?

---

[1] Kurland HD "Treatment of headache pain with auto-acupressure" Dis Nerv Syst 1976;37(3):127-9
[2] for a detailed description see www.homebackpainacupressure.com/acupressure-for-sea-sickness.html
[3] Allais G et al "Acupressure in the control of migraine-associated nausea" Neurol Sci 2012;33 Suppl1:S207-10

A review in 2012 found evidence from several studies that *peppermint* and *ginger* scents are helpful for nausea and vomiting.[1] *Lavender* is helpful for sleepless 45-55 year-old Chinese girls, as measured by the Pittsburgh Sleep Quality Questionnaire (in its Chinese version, of course).[2]

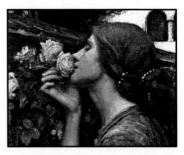

Lavender is also used to cool down cantankerous oldies with dementia[3] and there are enough studies for a systematic review about aromatherapy's efficacy.[4] When, however, scrutinized by medical researchers under the criteria for drug trials, aromatherapy comes out empty-handed.[5]

Korean school girls got better period-pain relief from a *tummy massage*—with clary sage, marjoram, cinnamon, ginger, and geranium in a base of almond oil—than they got from *acetaminophen* (= paracetamol; e.g. Tylenol®, Panadol®). They couldn't say what contributed more, the massage or the essential oils; but I'd prefer a smelly belly over the drug that causes the most liver failures in the Western world.[6] To me, aromatherapy makes a lot of scents!

"Bio Feedback", quantum style

The name "Bio Feedback" is *deceptively* similar to the established and well-researched field of biofeedback, which is the underlying principle of applied psychophysiology (see ch. 25). In contrast, "Bio Feedback" and *"quantum bio-feedback"* are less often the subject of research, rather the focus of criminal investigations.

When you google the infamous names of these devices—like Xrroid, QXCI, SCIO, EFPX, Indigo, LIFE system—you quickly arrive at websites of quackwatch and newspapers that reveal that these very '*promising*' methods represent the prime example of an ongoing *scam* which earned its fugitive mastermind millions.[7]

---

[1] Lua PL et al "A brief review of current scientific evidence involving aromatherapy use for nausea and vomiting" J Altern Complement Med 2012;18(6):534-40
[2] Chien LW et al "The effect of lavender aromatherapy on autonomic nervous system in midlife women with insomnia" Evid Based Complement Alternat Med 2012;2012:740813
[3] Lee SY "The effect of lavender aromatherapy on cognitive function, emotion, and aggressive behavior of elderly with dementia" Taehan Kanho Hakhoe Chi 2005;35(2):303-12
[4] Fung JK et al "A systematic review of the use of aromatherapy in treatment of behavioral problems in dementia" Geriatr Geront Int 2012;12(3):372-82
[5] Lee MS et al "Aromatherapy for health care: an overview of systematic reviews" Maturitas 2012;71(3):257-60
[6] Daly F et al "Guidelines for the management of paracetamol poisoning in Australia and New Zealand--explanation and elaboration. A consensus statement from clinical toxicologists consulting to the Australasian poisons information centres" Med J Aust 2008;188(5):296-301
[7] Seattle Times, 2009 Sep 3:"MIRACLE MACHINES:The 21st-Century Snake Oil" http://seattletimes.nwsource.com/html/medicaldevices/

This type of fraud is comparably easy to spot: The inventor is an alleged genius with multiple doctor titles, the machines are said to detect everything aberrant in the body from a frequency scan and a multitude of built-in therapies cure everything in no time. If things sound too good to be true, they usually are. More damaging is the systematic *medical swindle* that tells migraineurs that **MIGRAINE IS A GENETIC HEADACHE-DISEASE OF SWELLING AND INFLAMMATION** for which it's best to rely on drugs. This ongoing scam earns its masterminds *billions*.

Chirotherapy

I myself am a huge fan of chirotherapy for *blockages, subluxations* or *fixations* or whatever you like to call the disturbances and restrictions of movements of vertebrae. There are neither evidence nor clues that migraine is usually caused by blockages. Therefore it is not likely that trials researching the benefit of chirotherapy for migraine come up with staggering results.

An Australian study in 2000 described that after two months and up to 16 sessions of spinal manipulation treatment, 22% of the participants reported a reduction of more than 90% in migraine frequency. Moreover, another 50% saw significant improvements in the intensity of their migraine episodes.[1]

A comparison between spinal manipulation and amitriptyline, a medication against depression, found equally modest benefits for either, but no advantage from combining them.[2]

In summary, the scientific evidence for chirotherapy as treatment for migraine is called "moderate" even by chirotherapists.[3]

Here is my take. Think of the 'copper-boy' in chapter 15: Stopping the copper-exposure plus a zinc pill cured his migraine, although neither *copper-avoidance* nor *zinc* are effective migraine treatments; but effective for *migraine due to copper toxicity*!

Logically, magnesium can only be helpful for migraine due to magnesium deficiency and chirotherapy can only be helpful for *migraine due to spinal blockages*. There is no point in researching *chirotherapy for migraine*, but those migraineurs with a serious blockage, e.g. in the cervical spine, could actually benefit big time.

---

[1] Tuchin PJ et al "A randomized controlled trial of chiropractic spinal manipulative therapy for migraine" J Manipulative Physiol Ther 2000;23(2):91-5
[2] Nelson CF et al "The efficacy of spinal manipulation, amitriptyline and the combination of both therapies for the prophylaxis of migraine headache" J Manipulative Physiol Ther 1998;21(8):511-9
[3] Bryans R et al "Evidence-based guidelines for the chiropractic treatment of adults with headache" J Manipulative Physiol Ther 2011;34(5):274-89

Lidocaine nasal spray

Even the best revolution takes its time and even the highly motivated and diligent volleyball-crack Irene (see ch. 9) needed a crutch for a while. Lidocaine is a comparably benign local anesthetic that can be surprisingly effective in roughly every second migraine sufferer. It's anti-seizure effect at low doses is well known and so is the seizure-promoting effect at high doses.[1]

For migraine attack abortion a 4% nasal spray was tested. During the double-blind phase of the trial, it worked well for more than a third of the attacked patients and during the open-label period more than half had decent symptom relief,[2] but one fifth of the responders had a relapse. Still, not too bad.

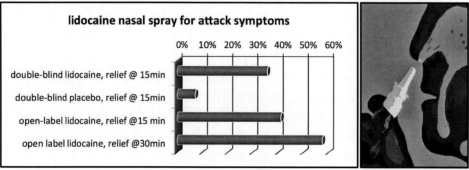

An earlier study by the same authors found a similar effect for the spray: roughly one half of the attack victims experience at least a 50% reduction in symptoms.[3] In contrast, a lidocaine trial in an emergency department failed bitterly with only 7.4% response rate, almost identical with the placebo spray.[4]

Lidocaine nasal spray is one of the acute treatment options listed by the American Academy of Family Physicians (AAFP).[5] Apart from conditions of slow or 'unreliable' heartbeat, lidocaine has no general contraindications and few side effects when used as a local anesthetic. A 4% lidocaine nasal spray is available at compounding pharmacies. For those who do respond to it, it could be a very economical alternative to expensive triptans and thereby save money for the weapons of the tyranny-ending revolution.

---

[1] DeToledo JC "Lidocaine and seizures" Ther Drug Monit 2000;22(3):320-2
[2] Maizels M et al "Intranasal lidocaine for migraine: a randomized trial and open-label follow-up" Headache 1999;39(8):543-51
[3] Maizels M et al "Intranasal lidocaine for treatment of migraine: a randomized, double-blind, controlled trial" JAMA 1996;276(4):319-21
[4] Blanda M et al "Intranasal lidocaine for the treatment of migraine headache: a randomized, controlled trial" Acad Emerg Med 2001;8(4):337-42
[5] Gilmore B et al "Treatment of acute migraine headache" Am Fam Physician 2011;83(3):271-80

Massage

Wouldn't it be nice, if regular massage led to a meaningful reduction in migraine attacks? Two studies tested the idea with control groups and the outcome wasn't too shabby: It would take 200mg of the anti-seizure drug Topiramate® to get the same attack rate reduction just shy of 30%.[1,2,3,4] Sure, that is still 70% off our goal to end the migraine tyranny, but expressed in the words of the researchers who tested the *drug*: Massage "showed a significant efficacy in migraine prevention".

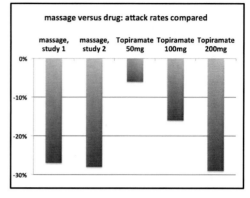

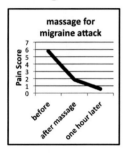

It would be even better, if massage could also abort migraine attacks or at least relieve the head and neck pain. One study found a drastic reduction in pain scores (0 to 10) from 5.8 via 1.8 right after the treatment to 0.6 one hour later. Okay, it was more of a chiropractic treatment on ten Iranian men only, but it seems for eight of them the migraine attack had a *happy ending*.[5]

Oxytocin

The mechanism for the respectable effect of massage is not clear, but massage is known to stimulate the release of oxytocin.[6] Messenger substances are called *hormones* in the body and *neuromodulators* in the brain. Like many other substances — e.g. estrogen, progesterone etc. — Oxytocin is both and acts in body and brain.

Many people love jazzy headlines and so you find lots of stock-phrases presenting oxytocin as the trust-, bonding-, cuddle-love- or birth-hormone. We don't have the time to elucidate these verbal stamps, we need weapons against the migraine terror.

---

[1] Hernandez-Reif M "Migraine Headaches are Reduced by Massage Therapy" Int J Neurosci 1998;1-2(96):1-11
[2] Lawler SP et al "A randomized, controlled trial of massage therapy as a treatment for migraine" Ann Behav Med 2006;32(1):50-9
[3] Chaibi A et al "Manual therapies for migraine: a systematic review" J Headache Pain 2011;12(2):127-33
[4] Brandes JL et al "Topiramate for migraine prevention: a randomized controlled trial" JAMA 2004;291(8):965-73
[5] Noudeh YJ et al "Reduction of current migraine headache pain following neck massage and spinal manipulation" Int J Ther Massage Bodywork 2012;5(1):5-13
[6] Bello D et al "An exploratory study of neurohormonal responses of healthy men to massage" J Altern Complement Med 2008;14(4):387-94

Let's cut to the chase. Pharma companies can't get a patent for natural substances (like hormones or neuromodulators) and so they are forced to research and sell *unnatural substances*. We can't blame them for that and even if we could, what's the point? What we *can* do is keep in mind that there may be biochemical glitches in our bodies and brains which no pharma-medical researcher gives a ... about, but which might have severe consequences for our health.

There is no evidence but strong hints that an *oxytocin deficiency* (in the sense of sub-normal oxytocin-based signaling) promotes seizure activity[1] and that oxytocin has an anti-migraine effect.[2] An oxytocin nasal spray was clinically tested as attack medication with decent results: Every second acute migraineur had at least 50% less pain, every fourth was pain-free after 4 hours. And so the question arises whether some migraineurs may be low in oxytocin.

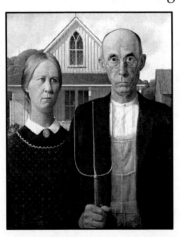

According to someone knowledgeable[3] these are some of the symptoms of an oxytocin deficiency: disturbed sleep, high pain-sensitivity, irritability, low mood, lack of affection, low libido, being distrustful/doubtful/suspicious, no joy and so on. With an oxytocin-deficiency it may seem as if **THE WORLD IS A HOSTILE PLACE**.

Therefore, if you feel like these two ← look and the list of symptoms rings a bell, you might want to consider giving *oxytocin supplementation* a go.

Oxytocin forms attachment and surges in mother and child during breastfeeding,[4] an activity that reduces migraine attacks.[5] Low oxytocin is connected to fibromyalgia,[6] anxiety, depression[7] and suicide[8] and is likely involved in overbreathing[9] (see ch. 12). One could write a whole book about oxytocin's therapy potential.

---

[1] Sala M et al "Pharmacologic rescue of impaired cognitive flexibility, social deficits, increased aggression, and seizure susceptibility in oxytocin receptor null mice: a neurobehavioral model of autism" Biol Psychiatry 2011;69(9):875-82
[2] Phillips WJ et al "Relief of acute migraine headache with intravenous oxytocin: report of two cases" J Pain Palliat Care Pharmacother 2006;20(3):25-8
[3] Dr. Thierry Hertoghe (MD) President of the International Hormone Society (www.intlhormonesociety.org)
[4] Nagasawa M "Oxytocin and mutual communication in mother-infant bonding" Front Hum Neurosci 2012;6:31
[5] Serva WA et al "Exclusive breastfeeding protects against postpartum migraine recurrence attacks?" Arq Neuropsiquiatr 2012;70(6):428-34
[6] Anderberg UM et al "Plasma oxytocin levels in female fibromyalgia syndrome patients" Z Rheumatol 2000;59(6):373-9
[7] Scantamburlo G et al "Plasma oxytocin levels and anxiety in patients with major depression" Psychoneuroendocrinology 2007;32(4):407-10
[8] Jokinen J et al "Low CSF oxytocin reflects high intent in suicide attempters" Psychoneuroendocrinology 2012;37(4):482-90
[9] de Oliveira DC et al "Oxytocin interference in the effects induced by inhalation of 7.5% CO_2 in healthy volunteers" Hum Psychopharm 2012;27(4):378-85

Since someone knowledgeable has done that, I recommend reading Dr. Thierry Hertoghe's book *"Passion, Sex and a Long Life - the incredible oxytocin adventure"*, which is packed with scientific references and practical advice about Oxytocin supplementation.[1] This much already: Oxytocin needs cooling; you get it from a *compounding pharmacist* and not from dubious internet sources.

Physical therapy or physiotherapy

There are studies which essentially assert that physiotherapy or physical therapy are pretty much useless for migraine,[2,3] but so are the articles, if they don't specify what kind of therapy was actually administered. Trigger point therapy, massage and spinal manipulations are inside or close to a physio's area of expertise. Beyond that, I'm sure that individual migraine patients swear by their physio's healing hands, but we just don't have any form of scientific clue or hypothesis that would allow for general advice.

Neck pain is a frequent symptom during migraine attacks[4] and so some patients believe that their migraine is *caused* by their neck, their *bad posture*, their *unevenly long legs* or some problem with their *feet*. In *individual* cases that may or may not be true. However, it is neither *plausible* nor *logical* nor *proven* that these factors play a mentionable role in migraine *in general*.

Tinted lenses

Visual stress is a factor in triggering some attacks in patients with migraine, particularly migraine with aura,[5] but there is a crutch for that too. A randomized controlled trial showed that some people benefit significantly from tinted glasses.[6] With the help of a so-called *intuitive colorimeter*, patients choose a lens-color that helps reduce pattern glare and distortions.[7] A second study showed that the chosen lens-tint indeed had a marginally better effect than the control glasses whose color was slightly off.[8] Sometimes it helps to see the world through rose-colored glasses.

---

[1] USA: www.antiaging-systems.com, $40; AUS: www.acpharm.com.au, AU$45; Europe: www.hertoghe.eu, €30.-
[2] Marcus DA et al "Nonpharma. treatment for migraine: incremental utility of physical therapy with relaxation and biofeedback" Cephalalgia 1998;18(5):266-72
[3] Biondi DM "Physical treatments for headache: a structured review" Headache 2005;45(6):738-46
[4] Calhoun AH et al "The prevalence of neck pain in migraine" Headache 2010;50(8):1273-7
[5] Hay KM et al "1044 women with migraine: the effect of environmental stimuli" Headache 1994;34(3):166-8
[6] Evans BJ et al "Optometric function in visually sensitive migraine before and after treatment with tinted spectacles" Ophthalmic Physiol Opt 2002;22(2):130-42
[7] Wilkins AJ et al "A colorizer for use in determining an optimal ophthalmic tint" Color Res Appl 2000;263:246–253
[8] Wilkins AJ et al "Tinted spectacles and visually sensitive migraine" Cephalalgia 2002;22(9):711-9

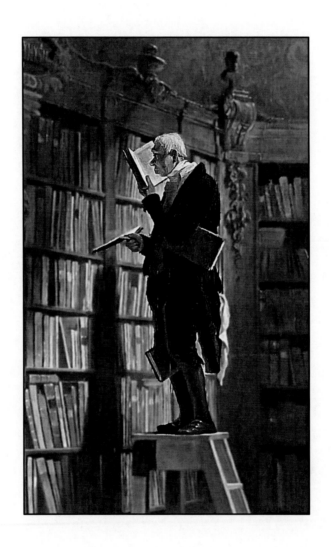

Section Two:

Weapons for the Mind

> "The greatest discovery of my generation is that a human being can alter his life by altering his attitudes of mind."
>
> William James

Are you out of your mind?

If you don't mind putting your mind to it, a mindboggling number of English idioms with "mind" can come to mind:
- *peace* of mind
- to *read* one's mind
- it *blows* your mind.

It is okay
- to *take* your mind *off* or
- to *change* your mind.

Recently it has become fashionable
- to adopt a new mind*set* or
- to be more *open*-minded, for instance towards
- mind-*body* therapies.

In short: The mind is trendy.

Bear in mind that for migraine mind therapies are fully evidence-based, established, and often curative treatments ("curative" = beating for good). So I think it's time that migraineurs make up their minds and decide that they've had enough of the mindless medication alone; time for a mindful migraine revolution; time to do what needs to be done to end the migraine tyranny.

Many complex and difficult cases won't mind seeking support from a trained mind coach in order to change their mind and adopt the new mindset of an ex-migraineur. Others are in two minds about it or it has never crossed their mind. Mind you, when things are tough, it is essential to keep an open mind.

In some migraineurs the brain seems to have a mind of its own. Mind therapies can help them to take that weight off their mind. I hope you don't mind that I continue to speak my mind. In case you think **"MIND YOUR OWN BUSINESS!"** I apologize. Never mind.

The mind and the brain

Isn't it amazing that every morning, when we wake up, our conscious mind comes back to life. Where was it at night?

Consciousness is a state of brain and subject to a lot of discussion in neuroscience.[1] Researchers are honing in on the mechanisms that create our conscious mind inside our brain.[2] The loss of consciousness during some forms of epileptic seizures, but also during sleep, shows that our *brain can change our mind*.[3]

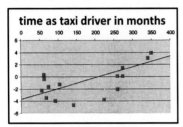

Less well known is that the *mind can change the brain*. For example, being a taxi driver in London, trains a certain area involved in memory formation; and so that area grows larger, similar to muscles after weight lifting.[4]

And so it shouldn't surprise us to learn, that therapies for the *mind* also lead to changes in function and structure of the *brain*. In this example the researchers found a changed activation of the prefrontal cortex as the expression of the improvements in depressive symptoms after 15 months of psychodynamic psychotherapy.[5]

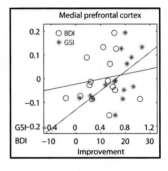

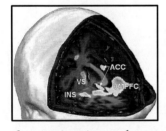

If you are in a hurry and don't have the time to do 15 months of psychotherapy, you can learn to change *brain and mind* with neurofeedback. In this study patients learnt to change the activation of some 'emotional' brain areas in the fMRI brain scanner, which reduced their depression in *four* sessions.[6]

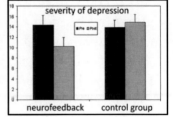

---

[1] Posner MI "Attentional Networks and Consciousness" Front Psychol 2012;3:6
[2] Greicius MD et al "Default network connectivity reflects the level of consciousness in non-communicative brain-damaged patients" Brain 2010 Jan;133(Pt 1):161-71
[3] Danielson NB et al "The default mode network and altered consciousness in epilepsy" Behav Neurol 2011;24(1):55–65
[4] Maguire EA et al "Navigation-related structural change in the hippocampi of taxi drivers" Proc Natl Acad Sci USA 2000;97(8):4398–4403
[5] Buchheim A, et al "Changes in prefrontal-limbic function in major depression after 15 months of long-term psychotherapy" PLoS One 2012;7(3):e33745
[6] Linden DE et al "Real-time self-regulation of emotion networks in patients with depression" PLoS One 2012;7(6):e38115

Chapter 21

Reflecting your Thoughts

"You are today where your thoughts have brought you; you will be tomorrow where your thoughts take you."

James Lane Allen

Cognitive Behavioral Therapy (CBT)

The improvement of skills for so-called stress management and coping, based on CBT (cognitive behavioral therapy), has long been recognized as an effective method in migraine rehabilitation;[1] studies show an average reduction of 50% in "headache activity".[2]

In a nutshell, CBT is based on the following premise: Our *thoughts* affect our feelings and actions. Bad thinking habits (see page 90) and unhelpful beliefs subsequently lead to 'bad' actions and negative feelings. This amplifies perceived stress and contributes to mood problems like anxiety and depression, but also to neuroticism, hopelessness[3] and even suicide.[4]

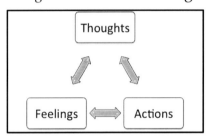

How thoughts create stress

When an event grabs our attention, our mind quickly comes up with an interpretation of its meaning, mostly based on already existing beliefs. In a second step, the mind then forms a prediction about the likely consequences of that situation. Hence the response is not really a result of the event itself, but of the mind's own thoughts and beliefs.

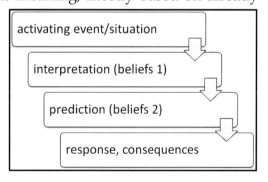

---

[1] Holroyd KA et al "Behavioral approaches to the treatment of migraine" Semin Neurol 2006;26(2):199-207
[2] Campbell K et al "Evidence-Based Guidelines For Migraine Headache: Behavioral and Physical Treatments" US Headache Consortium, available from the American Academy of Neurology, 2000; accessed March 10, 2012
[3] Becker-Weidman EG et al "Predictors of hopelessness among clinically depressed youth" Behav Cogn Psychother 2009;37(3):267-91
[4] Brent DA et al "Suicidality in affectively disordered adolescent inpatients" J Am Acad Child Adolesc Psychiatry 1990;29(4):586-93

In simple words: Our *thoughts* create the stress! Let's have a look at this example of two 'caring' moms with episodic migraine:

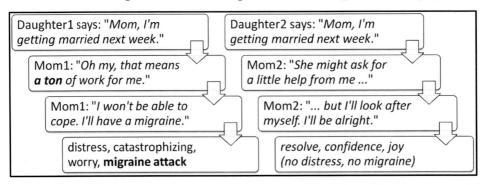

Mom1 jumps to the conclusion, that her daughter's wedding must inevitably mean a lot of work for her. Without really knowing anything about the young bride's plans and ideas, Mom1 is already convinced that she won't be able to cope with the 'immense workload', which her own mind has made up a split second ago. As a consequence Mom1 feels distressed, her mind predicts a grim future and so she has a good chance to self-trigger one migraine attack now and another one at the wedding. All in all, she perceives the wedding as a *threat*.

In contrast, although Mom2 is a bit of a mind-reader ("she might ask ...") she knows her limits and puts her own well-being first. For Mom2 the wedding is a *challenge*, but not a threat.

Let's make it worse

Many severe migraineurs are constantly in a state of terror, because they believe that "THE WORLD IS A HOSTILE PLACE" and "EVERYTHING CAN TRIGGER A MIGRAINE" (= stable-global external threats). Also they can't do anything about it, because they believe that "MIGRAINE IS GENETIC" and "MIGRAINE IS A NEUROLOGICAL DISEASE" (= stable-global internal defects). No wonder that they feel anxious and helpless.

The key to feeling helpless lies in the *explanation*. Is the alleged cause of the distress ...

- ... unstable or stable (= can or can't be changed)?
- ... internal or external (= inside or outside the person)?
- ... specific or global (= e.g. here/now or everywhere/always)?

Over time people develop a certain *style* in their explanations.

People with a *pessimistic explanatory style* tend to attribute unwanted outcomes to stable-global internal causes, for example: "OF COURSE, I FAILED THE EXAM. I'M A TOTAL FAILURE, BECAUSE I'M STUPID." Other people, with a more factual and *realistic* view, could come to a very different interpretation of exactly the same event: "I failed this exam, because I didn't take enough time to study for it." Not much drama here, ey?

Let's make it better

As we've seen, the stress is mainly caused by the thoughts and beliefs about a situation. In CBT the therapist and the client try to identify limiting unhelpful beliefs and practice correcting the bad thinking habits. One famous exercise is called the "ABCD method".

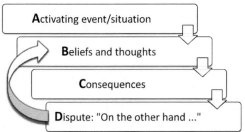

The task here is to question beliefs and thoughts about distressing events: "Is this a healthy, balanced and realistic view of the situation? Is there any evidence against my negative thoughts?"

Testing of one's own thoughts can be initiated by 1. scratching one's chin and then 2. speaking the magic formula: "*On the other hand ..., what if ...?*" Let's try it out on a hypothetical example:

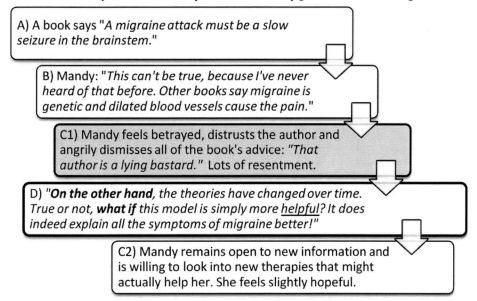

Mandy does benefit from fending off her negative thoughts, right?

That went well, let's look at another example:

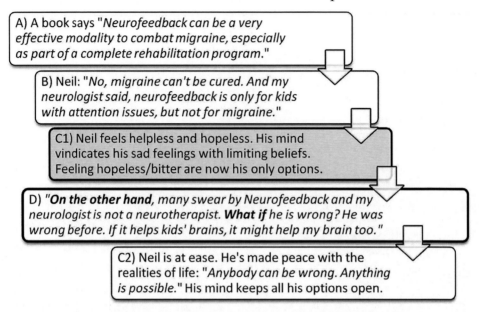

I hope Neil agrees with us, that wrestling with one's own negative thoughts is worthwhile to reduce self-made distress and despair. But a negatively tuned mind can be a formidable opponent. So we should develop our new skill with another example:

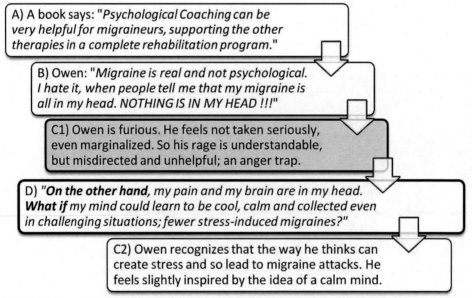

Please note that this is not about talking things up. It's about giving another, balanced view a shot at our mind's negativity bias.

I reckon you've got the idea and now you're eager to do one by yourself? Am I right? Okay, here we go:

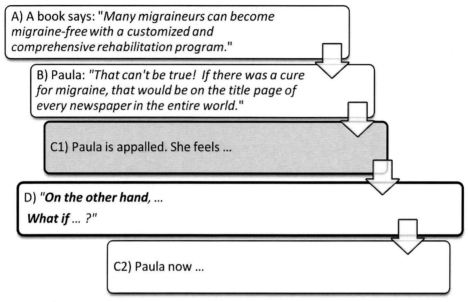

Of course, there is more to cognitive behavioral therapy than this one exercise, but I thought the ABCD method—also called reappraisal—represents CBT well enough to leave it at that.

Limitations of CBT

Psychology has a long tradition of excessive self-criticism and cantankerous combativeness amongst the different approaches. CBT is a well-established and well-researched therapy that helps people to feel better by thinking better. This strategy is not always the fastest way to deal with deep-rooted issues of people's personality, traumas and suffered abuses. *On the other hand* CBT is well-suited for stress management and as an entry point for those clients who are scared of ending up in a "touchy-feely" therapy (e.g. men!).

The 'inventor' of CBT, Aaron Beck, remarked in an article in 2008[1] that clients with deficits in the prefrontal cortex often have great difficulties with the re-appraisal strategy (ABCD method).[2] That's why many therapists prefer to first utilize neurotherapy on the PFC to speed up the process and to save time and money.

---

[1] Beck AT "The evolution of the cognitive model of depression and its neurobiological correlates" Am J Psychiatry 2008;165(8):969-77
[2] Siegle GJ et al "Increased amygdala and decreased dorsolateral prefrontal BOLD responses in unipolar depression: related and independent features" Biol Psychiatry 2007;61(2):198-209

Acceptance and Commitment Therapy (ACT)

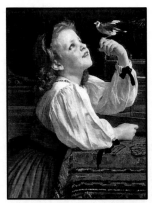

ACT is a newly developed approach and belongs to those mind therapies that aim at teaching skills to improve the client's capacity to cope with life's troubles despite the human mind's imperfections. For example, in chapter 5 we've discussed the negativity bias, our mind's tendency to overestimate potential threats ("You never know what's gonna happen!"). Another mechanism from our savannah past that tends to make us miserable is the *worry* about fitting in: To survive, we need to belong to a group and so our mind is afraid of being rejected.

This creates an abundance of worries, doubts and negative thoughts which our mind presents to us as '*inner chatter*', an almost constantly *admonishing voice* in our heads. So it is no wonder that we feel bad a lot, despite regular meals and the absence of lions.

The problem starts with the idea that we *should* be feeling better, that we *should* be happy all the time or at least contented. This now gets the vortex started: "Why am I so tense? The others seem to be way more relaxed. That makes me really nervous. I bet they think that I'm always tense."

When we try to suppress these anxious thoughts, chances are that they'll come back at us as physical complaints or 'medical' symptoms. Therapists may see those symptoms as 'psychosomatic', but with the help of doctors and the pharmaceutical industry, as suffering patients, we all manage to deny that insight successfully.

ACT teaches clients to *observe* and accept these thoughts and feelings with the awareness that their mind means well, but that's not always helpful. A-C-T even serves as an acronym for the method: 1. Accept your thoughts and feelings!
2. Connect with your values!
3. Take effective action!

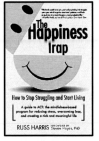

Although ACT has only been around since 1999 it is well established and researched.[1] The book "The Happiness Trap" by Russ Harris is recommended reading for interested migraineurs.

---

[1] Powers MB et al "Acceptance and commitment therapy: a meta-analytic review" Psychother Psychosom 2009;78(2):73-80

Chapter 22

Escaping your Traps

"I grew up to have my father's looks, my father's speech patterns, my father's posture, my father's walk, my father's opinions and my mother's contempt for my father."

Jules Feiffer

Schema Therapy

Imagine someone riding a bike along a very long road. Many years ago a tram or streetcar line occupied a certain part of that same road. Now there is only the old tram-track left, firmly embedded in the surface of the road. And although there is enough space for a smooth ride, sometimes when the wind blows, the cyclist can't help it but swerve off course a bit. And so occasionally his wheels get trapped in the tram-track, he loses his balance, falls and hurts himself.

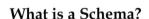

Some folks get trapped in their 'tram-track' more often than others. Some people get caught by their 'track-trap' a lot and some seem to be 'very trapped' and can barely ever enjoy a smooth ride.

A 'schema' or 'life-trap' is a bit similar to the out-of-service tram-track from the past: When the wind of life blows harshly into our face and we swerve off course, the trap can catch our wheels and control our experience; we lose our emotional balance, our mind falls over and our actions hurt ourselves and others.

What is a Schema?

A schema is a set of core beliefs, emotions and thoughts about oneself and the world; like a character in a play with distinct behaviors and attitudes. Everybody plays "The Child" in "The Childhood Drama". At the end of childhood that role ceases to exist — the play is over, end of season — but sometimes the character lives on.

That is normal to some extent, but when being that character poses problems, that role is called a *maladaptive* schema.

How maladaptive schemas emerge

As we are all aware, children have a lot of needs:

• safety	• stability	• predictability
• love	• nurturing	• attention
• acceptance	• praise	• empathy
• guidance	• protection	• validation

When these core needs are *not* met, the infantile mind draws certain conclusions about itself and the world. The child might also try to cope with its resulting emotional distress in a certain way, e.g. trying harder to attract attention, surrendering to loneliness or avoiding exploration due to a lack of encouragement.

These behaviors, including their driving beliefs and emotions, can persist into adulthood. Actually, they can become patterns that define a person's identity and personality. Sometimes they can become a life-long problem, a life-trap.

A list of common life-traps (schemas)

As you already know, I'm a sucker for concrete examples. So let's have a look at some of these life-traps (maladaptive schemas):

When a child experiences its parents as emotionally cold or distant, it may form the life-trap **Emotional Deprivation**, which is the deep-seated, *unconscious belief that one's emotional needs will never be met* by others. Depending on the coping style, this can lead to:

    1. overly demanding behaviors in relationships or
    2. a preference for emotionally cold partners or
    3. the avoidance of close relationships altogether.

It is obvious that none of these three strategies is capable of healing the emotional pain underlying the schema.

When the child experiences the parents as too critical, this may lead to feeling *unworthy of being unconditionally loved* and is called **Defectiveness/Shame**. As adults these children tend to:

    1. be very critical of others, while striving for perfection or
    2. put themselves down and choose judgmental friends or
    3. avoid being open and genuine.

When the child learns from a fearful parent that *the world is essentially a dangerous place*, this can lead to very stable beliefs about having a particular **Vulnerability to Harm and Illness** and the constant need for vigilance, caution and precautions. Adults with this maladaptive schema might:
1. do the exact opposite and seek dangerous 'adventures' or
2. accept the 'perilous-world' concept and be obsessed with real and potential hazards, adversities and disasters or
3. avoid unfamiliar (= unsafe) things, places and people.

Eighteen maladaptive schemas have been documented:

- abandonment/instability
- mistrust/abuse
- emotional deprivation
- defectiveness/shame
- social isolation/alienation
- dependence/incompetence
- vulnerability to harm or illness
- enmeshment/undeveloped self
- failure
- entitlement/grandiosity
- insuffficient self-control/self-discipline
- subjugation
- self-sacrifice
- approval-/recognition-seeking
- negativity/pessimism
- emotional inhibition
- punitiveness
- unrelenting standards/hypercriticalness

Healing schemas = Escaping life-traps

Schemas are very pervasive patterns and try to resist change *as if* the maladaptive 'character' from the childhood drama was fighting for its 'survival'. A powerful alliance is required between the adjusted parts of the client and a competent, trusted therapist:

➢ Step 1: identification, recognition, acknowledgment, observation of schemas
➢ Step 2: thinking about / arguing against schemas, changing core beliefs
➢ Step 3: feeling and building resistance, validation of one's true needs
➢ Step 4: actively exploring and practicing new behaviors in gradual steps
➢ Step 5: forgiving/making inner peace with those responsible for the schema

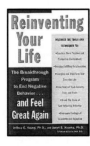 Read more about Schema Therapy in these highly recommended books

⬅ for laypeople: "Reinventing Your Life" by Jeffrey Young, PhD & Janet Klosko, PhD

➡ for therapists: Young, Klosko & Weishaar "Schema Therapy—A Practitioner's Guide"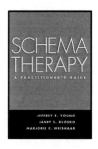

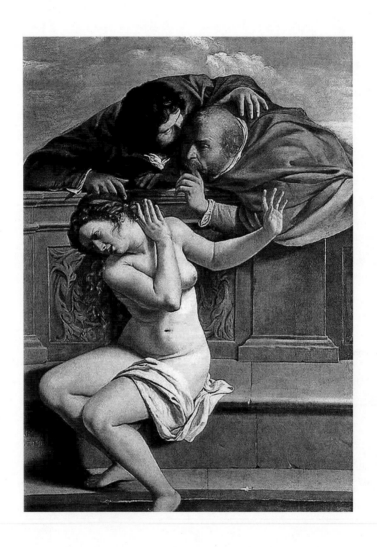

Chapter 23

Healing Shocks

> "Freedom is what you do
> with what has been done to you."
> Jean Paul Sartre

Trauma therapy

If we understand *resilience* as a person's capacity to recover from stress and adversity, then a *trauma* is a distressing experience, which exceeds a person's resilience. The long-term consequences of overwhelming distress are well researched thanks to the many military veterans with PTSD (= post-traumatic stress disorder).

Migraine and PTSD are not only comorbid to one another—which means they appear together more often than they should—they also share that the amygdala can get the better of the prefrontal cortex (see page 185), which is not desirable.

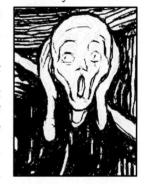

As we've seen in chapter 5, some form of childhood-maltreatment trauma is a frequent finding in severe migraineurs. What if most (if not all) migraineurs have faced *some* form of early life stress,[1] which exceeded their resilience at the time and which set them up to be an active 'migraine-volcano' in life?[2] In contrast, their migraine-free siblings and twins (with the same or similar genetic 'talent') get away without migraine-'eruptions', either due to a higher resilience at that time or due to less disturbing circumstances.[3]

Please keep in mind that 'distress' and 'trauma' lie in the eye of the beholder: It is not the event itself, but the *subjective experience* that counts and that leaves its traces. It doesn't take war, rape or natural disasters; persistent tension in close relationships, hurtful remarks or public ridicule can be traumatizing too.[4]

---

[1] Tietjen GE et al "Childhood abuse and migraine: epidemiology, sex differences, and potential mechanisms" Headache 2011;51(6):869-79
[2] New AS et al "A functional magnetic resonance imaging study of deliberate emotion regulation in resilience and posttraumatic stress disorder" Biol Psychiatry 2009;66(7):656-64
[3] Siniatchkin M et al "Migraine and asthma in childhood: evidence for specific asymmetric parent-child interactions in migraine and asthma families" Cephalalgia 2003;23(8):790-802
[4] Teicher MH et al "Sticks, stones and hurtful words: relative effects of various forms of childhood maltreatment" Am J Psychiatry 2006;163(6):993-1000

Shocking memories

When our mind *remembers* an event from the past, it feels to us like reading a technical description: The brain reassembles the facts, but not the emotions; nor do we precisely recall sensory details like images, sounds, smells or bodily feelings. We might even *know about* the emotions at the time, for instance "I was scared to death, before the bungee jump", but we don't re-experience that fear.

When memories are *re-lived* with strong emotions and the revival of sensory details, we call that a traumatic memory; the brain re-experiences the event, as if it were happening now: "I'm still shaking, when I think of that incident in the car park."

When the brain is overwhelmed and too distressed, it stores events as memories without 'cleaning' them from the emotional experience and without stamping them as "PAST". That's why they can get triggered and re-experienced and give us a lot of grief and stress. Moreover, the mind adds an interpretation like "I'm not safe", which may have been true at the time, but now creates a general sense of un-safety (e.g. "EVERYTHING CAN TRIGGER A MIGRAINE ATTACK")

Since those trauma-induced feelings and unconscious thoughts keep us on our toes all the time, which translates into hypervigilance, anxiety and disturbing thoughts, we need to heal these distressing memories by giving the brain an opportunity to process the events properly and turn them into factual memories.

Fortunately, we have helpful therapies for that and the process is actually quite simple, although not always easy. In any case it's well worth the effort and amazingly liberating.[1]

Eye Movement Desensitization Reprocessing (EMDR)

In order to re-process a traumatic memory, the client needs to recollect it and simultaneously maintain an awareness of the "here and now" in the role of an adult observer. Since these upsetting memories typically try to pull the entire mind into the recalled experience, various techniques are employed to 're-mind' both brain hemispheres (= halves) of the difference between the *experienced present* of the past trauma and the *real present* of the session in the therapist's office.

---

[1] Ponniah K et al Empirically supported psychological treatments for adult acute stress disorder and posttraumatic stress disorder: a review" Depress Anxiety 2009;26(12):1086-109

One of those 're-minding' techniques are side-to-side eye movements, which became part of the name for this very structured approach. Other forms of bi-lateral stimulation are alternating taps on the knees, hand-held devices or audio-files with left-right sound patterns.

The difference between the two sides of the brain is often *characterized* in word pairs like so:

left hemisphere	right hemisphere
analytic	wholistic
language	music
conscious	subconscious
thoughts	emotions
'adult'	'child'

Some clients, especially those abused in childhood, have great difficulty letting go of the traumatic experience, possibly because they are stuck in a state of *infantile appeal* ("Help me, daddy!"), which corresponds with excessive 'doctor shopping' ("One day, he'll come to my rescue"). In those cases the adult parts of the ego (see page 129) need to learn how to take better care of themselves and give their own pleading 'Inner Child' ("HEAL ME") a sense of nurturance and protection ("Daddy won't come, but I am here for you—always").

Energy Psychology for trauma resolution

Over the last couple of years a number of weird and wonderful methods have emerged that claim to promote emotional healing by "unblocking" or "correcting" subtle energies in the body. Allegedly and against any healthy common sense, odd rituals of tapping on meridian points called "Emotional Freedom Technique" or "Tapa's Acupressure Technique" are supposed to help overcome trauma, phobias and other unsettling issues.

The kicker is, that these peculiar methods work like a charm[1] and exceptionally well for intensely upsetting traumatic memories. As a therapist, I don't really care whether a good effect is caused by *"bilateral stimulation of the sensory cortex"* or by *"unblocking an energy meridian"*, as long as it helps my clients. And that it does.

---

[1] Salas MM et al "The immediate effect of a brief energy psychology intervention (Emotional Freedom Techniques) on specific phobias: a pilot study" Explore (NY) 2011;7(3):155-61

Alpha-Theta neurofeedback

When we want to go to sleep, we deliberately slow our brain down in order to change from the 'awake-state' to the 'asleep-state'. During that process, we transit to an *'in-between-state'*, which we call trance. In trance, most parts of the brain have calmed down, but our 'Reflective Self', located in the prefrontal cortex[1], hasn't completely switched off yet.

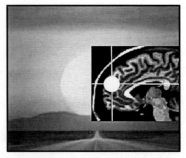

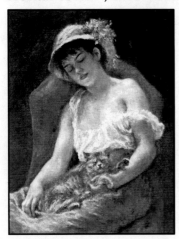

We can see the onset of trance in the EEG, when the main energy at the back of the brain starts shifting from the alpha towards the theta range. Alpha-theta neurofeedback[2] can guide the brain into this trance-state, [3] in which the "Reflective Self" can look at scenes from the past without distress or distraction. This allows for the processing of traumatic imagery[4] and the drama-free release of the associated emotional discomfort in a safe environment.

Alpha-theta neurofeedback combines 'brainwave-training' with a very strong guidance tool for trauma therapy. It is traditionally used for very severe PTSD[5] and therapy-resistant addictions[6,7,8,9,10] with outstanding success.

---

[1] D'Argembeau A et al "Distinct regions of the medial prefrontal cortex are associated with self-referential processing and perspective taking" J Cogn Neurosci 2007;19(6):935-44

[2] Egner T et al "The temporal dynamics of electroencephalographic responses to alpha/theta neurofeedback training in healthy subjects" J Neurotherapy 2004;8(1):43-57

[3] Egner T et al "EEG signature and phenomenology of alpha/theta neurofeedback training versus mock feedback" Appl Psychophysiol Biofeedback 2002;27(4):261-70

[4] Moore et al "Comparison of Alpha-Theta, Alpha and EMG Neurofeedback in the Production of Alpha-Theta Crossover and the Occurrence of Visualizations" J Neurotherapy 2000;4(1):29-42

[5] Peniston EG et al "Alpha-theta brainwave neurofeedback for Vietnam veterans with combat-related post-traumatic stress disorder" Medical Psychotherapy 1991;4(1):47-60

[6] Peniston EG et al "Alpha-theta brainwave training and beta-endorphin levels in alcoholics" Alcohol Clin Exp Res 1989;13(2):271-9

[7] Saxby E, et al "Alpha-theta brainwave neurofeedback training: an effective treatment for male and female alcoholics with depressive symptoms" J Clin Psychol 1995;51(5):685-93

[8] Scott WC et al "Effects of an EEG biofeedback protocol on a mixed substance abusing population" Am J Drug Alcoh Abuse 2005;31(3):455-69

[9] Fahrion SL et al "Alterations in EEG amplitude, personality factors, and brain electrical mapping after alpha-theta brainwave training: a controlled case study of an alcoholic in recovery" Alcohol Clin Exp Res 1992;16(3):547-52

[10] Sokhadze TM et al "EEG biofeedback as a treatment for substance use disorders: review, rating of efficacy, and recommendations for further research" Appl Psychophysiol Biofeedback 2008;33(1):1-28

Other scientifically validated applications are the therapy of mood disorders[1,2,3] and the enhancement of artistic performance of dancers and musicians.[4,5,6]

For therapists who pay attention not only to officially recognized trauma events (war, rape, tsunami etc.), but also to the seemingly pathetic, yet personality-forming little hurts and humiliations, it is reassuring to have alpha-theta neurofeedback as an option; for instance for those clients, who simply don't feel comfortable in any form of talk therapy and can't at all imagine to tell their stories to a therapist; but also in those cases, where there are more *feelings* of hurt than concrete traumatic memories. All this might only apply to a minority of migraineurs anyway.

The last group of migraine patients who could potentially benefit from alpha-theta neurofeedback is hopefully even smaller: I'm thinking of those, who have become addicted to opioid-containing pain medication.[7]

Therapists who offer alpha-theta neurofeedback therapy can be found in the directory at www.TheMigraineRevolution.com.

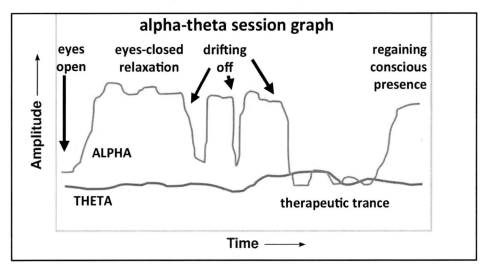

---

[1] Vanathy S et al "The efficacy of alpha and theta neurofeedback training in treatment of generalized anxiety disorder" Indian J Clin Psych 1998;25(2):136-43
[2] Moore NC "A review of EEG biofeedback treatment of anxiety disorders" Clin Electroencephalogr 2000;31(1):1-6
[3] Raymond J et al "The effects of alpha/theta neurofeedback on personality and mood" Brain Res Cogn Brain Res 2005;23(2-3):287-92
[4] Egner T et al "Ecological validity of neurofeedback: modulation of slow wave EEG enhances musical performance" Neuroreport 2003;14(9):1221-4
[5] Gruzelier J "Validating the efficacy of neurofeedback for optimising performance" Prog Brain Res 2006;159:421-31
[6] Gruzelier J "A theory of alpha/theta neurofeedback, creative performance enhancement, long distance functional connectivity and psychological integration" Cogn Process 2009;10 Suppl 1:S101-9
[7] Arani FD et al "Effectiveness of neurofeedback training as a treatment for opioid-dependent patients" Clin EEG Neurosci 2010;41(3):170-7

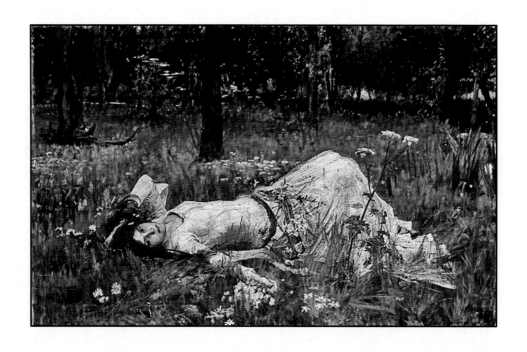

Chapter 24

Feeling Heavy and Warm

> "Energy and persistence conquer all things."
> Benjamin Franklin

Autogenic Training

The bad news right upfront: Autogenic Training (AT) requires diligent and persistent practice over weeks and months in order to reach its full potential. *AT alone* is probably insufficient to stop migraine attacks within a few weeks in complex and difficult cases. However, this is where the negatives end.

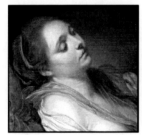

On the *entry level*, AT is a form of arranged self-hypnosis for calming body, mind and brain. Autogenic means 'self-generated' and refers to the fact that the clients actively regulate their autonomic nervous system by repeating the suggested phrases in their head. They also need to observe the body's subtle responses and amplify them with their imagination. Mastering the six basic sessions takes persistent practice.

The *intermediate level* adds positive auto-suggestions, self-selected phrases to purposely change one's experience (for instance "I always remain calm and collected") or unwanted behaviors (e.g. "Cigarettes have no power over me").

The *advanced level* of AT contains psycho-dynamic elements like working with colors and symbols, or questions for the subconscious. Whilst this deeply analytical level requires guidance and supervision by a qualified psychotherapist, the exercises of the intermediate and entry level can (and should) be used as a very sophisticated 'relaxation' training, leading to profound changes.

I've never heard of it, is it any good?

Autogenic Training was developed in the 1920s by the Berlin psychiatrist J. H. Schultz and is popular and widely applied in German-speaking Europe, primarily taught by psychologists. In Austria, AT is listed as an officially recognized psychotherapy.

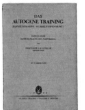
Autogenic Training[1] is less well-known in most English-speaking countries, but it has quite a good reputation in the medical community. The number of scientific papers is actually quite impressive; and so are the results for patients with migraine:

A meta-analysis of 60 studies of the effects of AT in all sorts of disorders found *significantly positive* outcomes for migraine,[2] similar to other 'mind therapies'. The impact of AT on mood, cognitive performance and quality-of-life was found to be even stronger.[1] So it's no surprise that the consumption of pain medication and migraine drugs shows a *substantial, long-term reduction* under the influence of the persistent practice of AT.

AT also works well for children; 50% of them ended up totally migraine-free without any medication with AT alone (Only thermal biofeedback was stronger with 80% migraine-free kids).[3]

Autogenic Training as 'relaxation' technique?

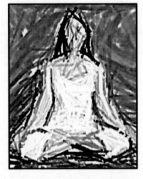

'Relaxation' exercises are highly endorsed by official, evidence-based treatment guidelines, but that's like putting apples and oranges in one pot and calling it fruit. 'Relaxation' exercises have very specific effects.[4] A CD with spacey music that makes you doze off is not necessarily an effective therapy. The goal of all 'relaxation' exercises is to acquire and to improve the skill of controlling the body's stress response in daily life; and that needs participation and regular practice.

My stern advice for everyone plagued by migraine is to consider adopting and cementing the habit of regular 'relaxation' exercises: 1. start with breathing retraining (see chapter 12), after a few weeks move to 2. progressive muscle relaxation (see chapter 13) and finally 3. Autogenic Training. Detailed instructions can be found for free on many websites, e.g. on youtube.com.

---

[1] Book "Das Autogene Training - Konzentrative Selbstentspannung" by J. H. Schultz, 1932; photo by H.-P. Haack
[2] Stetter F et al "Autogenic training: a meta-analysis of clinical outcome studies" Appl Psychophysiol Biofeedback 2002;27(1):45-98
[3] Labbé EE "Treatment of childhood migraine with autogenic training and skin temperature biofeedback: a component analysis" Headache 1995;35(1):10-3
[4] Lehrer PM et al "Stress management techniques: are they all equivalent, or do they have specific effects?" Biofeedback Self Regul 1994;19(4):353-401

Chapter 25

When the Mind Sees what the Body Does

> "Your body is your subconscious mind."
> Candace Pert

Applied psychophysiology

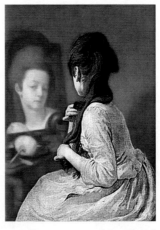

Psyche—e.g. in psychology—simply means mind or soul. *Physiology* is the study of the function of living organisms. Ergo psychophysiology is about the interactions between mind and body.

When scientific fields turn out to be helpful for people, the therapeutic branch of that domain adds the label '*applied*' to it, as in Applied Neuroscience and Applied Psychophysiology.

Nowadays every academic discipline needs to use big and complicated words, to make it harder for *angry rivals* to be critical and scornful. As a reader of migraine books you can judge how ferocious the competition for patients' attention is by how condescending and dismissive the authors are, when they write about therapies that they themselves don't make money from.

It is therefore unfortunate for patients that most migraine books are written by medical doctors, who naturally push their own barrow with drugs and surgery and banalize non-medical therapies as 'alternative' or 'complementary'. Another reason for glibness is the inability to admit:

"I don't know much about it and therefore don't have an opinion."

Patients often expect their doctors to provide competent and sensible guidance for everything, but why would a doc say

"Drugs don't end the tyranny; go and start your migraine revolution"?

In all disorders that involve body, mind and brain, applied psychophysiology is a valuable therapy field to give patients the understanding and experience of how thoughts and emotions affect the body, and how bodily functions, like muscle tension, posture or breathing, have an impact on the state of mind.

In my experience, migraine patients benefit greatly and typically are very excited about the insights, increased awareness and skills they gain in a few sessions of *applied mind-body study*.

Thanks to sanitation, hygiene, germ-free drinking water, antibiotics and vaccinations, diseases are somewhat under control in the Western world. Instead we're struggling with disorders, which make us miserable throughout our extended lifespan. Thus it would be appropriate not only for patients with a disorder, but especially for doctors and other healthcare providers to study a few semesters at a *mind-body university*.

Those black-and-white thinkers (see page 91) who still insist that migraine is a 'medical' disease and *not at all* a mind issue, are recommended to study the emerging discipline of psychoneuro-immunology and be amazed by scientific discoveries of puzzling mind-body interactions, like—for example, but not limited to—the mind's contribution to wound healing.[1]

The practice of applied psychophysiology does not replace abortive migraine medication, but it can teach and hone the skills, which can help end the migraine tyranny altogether.

Good feedback

If you are female, please imagine that, for a special occasion, you need to put a lot of make-up on, the whole shebang. If you are a man, please imagine shaving your facial hair with a barber's knife and if you are a teenager, imagine yourself squeezing several ripe pimples on your face. Are you imagining it? Are you doing it in front of a mirror? Why?

Your answer is probably something like: "So that I can see what I'm doing." Exactly, a mirror gives us good feedback, what exactly our hands are doing in our face and without it we wouldn't even start to squeeze, to shave or to paint our face on.

Serious language students need to listen to recordings of themselves talking, in order to match their pronunciation to that of their teacher. Easy to understand if you think of the Swedish word for nurse ("sjuksköterska"), the elegant Hungarian word for flatulence ("hátvágánygáz") or the 21 click sounds in the Xhosa language of Southern Africa (sing "Qongqothwane"!).

---

[1] Broadbent E et al "The psychology of wound healing" Curr Opin Psychiatry 2012;25(2):135-40

Proper chefs taste every dish they're cooking, so that they aren't surprised by their customers' negative feedback. Engaged ski

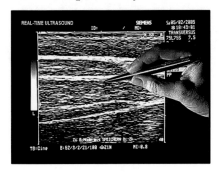

instructors take videos of their students to show them how they're skiing and thereby make learning easier. Patients with low back pain can re-learn to activate their deep abdominal muscles to re-normalize their muscular spinal stabilization with the help of visual feedback, provided by real-time ultrasound.

Feedback of function

So far we've looked at people receiving visual, auditory or taste feedback about details of their actions: face painting, shaving, squeezing, speaking foreign, cooking, skiing and stabilizing their back. The additional information delivered by the feedback helped all of them to improve the quality of their actions: make-up precision, exotic pronunciation, gourmet excellence and efficiency of muscle activity.

When this principle is used to feed back signals from the body, e.g. heartbeat, blood flow, muscle activity, CO_2 in the lungs and the like, it's called *biofeedback* in order to emphasize that a *biological* signal is observed. Since the necessary measurement devices are expensive, this field absolutely deserves its own name.

After knee surgery, biofeedback of the electrical activity of the various knee-stabilizing muscles can help a lot to get the muscle balance right and speed up the rehabilitation process.[1] For that you need an EMG (= electromyography) device. We already know "graphy" from EEG, 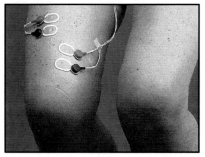 "myo" means muscle and "electro" is obvious: EMG records the electrical activity in muscles, and that's what you would want to feed back in order to help the knee patient to get back on their feet.[2]

---

[1] Wild JJ Jr et al "Patellar pain and quadriceps rehabilitation. An EMG study" Am J Sports Med 1982;10(1):12-5
[2] Basmajian JV "Research foundations of EMG biofeedback in rehabilitation" Biofeedback Self Regul 1988;13(4):275-98

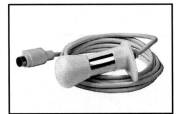
EMG biofeedback is also used for *pelvic floor rehabilitation*, which those women appreciate who leak a bit after giving birth to bigheaded offspring. The same kind of EMG sensor is used for the treatment of chronic pelvic pain due to overly tense pelvic muscles,[1] a condition that can affect men too.

With the help of EMG biofeedback, patients after *spinal cord injury* (e.g. paraplegics) can sometimes regain control over their supposedly paralyzed leg muscles to a degree that makes walking possible.[2,3] *Stroke patients* too can re-establish lost motor functions, when the process is supported by instant information about electrical muscle activity.[4]

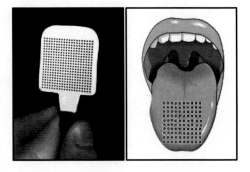

Stroke victims can also repair their sense of balance with a mouthpiece whose tiny pins draw tactile patterns onto the tongue to inform about body sway.[5,6] The same type of mouthpiece can give blind people a substitute for vision.[7,8]

Strictly speaking this is not biofeedback, because the observed signal is derived from visual contrast or wobbly posture and not from an internal *physiological* source; but isn't it interesting how a nervous system can re-learn or substitute lost functions when it gets good feedback about the effects of its own actions?

The basis for that is *neuroplasticity*, the ability of the brain and nervous system to adapt and change: People who learn all the streets of London for the taxi driver exam, change the structure of their brain. If their brain does *not* change, they fail the exam.[9]

---

[1] Ye ZQ et al "Biofeedback therapy for chronic pelvic pain syndrome" Asian J Androl 2003;5(2):155-8
[2] Brucker BS et al "Biofeedback effect on electromyography responses in patients with spinal cord injury" Arch Phys Med Rehab 1996;77(2):133-7
[3] Houldin A et al "Locomotor adaptations and aftereffects to resistance during walking in individuals with spinal cord injury" J Neurophysiol 2011;106(1):247-58
[4] Doğan-Aslan M et al "The effect of electromyographic biofeedback treatment in improving upper extremity functioning of patients with hemiplegic stroke" J Stroke Cerebrovasc Dis 2012;21(3):187-92
[5] Danilov YP et al "Efficacy of electrotactile vestibular substitution in patients with peripheral and central vestibular loss" J Vestib Res 2007;17(2-3):119-30
[6] Badke MB et al "Tongue-based biofeedback for balance in stroke: results of an 8-week pilot study" Arch Phys Med Rehabil 2011;92(9):1364-70
[7] Ptito M et al "Cross-modal plasticity revealed by electrotactile stimulation of the tongue in the congenitally blind" Brain 2005;128(Pt 3):606-14
[8] Liu J et al "Recognition of Chinese character on electrotactile vision substitution system" Zhongguo Yi Liao Qi Xie Za Zhi 2010;34(5):313-6
[9] Woollett K et al "Acquiring "the Knowledge" of London's layout drives structural brain changes" Curr Biol 2011;21(24):2109-14

Biofeedback for migraine?

After all these fascinating examples of what brains are capable of in terms of learning, changing and repairing when supported with informative feedback, one wonders whether it is possible to teach a migraine brain, *not to produce migraine episodes* any longer. The precondition would be that the measured signal somehow represents the mechanisms that lead to the dreaded attack.

If there was a detectable signal showing the quality of brain function, then it should be possible—with the right biofeedback—to train the brain to do a better job and not produce the exploding seizure activity in the brainstem. Can you think of a way to record *electrical brain activity*, which one could use for some kind of 'brain biofeedback' to harvest the potential of neuroplasticity and applied neuroscience? It would have to be somehow similar to EMG biofeedback, but with "brain" instead of "myo". Any ideas?

The most popular migraine books and websites don't mention the enticing concept of brain biofeedback. It seems migraineurs are supposed to live in fear, watch out for triggers and swallow drugs. According to these sources biofeedback is used to *control stress*. That is a great idea, stress is the number one 'trigger' for migraine attacks and surely needs to be controlled, but what does that mean "control stress"? Does that refer to distressing situations or to the stress response of body and brain?

We've seen that biofeedback is neither a *method* nor a *therapy*, but merely a *technical principle* to inform someone about certain body functions, preferably those that they can't see, hear or precisely feel. We can't feel where exactly the mascara or the blade are going to hit our face, that's why we need the mirror. And the patients after knee surgery, spinal cord injury, stroke, as well as the leaking ladies, can't feel what their half-dead muscles are doing.

It may well be that there are methods using the biofeedback principle, which help people to cope better with distressing situations by teaching and practicing the ability to dampen the stress response. I suppose *those* people could benefit, who have difficulties feeling how revved up they really are. That is quite likely in migraineurs with alexithymia (see page 87) and a better sense of one's own stress response allows for an informed decision whether the distressing situation is actually worth it.

The stress response

Let's not forget that—biologically—humans are designed to live on the savannah as hunters and gatherers. When we did, it could easily happen that during a playful rabbit hunt we were surprised by a hungry lion or a pack of hyenas. For such a lethal threat it would be awesome to have a capable nervous system which recognizes the urgency of the situation and enables us to run as fast as humanly possible to the next tree and climb it.

There are two bits of good news: First, we do indeed have such a nervous system and second, we don't have to outrun the lion, we only have to be faster than the other tribe members!

The autonomic nervous system (ANS) with its activating *"sympathetic"* branch gets the body ready for an emergency escape as soon as the limbic system rings the alarm bell. The amygdala even has a special cable from the optic nerve, so that in cases of imminent danger, our alarm reaction is immediate and not delayed by visual processing. Simply put: We're ready before we know it.[1]

Once the danger is over, the deactivating *"parasympathetic"* branch of the ANS needs to switch off the alarm systems in the body, so that we don't waste precious resources and instead start healing and recovery: We might have suffered an injury during our lucky escape and we might have to run again tomorrow or tonight.

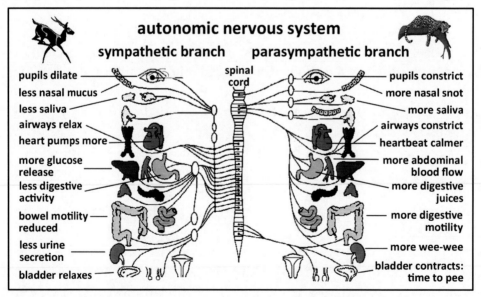

[1] Liddell BJ et al "A direct brainstem-amygdala-cortical 'alarm' system for subliminal signals of fear" Neuroimage 2005;24(1):235-43

The stress response is designed to prepare us for *physical* "fight or flight". It serves to aid our efforts to *survive* threatening situations. A decent level of activity in the amygdala (limbic system) activates the stress alarm, the body responds with faster heartbeat, narrower blood vessels, faster and deeper breathing, higher blood sugar and so on in preparation for running and climbing. The brain gets ready with *vigilant attention* and interprets the incoming body sensations in the context of the threatening situation as fear.[1] During a *bungee jump* the brain might interpret the same sensations as 'excited joy' (perhaps not during the first jump though). The emotional experience depends on *what the mind knows and thinks* about a certain situation.[2,3]

The closer the threat comes, (1) the more brain activity shifts away from the prefrontal cortex and towards the PAG[4] in the brainstem, (2) the more the behavioral choices (fight or flight?) are restricted to run or freeze,[5] and (3) the more fear and anxiety change into panic and sheer terror:[6]

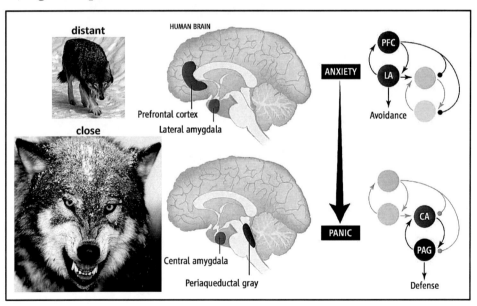

And that is not even a lion!

---

[1] James W "The physical bases of emotion. 1894" Psychol Rev 1994;101(2):205-10
[2] Schachter S "Cognitive, social, and physiological determinants of emotional state" Psychol Rev 1962;69:379-99
[3] Gray MA et al "Modulation of emotional appraisal by false physiological feedback during fMRI" PLoS One 2007;2(6):e546
[4] Mobbs D et al "When fear is near: threat imminence elicits prefrontal- shifts in humans" Science 2007;317(5841):1079-83
[5] Graeff FG et al "Role of the amygdala and periaqueductal gray in anxiety and panic" Behav Brain Res 1993;58(1-2):123-31
[6] Maren S "Neuroscience. The threatened brain" Science 2007;317(5841):1043-4 (Photo of the distant wolf by Daniel Mott)

In the unlucky case that we are the slowest runner of our tribe and the predator gets hold of us, the autonomic nervous system (ANS) may have to use the last resort, which is *feigning death* or 'freezing/fainting':[1] A special division of the parasympathetic[2] (deactivating) ANS induces a behavioral paralysis and dissociation, a state of relatively pain-free absent-mindedness. At least the ANS has mercy with us, in case the lion does not.

Hunter-gatherers in Sydney, London and New York

Imagine the boss of a company makes the announcement:

> "Business is down 50%, I'll have to sack half of you guys. To make it fair to everybody, we'll play rock-paper-scissors to decide who stays and who goes."

Understandably all the employees with a car loan and a fat mortgage perceive this announcement as a threat to their livelihood and their nervous system triggers a stress response, which means they are *ready to run away and climb a tree*. But nobody does.

Instead they have to stay and put on a brave face during a humiliating procedure that will decide their occupational fate, at least for now. It is somehow likely that the stress-sensitive of the migraineurs amongst them will have an attack soon, right? The ones with neck pain will probably have more neck pain. What's your vision for the employees with irritable bowel syndrome (IBS)?

Unfortunately we've inherited certain biological mechanisms for emergencies from our ancestors, which aren't particularly helpful for most of the distressing situations in the modern world. Running away and climbing trees simply doesn't cut it anymore.

As a result, the frequent igniting of the stress response elicits a plethora of symptoms in various body systems: gastrointestinal, cardiovascular, musculoskeletal, respiratory, mood regulation, arousal regulation/sleep, concentration/memory and so forth.

If it were true that modern disorders (like IBS, chronic fatigue syndrome etc.) can largely be explained with the stress response, then people, who are *more distressed*, would have to have *more symptoms*, right? And that is exactly the case.[3]

---

[1] Bracha HS "Freeze, flight, fight, fright, faint: adaptationist perspectives on the acute stress response spectrum" CNS Spectr 2004;9(9):679-85

[2] Porges SW "The polyvagal theory: New insights into adaptive reactions of the autonomic nervous system" Cleve Clin J Med 2009;76(Suppl 2):S86–S90

[3] Fink P et al "Symptoms and syndromes of bodily distress: an exploratory study of 978 internal medical, neurological, and primary care patients" Psychosom Med 2007;69(1):30-9

Danish scientists could impressively prove that patients' so-called "functional" symptoms simply don't support the common diagnostic criteria, because the patient with the label '*chronic fatigue syndrome*' is just as disposed to diffuse muscle pain as is the declared '*fibromyalgia*' patient to '*insomnia*' and a 'lack of energy'. And both are prone to the same gastrointestinal symptoms that make up the '*irritable bowel syndrome*' in the patient with the additional frequent headaches. The Danish authors suggest calling it *bodily distress syndrome*. It explains at least ten disorders. [1,2]

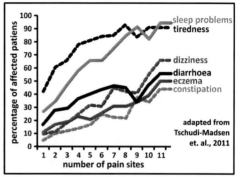

Investigators in Norway found in patients a strong linear connection between the number of painful body sites and the number of other complaints, which convincingly supports the Danish conclusions. [3] All these Scandinavian studies were done on very large groups.

The ensuing diagnoses are considered a result of the fact that patients tend to take one symptom more seriously than others and doctors usually stick to their diagnostic guns: e.g. the gastro-enterologist discovers the '*irritable bowel syndrome*' and ignores the overbreathing, the mood issues and the trauma history of the patient.[4] Patients are typically elated that the doctor found something apparently '*real*', because they were concerned that they would be dismissed with a condescending "It's all in your head".

Sadly, not many patients say to their gastroenterologist:

> "Well, doc, I'm glad that you could rule out cancer and parasites in my gut and I'm deeply grateful that you've stuck your funky camera up my rectum, but your diagnostic label 'irritable bowel syndrome' is nothing more than a summary of the symptoms I've told you about, mate. Given my personal history and my other stress-related symptoms, I'm beginning to think I should talk to therapists who deal with stress and trauma. What do you reckon, doc?"

---

[1] Fink P et al "One single diagnosis, bodily distress syndrome, succeeded to capture 10 diagnostic categories of functional somatic syndromes and somatoform disorders" J Psychosom Res 2010;68(5):415-26
[2] Fink P et al "New unifying diagnosis of functional diseases" Ugeskr Laeger 2010;172(24):1835-8
[3] Tschudi-Madsen H et al "A strong association between non-musculoskeletal symptoms and musculoskeletal pain symptoms: results from a population study" BMC Musculoskelet Disord 2011;12:285
[4] Wessely S et al "Functional somatic syndromes: one or many?" Lancet 1999;354(9182):936-9

Although for different reasons, doctor and patient are often complicit in explaining a symptom as a '*medical*' problem, so that it requires medication, surgery or other '*medical*' treatments. Both parties are more than willing to ignore and deny the origin of the complaints: One of them is fearful, the other has no clue. I wonder who can tell me, who is who?

A horrible mismatch

Modern medicine can be proud of many spectacular achievements. Antibiotics, vaccinations, anesthesia, organ transplants, prosthetics, stem cell research, gene therapy, emergency medicine and plenty more deserve awe and admiration. On the other hand, modern medicine is ignorant and ruthless when it comes to health issues that simply don't fit into the Newtonian model and Descartes' contract with the Pope (see page 156), which still today seems to oblige medics to ignore dysfunctions of the *regulatory* systems.[1] The human stress response sits exactly at the intersection of body, mind and brain and its frequent activation of the sympathetic branch of the autonomic nervous system is undoubtedly the foundation of the majority of symptoms that define a multitude of life-destroying disorders.[2]

It is neither my intention nor would it be fair to put the blame for this horrible mismatch solely on doctors and conventional medicine. Human beings have plenty of needs: security, intimacy, love, friendship, status within a group, social support, respect, sense of competence and achievement, meaning and purpose in life, autonomy and control over one's own destiny. Yet we have allowed ourselves to give most of it up for a take-away pizza, a flatscreen TV and pills for depression and acid reflux.

It will take more than a book to change this inhumane complicity, that exploits patients' need for help to their own detriment. Interestingly, severe migraineurs are probably the most disillusioned and disappointed patient group of all, considering that more than half of them can't be bothered to even consult with a doc anymore, despite very severe symptoms (see page 39). Perhaps it's them who have the guts to ignite a change, to start a revolution.

---

[1] Williams N et al "Functional illness in primary care: dysfunction versus disease" BMC Fam Pract 2008;9:30
[2] Bakal D et al "Somatic awareness in the clinical care of patients with body distress symptoms" Biopsychosoc Med 2008;2:6

Checking the ANS

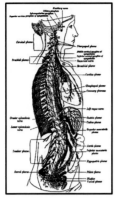

It has become clear that the autonomic nervous system has enormous power over our health and wellbeing. Furthermore, we have discovered that we are essentially confused and irritated hunter-gatherers in a relatively safe, but brutally alarming and distressing environment. Now it's not the slow runners who need to be concerned, but all those who are less resistant, whose bodies, minds and brains are more reactive, who are more alert, observant and vigilant.[1]

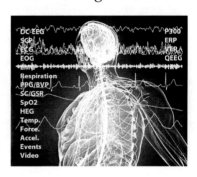

Perhaps one should think about checking a patient's ANS for imbalance, for stronger responses and for delayed recovery. This is the task of applied psychophysiology and called a *psychophysiological stress profile* (PSP).[2,3] A PSP is a recording of several parameters that represent the behavior of the *autonomic nervous system* during self-induced relaxation and during slightly challenging tasks.[4]

The signals of ANS-influenced body functions that therapists in clinical practice commonly measure and record are listed here:

measured parameter	biological function	informs about
surface EMG	muscle activity	involuntary tension
electrodermal activity[5]	sweat gland activity	sympathetic arousal
skin temperature	blood perfusion	vascular ANS balance
blood volume pulse	vasoconstriction/dilation	vascular ANS activity
respiratory expansion	thoracic/belly breathing	breathing pattern/rate
ECG	heart rate variability	cardiac ANS tone
end-tidal CO_2	alveolar CO_2 exchange	overbreathing

---

[1] Meyer GA "The art of watching out: vigilance in women who have migraine headaches" Qual Health Res 2002;12(9):1220-34
[2] Berman PS et al "A psychophysiological assessment battery" Biofeedback Self Regul 1985;10(3):203-21
[3] Diaz MI et al "Development of a multi-channel exploratory battery for psychophysiological assessment: the Stress Profile" Clin Neurophysiol 2003;114(12):2487-96
[4] Crocetti A et al "Psychophysiological Stress Profile: A Protocol to Differentiate Normal vs Pathological Subjects" Act Nerv Super Rediviva 2010; 52(4): 241–245
[5] EDA = electrodermal activity is the correct term for 'galvanic skin response', can be measured as conductance or resistance

High-quality multi-channel data acquisition systems for research and therapy are available for professional psychophysiology experts, including a wide range of measurement sensors. (The photo shows the best device currently.[1])

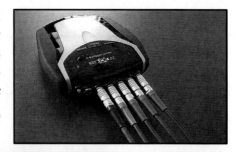

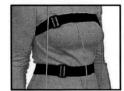 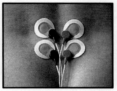 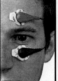 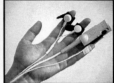

Special belts quantify the expansion of the chest and the abdomen during breathing, adhesive EMG electrodes detect the activity in suspicious muscle groups, EOG[2] electrodes record eye blinks and a heap of sensors get attached to the hand.

The graph of such a PSP looks somewhat like this:

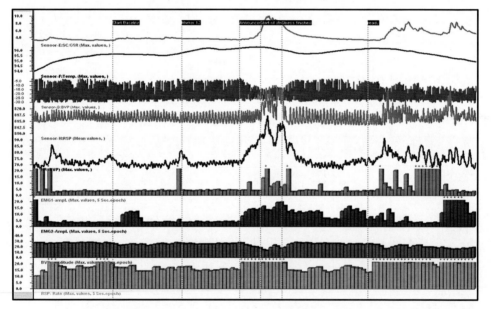

Psychophysiologists can make sense of this and ascertain which of the biological systems express the client's stress response overly strongly and which ones don't recover well.

---

[1] Nexus10 from the Dutch company MindMedia (www.mindmedia.nl)
[2] "EOG" is short for electrooculography; 'oculus' is Latin for eye, so EOG measures eye movements; involuntary eye blinks are regulated by the brainstem and frequent blinking is a sign of a 'jumpy brainstem'

People's bodies react very individually to 'stress'. Some tense up certain muscles involuntarily without noticing or they 'forget' to relax them afterwards. Others display their hunter-gatherer heritage predominantly in their cardiovascular system.[1]

These objective measures of the stress response are not only fascinating for patients, who *experience and sense* a lot of emotional distress (labeled neuroticism), but also for those, who *do not feel* the level of distress that their body endures (labeled alexithymia).[2,3] This discrepancy between the mind's opinion ("I'M NOT DISTRESSED") and the body's 'stress data', can be an indicator for *dissociation;* or in other words: a bit of a freeze response,[4,5,6] which mildly indicates some childhood adversities and aversive life events.[7,8]

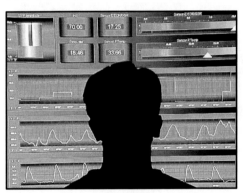

Clients are usually rapt to see their personality and 'scars of life' reflected in their body's reactions and eager to learn and practice managing their edgy nervous system as a resource to *master and control their 'stress'*. Progress is visible and empowers the client's self-efficacy, the best *antidote to helplessness*.

Biofeedback applied to psychophysiology

We've said earlier that biofeedback is neither a *method* nor a *therapy*, but a *technical principle* to inform us about certain body functions, preferably those that we can't see, hear or precisely feel. While the stress response is preparing us for 'fight or flight', we're probably busy paying attention to something scary, e.g. a lion, a wolf or the boss at work, and so we won't have the time or nerves to stop our ANS from freaking out our body.

---

[1] Cohen MJ et al "Evidence for physiological response stereotypy in migraine headache" Psychosom Med 1978;40(4):344-54
[2] Martin JB et al "Influence of alexithymic characteristics on physiological and subjective stress responses in normal individuals" Psychother Psychosom 1986;45(2):66-77
[3] Kanbara K et al "Paradoxical results of psychophysiological stress profile in functional somatic syndrome: correlation between subjective tension score and objective stress response" Appl Psychophysiol Biofeedback 2004;29(4):255-68
[4] Irwin HJ et al "Alexithymia and dissociative tendencies" J Clin Psychol 1997;53(2):159-66
[5] Majohr KL et al "Alexithymia and its relationship to dissociation in patients with panic disorder" J Nerv Ment Dis 2011;199(10):773-7
[6] Linden W et al "Alexithymia, defensiveness and cardiovascular reactivity to stress" J Psychosom Res 1996;41(6):575-83
[7] Kooiman CG et al "Childhood adversities as risk factors for alexithymia and other aspects of affect dysregulation in adulthood" Psychother Psychosom 2004;73(2):107-16
[8] Hagenaars MA et al "Aversive life events enhance human freezing responses" J Exp Psychol Gen 2012;141(1):98-105

And whilst our ancestors could probably feel their racing heart once they were up the tree, nowadays it is rather difficult to notice the more subtle changes in our bodies as they occur *without* the sprint. Thus it is clever to exploit modern technology for biofeedback to achieve 'ANS mastery' when 'stress' is an issue.

When clients want to learn to influence their body's automatic reactions, biofeedback is an invaluable tool to make their conscious mind *see what exactly it is doing*, when it itself regulates the body (= self-regulation). With a bit of practice and by weaning off the external biofeedback, the mind becomes more perceptive of the 'internal feedback' from the body;[1] and over time the moderation of the ANS becomes increasingly automatic (= auto-regulation).

People often don't feel the tension they create, when someone is *breathing down their neck*.[2] Whatever makes the hair on the back of their neck stand up, could become *a pain in the neck*.[3] Practicing poise with EMG biofeedback can ease the pain and save their neck.[4]

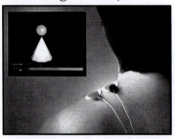

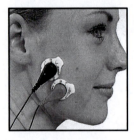

When people need to *grit their teeth* or *bite their tongue* most of the time, they might find themselves grinding their teeth at night. One can call it "bruxism" or "temporomandibular disorder", but in the end it is still *withheld anger*. Psychophysiologists can help clients to change this painful habit with EMG biofeedback.[5]

There is a reason that we say 'holding your breath' or 'with bated breath': Our breathing gives away our emotions ("sigh") and so we stop the natural respiratory flow to hide them. Psychophysiological therapy often starts with exercises to renormalize breathing action and frequency.

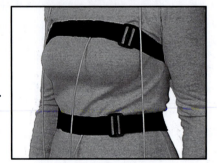

---

[1] Bakal D et al "Somatic awareness in the clinical care of patients with body distress symptoms" Biopsychosoc Med 2008;2:6
[2] Rissén D et al "Surface EMG and psychophysiological stress reactions in women during repetitive work" Eur J Appl Physiol 2000;83(2-3):215-22
[3] Kumar S et al "Cervical EMG profile differences between patients of neck pain and control" Disabil Rehabil 2010;32(25):2078-87
[4] Middaugh SJ et al "Biofeedback-assisted relaxation training for the aging chronic pain patient" Biofeedback Self Regul 1991;16(4):361-77
[5] Crider AB et al "A meta-analysis of EMG biofeedback treatment of temporomandibular disorders" J Orofac Pain 1999;13(1):29-37

The sympathetic ('gas pedal') and the parasympathetic branch ('brake') of the ANS are in balance, when the heart rate resonates well with the breathing rhythm. During inspiration the ANS' 'gas pedal' speeds up the 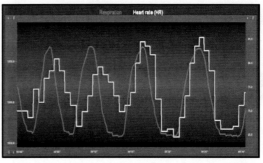 heartbeat, impatiently pumping blood into the lungs to pick up some fresh oxygen. During expiration the autonomic 'brake' slows the heartbeat down again, since the lungs are busy letting air out anyway. The variability in the heart rate exhibits not only this alternating impact of the breathing pattern, but also of what else the limbic system is throwing at the body.

The heart rate variability (HRV) has been subject to a lot of research in psychology,[1,2] psychophysiology[3,4,5,6] and many areas of medicine.[7] In cardiology it is used to predict fatal difficulties,[8] since a reduced HRV is associated with clogged arteries and acute heart attacks.[9,10,11] Even the intake of omega-3 FA shows up in the heart rate variability.[12]

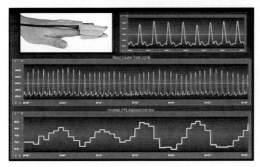

In recent years the HRV has also become very popular as a biofeedback parameter for distress management and autonomic mastery.

---

[1] Kop WJ et al "Autonomic nervous system reactivity to positive and negative mood induction: the role of acute psychological responses and frontal electrocortical activity" Biol Psychol 2011;86(3):230-8
[2] Dobkin PL et al "Measurement of psychological and heart rate reactivity to stress in the real world" Psychother Psychosom 1992;58(3-4):208-14
[3] Buccelletti F et al "Linear and Nonlinear Heart Rate Variability Indexes in Clinical Practice' Comput Math Methods Med 2012;doi: 10.1155/2012/219080
[4] Terkelsen AJ et al "Heart rate variability in complex regional pain syndrome during rest and mental and orthostatic stress" Anesthesiology 2012;116(1):133-46
[5] Reyes Del Paso GA et al "Aberrances in autonomic cardiovascular regulation in fibromyalgia syndrome and their relevance for clinical pain reports" Psychosom Med 2010;72(5):462-70
[6] Mazurak N et al "Heart rate variability in the irritable bowel syndrome: a review of the literature" Neurogastroenterol Motil 2012;24(3):206-16
[7] Ranpuria R, et al "Heart rate variability (HRV) in kidney failure: measurement and consequences of reduced HRV" Nephrol Dial Transplant 2008;23(2):444-9
[8] Kudaiberdieva G et al "Heart rate variability as a predictor of sudden cardiac death" Anadolu Kardiyol Derg 2007;7 Suppl1:68-70
[9] Neves VR et al "Linear and nonlinear analysis of heart rate variability in coronary disease" Clin Auton Res 2012;22(4):175-83
[10] Kunz VC et al "The relationship between cardiac autonomic function and clinical and angiographic characteristics in patients with coronary artery disease" Rev Bras Fisioter 2011;15(6):503-10
[11] Heikki V et al "Clinical Application of Heart Rate Variability after Acute Myocardial Infarction" Front Physiol 2012;3:41
[12] Christensen JH "Omega-3 polyunsaturated Fatty acids and heart rate variability" Front Physiol 2011;2:84

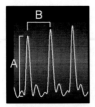Heart rate variability is very responsive to changes in the autonomic balance. The density of information encoded in the HRV allows for sophisticated data analysis, for instance a frequency *power spectrum* that reveals a lot about the ANS.

The various frequencies and indices give experts in their respective fields at least some pointers, e.g. when an epileptic seizure is about to strike,[1] how comfortable someone in a coma is after a severe head injury,[2] when a baby wants to be born[3] or when someone's life is coming to an end,[4] but also whether a conscious ferret sniffed cocaine![5]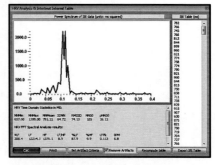

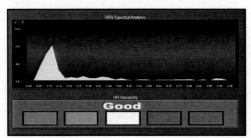Clients don't have to study human physiology, mathematics and chaos theory in order to benefit from HRV biofeedback. Their brain can figure out by itself, what it is supposed to do to the ANS so that the shape of the HRV power spectrum indicates a good balance: The body's echo's of fears, doubts and worries typically show up in a certain frequency range.[6,7]

Although psychophysiological therapy with HRV biofeedback does *not* target 'diseases' or 'disorders', it provides clients with a powerful learning tool to reduce and minimize the damaging effects of an imbalanced and edgy ANS and the self-perpetuating effects of emotional distress. *As an added bonus* most patient groups report marked improvements not only in HRV, but also in mood, sleep and self-efficacy, as well as in their specific symptoms.

---

[1] Jeppesen J et al "Detection of epileptic-seizures by means of power spectrum analysis of heart rate variability" Techn Health Care 2010;18(6):417
[2] Hildebrandt H et al "Differentiation of autonomic nervous activity in different stages of coma displayed by power spectrum analysis of heart rate variability" Eur Arch Psychiatry Clin Neurosci 1998;248(1):46-52
[3] van Laar JO et al "Power spectrum analysis of fetal heart rate variability at near term and post term gestation during active sleep and quiet sleep" Early Hum Dev 2009;85(12):795-8
[4] Arzeno NM et al "Heart rate chaos as a mortality predictor in mild to moderate heart failure" Conf Proc Eng Med Biol Soc2007;2007:5051-4
[5] Stambler BS et al "Cocaine alters heart rate dynamics in conscious ferrets" Yale J Biol Med 1991;64(2):143-53
[6] McCraty R et al "The effects of emotions on short-term power spectrum analysis of heart rate variability" Am J Cardiol 1995;76(14):1089-93
[7] Kop WJ et al "Autonomic nervous system reactivity to positive and negative mood induction: the role of acute psychological responses and frontal electrocortical activity" Biol Psychol 2011;86(3):230-8

Studies investigating the clinical effect of therapy utilizing HRV biofeedback-based methods reported positive results with groups of people with these conditions:

- coronary artery disease[1]
- anxiety and depression in coronary artery disease[2]
- heart failure[3]
- high blood pressure (hypertension)[4]
- mildly elevated blood pressure (pre-hypertension)[5]
- major depression[6,7]
- anxiety[8]
- test anxiety[9]
- post-traumatic stress disorder (PTSD)[10,11]
- chronic neck pain[12]
- fibromyalgia[13]
- asthma[14,15]
- psychiatric conditions[16]
- common mental health problems in children[17]

It also improved movement skills in basketball players.[18]

---

[1] Del Pozo JM et al "Biofeedback treatment increases heart rate variability in patients with known coronary artery disease" Am Heart J 2004;147(3):E11

[2] Nolan RP et al "Heart rate variability biofeedback as a behavioral neurocardiac intervention to enhance vagal heart rate control" Am Heart J 2005;149(6):1137

[3] Swanson KS et al "The effect of biofeedback on function in patients with heart failure" Appl Psychophysiol Biofeedback 2009;34(2):71-91

[4] Nolan RP et al "Behavioral neurocardiac training in hypertension: a randomized, controlled trial" Hypertension 2010;55(4):1033-9

[5] Lin G et al "Heart rate variability biofeedback decreases blood pressure in prehypertensive subjects by improving autonomic function and baroreflex" J Altern Complement Med 2012;18(2):143-52

[6] Karavidas MK et al "Preliminary results of an open label study of heart rate variability biofeedback for the treatment of major depression" Appl Psychophysiol Biofeedback 2007;32(1):19-30

[7] Siepmann M, et al "A pilot study on the effects of heart rate variability biofeedback in patients with depression and in healthy subjects" Appl Psychophysiol Biofeedback 2008;33(4):195-201

[8] Henriques G et al "Exploring the effectiveness of a computer-based heart rate variability biofeedback program in reducing anxiety in college students" Appl Psychophysiol Biofeedback 2011;36(2):101-12

[9] Bradley RT et al "Emotion self-regulation, psychophysiological coherence, and test anxiety: results from an experiment using electrophysiological measures" Appl Psychophysiol Biofeedback 2010;35(4):261-83

[10] Zucker TL et al "The effects of respiratory sinus arrhythmia biofeedback on heart rate variability and posttraumatic stress disorder symptoms: a pilot study" Appl Psychophysiol Biofeedback 2009;34(2):135-43

[11] Tan G et al "Heart rate variability (HRV) and posttraumatic stress disorder (PTSD): a pilot study" Appl Psychophysiol Biofeedback 2011;36(1):27-35

[12] Hallman DM et al "Effects of heart rate variability biofeedback in subjects with stress-related chronic neck pain: a pilot study" Appl Psychophysiol Biofeedback 2011;36(2):71-80

[13] Hassett AL et al "A pilot study of the efficacy of heart rate variability (HRV) biofeedback in patients with fibromyalgia" Appl Psychophysiol Biofeedback 2007;32(1):1-10

[14] Lehrer P et al "Heart rate variability biofeedback: effects of age on heart rate variability, baroreflex gain, and asthma" Chest 2006;129(2):278-84

[15] Giardino ND et al "Combined heart rate variability and pulse oximetry biofeedback for chronic obstructive pulmonary disease: preliminary findings" Appl Psychophysiol Biofeedback 2004;29(2):121-33

[16] Servant D et al "Heart rate variability. Applications in psychiatry" Encephale 2009;35(5):423-8

[17] Nada PJ "Heart rate variability in the assessment and biofeedback training of common mental health problems in children" Med Arh 2009;63(5):244-8

[18] Paul M, et al "Role of biofeedback in optimizing psychomotor performance in sports" Asian J Sports Med 2012;3(1):29-40

HRV biofeedback and migraine comorbidities

We've already seen that developing better auto-regulation skills with methods based on HRV biofeedback leads to decreased symptoms in patients with anxiety or depression, which are also common comorbidities of migraine (see chapter 1). Furthermore, PTSD and chronic neck pain, as well as fibromyalgia patients benefit from 'ANS mastery' achieved with HRV biofeedback.

Irritable bowel syndrome (IBS) is another popular diagnosis collected by migraine sufferers. Not at all surprisingly, IBS is connected to dysregulations of the autonomic nervous system (ANS),[1,2] which can be seen in the spectral analysis of the heart rate variability (HRV).[3,4] It's the same in kids with IBS or abdominal pain. Even better, studies revealed how exactly the ANS freaks out the bowel walls[5] and explain: *the worse the HRV, the worse the IBS*.[6]

Knowing what we now know about IBS and HRV and being aware of the effects of therapy with HRV biofeedback, one would think that there are probably dozens of trials showing the roaring success of HRV biofeedback with IBS patients, right?

Oddly, there is not a single such study published by May 2012. Isn't this weird? One could almost think, there is *no interest* in helping IBS patients to control their 'stress' levels and so reduce their IBS. However, an unpublished dissertation analyzed a trial comparing HRV biofeedback training to cognitive behavioral therapy (CBT) for women with IBS. Both these behavioral therapies came out with flying colors and both did equally well:[7]

> "...improvements in symptom frequency and severity, reduced maladaptive cognitions and increases in quality of life as it relates to IBS."

The good news: HRV biofeedback therapy and CBT combined yield even better results, at least in 'teeth grinding pain'.[8] The bad news is that there are no studies about HRV in migraine. Weird.

---

[1] Heitkemper M et al "Evidence for autonomic nervous system imbalance in women with irritable bowel syndrome" Dig Dis Sci 1998;43(9):2093-8
[2] Heitkemper M et al "Autonomic nervous system function in women with irritable bowel syndrome" Dig Dis Sci 2001;46(6):1276-84
[3] Karling P et al "Spectral analysis of heart rate variability in patients with irritable bowel syndrome" Scand J Gastroenterol 1998;33(6):572-6
[4] Dobrek L et al "Autonomic nervous system activity in IBS patients estimated by heart rate variability (HRV)" Przegl Lek 2006;63(9):743-7
[5] Mazur M et al "Dysfunction of the autonomic nervous system activity is responsible for gastric myoelectric disturbances in the irritable bowel syndrome patients" J Physiol Pharmacol 2007;58 Suppl3:131-9
[6] Cain KC et al "Heart rate variability is related to pain severity and predominant bowel pattern in women with irritable bowel syndrome" Neurogastroenterol Motil 2007;19(2):110-8
[7] Thompson M "Heart rate variability biofeedback therapy versus cognitive therapy for irritable bowel syndrome: a study of attendance, compliance and symptom improvement" 2010 Dissertation at the California Professional School of Psychology, University UMI Number: 3401769
[8] Gardea MA et al "Long-term efficacy of biobehavioral treatment of temporomandibular disorders" J Behav Med 2001;24(4):341-59

A study with fMRI (functional magnetic resonance imaging) showed "a robust relationship" between a *dysregulated limbic system* and the heart rate variability in subjects with high trait anxiety.[1] This finding, although not unexpected, completes our understanding why HRV biofeedback is such an amazingly powerful therapy tool to teach clients *the skills that enable them* to reduce their 'stress' and anxiety levels.

Is biofeedback an effective treatment for migraine?

As an intelligent and attentive reader you already know the answer: Biofeedback is neither a treatment nor a therapy, it's a technical principle. Once a competent therapist has determined which one of the many available biological signals he wants to use with a particular client, you can speak of it as a tool; e.g. EMG biofeedback and HRV biofeedback are the *therapist's tools*, analogue to the school teacher's blackboard and chalk. Therapists who use 'biofeedback' often perform an assessment first, a psychophysiological stress profile (PSP), in order to pick the best tool for the individual client. The tool, the goals, the methods and the concrete content define the therapy. For instance, the EMG biofeedback tool can be used on any muscle that one can access. Most 'biofeedback' therapists restrict their work to muscles near the skin. That means they use surface electrodes (sEMG) and not EMG needles.

But even EMG biofeedback for the same muscle can be done in several different ways to pursue different goals with different methods. Some even use biofeedback instruments only to monitor general relaxation exercises, meditation or autogenic training.

Lets get back to the question and rephrase it: Are therapies that utilize biofeedback-based methods *effective for migraine?*

This innocuous question sums up the problem that modern medicine has with *disorders*: The questions and the answers are *not* about the patient, the client, the suffering human being, but about the *ailment*. This viewpoint works well with *diseases* or injuries, because the patient's unique individuality in body, mind and brain are pretty much irrelevant in the treatment of pneumonia, leukemia, Creutzfeldt-Jakob disease or Ebola virus.

---

[1] Tolkunov D et al "Power spectrum scale invariance quantifies limbic dysregulation in trait anxious adults using fMRI: adapting methods optimized for characterizing autonomic dysregulation to neural dynamic time series" Neuroimage 2010;50(1):72-80

Disorders are the exact opposite. They are the result of very individual nutritional deficiencies, hormone imbalances, breathing patterns, attachment and early life experiences, PFC development, toxic exposures, traumas and injuries, behaviors and habits on all levels of body, mind and brain, especially the ANS,[1] in a complex interplay with genetic predispositions and epigenetic mechanisms. That's why I consider conventional medicine's narrow-minded insistence on the failed pharmaco-medical model for *disorders* a cruel continuation of the physical and emotional abuse and neglect that many patients with life-destroying disorders have experienced in their past (see page 105). [2,3,4,5,6,7,8]

Psychophysiological therapy doesn't kill '*migraine bacteria*' or cut out '*migraine tumors*' and doesn't see the client as a *walking diagnosis*. This approach is supportive of *people* who get tormented by their own stress response, which mediates or aggravates their condition. It teaches clients *the skills that enable them* to reduce their 'stress' levels[9] and emotional burden[10] and might help to protect them from going nuts.[11] *As an added bonus* most patients report marked improvements not only in mood, sleep and self-efficacy, but also in their specific symptoms. Experience shows that most migraineurs have fewer attacks when they are less distraught.[12] Some change even more and terminate the tyranny.

In migraine cases where 'stress' levels and the ANS don't play a role at all, neither precipitate attacks nor aggravate comorbidities, it may well happen that biofeedback-based therapies don't have any impact whatsoever; but they don't cause any harm either.

---

[1] Clauw DJ et al "Heart rate variability as a measure of autonomic function in patients with fibromyalgia (FM) and chronic fatigue syndrome (CFS)" J Musculoskeletal Pain 1995;3:78
[2] Tietjen GE et al "Childhood maltreatment and migraine (part I). Prevalence and adult revictimization: a multicenter headache clinic survey" Headache 2010;50(1):20-31
[3] Tietjen GE et al "Childhood maltreatment and migraine (part II). Emotional abuse as a risk factor for headache chronification" Headache 2010;50(1):32-41
[4] De Benedittis G et al "The role of stressful life events in the onset of chronic primary headache" Pain 1990;40(1):65-75
[5] Tietjen GE et al "Adverse Childhood Experiences Are Associated With Migraine and Vascular Biomarkers" Headache 2012;52(6):920-9
[6] Kendall-Tackett KA "Physiological correlates of childhood abuse: chronic hyperarousal in PTSD, depression, and irritable bowel syndrome" Child Abuse Negl 2000;24(6):799-810
[7] Berenbaum H "Childhood abuse, alexithymia and personality disorder" J Psychosom Res 1996;41(6):585-95
[8] Harkness KL et al "Childhood Maltreatment and Differential Treatment Response and Recurrence in Adult Major Depressive Disorder" J Consult Clin Psychol 2012;80(3):342-53
[9] Roditi D et al "The role of psychological interventions in the management of patients with chronic pain" Psychol Res Behav Manag 2011;4:41–49
[10] Ode S et al "Neuroticism's importance in understanding the daily life correlates of heart rate variability" Emotion 2010;10(4):536-43
[11] Di Simplicio M et al "Decreased heart rate variability during emotion regulation in subjects at risk for psychopathology" Psychol Med 2011:1-9
[12] Blanchard EB "Psychological treatment of benign headache disorders" J Consult Clin Psychol 1992;60(4):537-51

Biofeedback-based therapy and migraine

Once upon a time when computers were expensive, huge and slow and even smart people believed that migraine was caused by blood vessels running amok, a two-pronged approach of biofeedback therapy for migraine was popular and reasonably successful. Patients learned and practiced to dominate their rambunctious arteries to the head and to the rest of the body, e.g. a hand or a foot. Additionally, voluntary control over this otherwise automatic function was practiced in both directions: *Vasoconstriction* is the narrowing and *vasodilation* is the widening of blood vessels, executed by smooth muscle tissue in the arterial wall. Either one of these "vasomotor" actions can be observed and fed back to the client by measuring the blood flow directly or indirectly.

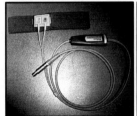
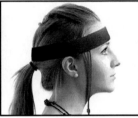
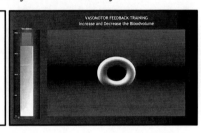

It is typical for this type of biofeedback of the "*superficial temporal artery*" that the measured vasodilation is represented by the expansion of a ring and the vasoconstriction action by its shrinking, possibly accompanied by equally intuitive sound effects.

The blood flow to the hand and thereby vasomotor action is measured with a similar sensor ("photoplethysmograph") and as visual feedback for vasoconstriction and vasodilation we've picked a little animation:

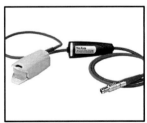
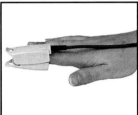
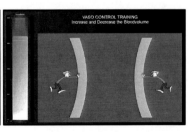

It is advisable to practice voluntary control over vasoconstriction and vasodilation in both locations (head and hand), as well as during mental tasks and other challenging conditions.

As homework assignment it is common practice to do daily relaxation exercises, like slow abdominal breathing, progressive muscle relaxation and autogenic training, and monitor the achieved vasodilation as increased finger tem- 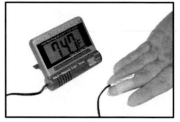 perature with a good digital thermometer. Some can so abort attacks, but once the headache starts, handwarming rarely helps.

Patients, who want to make the most of it, *complement* the professional psychophysiological therapy with the purchase of a basic biofeedback home system. *Between* attacks they practice vasodilation with handwarming exercises as their regular biofeedback-assisted relaxation training. Here is a display that appears to open a flower with increasing relaxation/vasodilation:

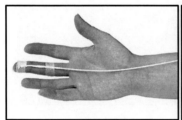 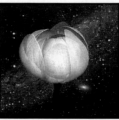 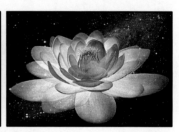

The advantage of this two-pronged approach is the possibility to reduce the migraine headache *during an attack*: Those patients, who gain mastery over the vasomotor action of their superficial temporal artery can reduce their headache *significantly* without medication with active vasoconstriction during an attack,[1] whereas vasodilation, even handwarming, generally leads to more pain.[2]

That does *not* prove that the headache is caused by the blood vessels: The vasomotor center of the brain is located in the brainstem[3,4] and the effectiveness of vasomotor biofeedback is believed to result from improved neuronal regulation. Also, whilst vasoconstriction is ruled by the sympathetic ANS, a very strong vasodilating effect comes from our good old friend CO_2.[5]

---

[1] Allen RA et al "The effects of unilateral plethysmographic feedback of temporal artery activity during migraine head pain" J Psychosom Res 1982;26(2):133-40
[2] Lisspers J et al "BVP-biofeedback in the treatment of migraine. The effects of constriction and dilatation during different phases of the migraine attack" Behav Modif 1990;14(2):200-21
[3] Zanutto BS et al "Neural set point for the control of arterial pressure: role of the nucleus tractus solitarius" Biomed Eng Online 2010;9:4
[4] Geppetti P et al "Antidromic vasodilatation and the migraine mechanism" J Headache Pain 2012;13(2):103–111
[5] Willie CK et al "Regional Brain Blood Flow in Man during Acute Changes in Arterial Blood Gases" J Physiol 2012;590(Pt14):3261-75

That means that the two-pronged vasomotor biofeedback training indirectly encourages a renormalization of CO_2 levels.

Vasomotor biofeedback is still popular in Europe, but less so in the English-speaking world. It is a bit more difficult to learn, but beginning with handwarming biofeedback isn't always easy either. Migraineurs with *strictly bilateral*[1] head pain during attacks, should —theoretically—benefit the most from the skill to voluntarily constrict their superficial temporal artery, because their brainstem is particularly keen on vasodilation in response to head pain.[2] In contrast, migraineurs who always have their head pain on the same side (= *strictly unilateral*), especially on the right,[3] may not be able to abort an attack with voluntary vasoconstriction. There are, however, no published data about different success rates of this abortive maneuver, sorted by head pain location.

Another signal that psychophysiologists measure and observe comes with some name confusion:[4] Electrodermal activity (EDA) or galvanic skin response (GSR) refer to sweat gland activity, which is only under *sympathetic* command ('gas pedal') and not influenced by the *parasympathetic* ANS branch ('brake'). Typically, when people are distressed, their hands are sweaty and slightly cold, because the sympathetic mobilization prepares for the dash to the tree by constricting blood vessels (to raise the blood pressure) and by producing sweat (to cool the runner). So we can use the sweat gland output to gather information about the sympathetic 'running readiness' and thus for biofeedback purposes:

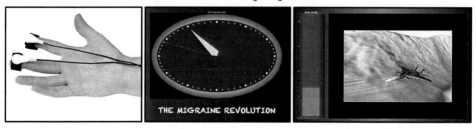

Spoilt for choice, I've picked two cool biofeedback displays: a revolutionary meter and a video screen that shrinks or stops, when the GSR level doesn't move in the currently trained direction.

---

[1] "bilateral" from Latin 'latus"=side, means both-sided, left and right together
[2] Avnon Y et al "Different patterns of parasympathetic activation in uni- and bilateral migraineurs" Brain 2003;126(7):1660-70
[3] Avnon Y et al "Autonomic asymmetry in migraine: augmented parasympathetic activation in left unilateral migraineurs" Brain 2004;127(9):2099-108
[4] GSR = old term for EDA, can refer to either skin conductance **or** resistance measurements, conductance = 1/resistance, SCR vs SCL = skin conductance response vs level; for details: Boucsein W "Electrodermal Activity" Plenum Press 1992

At this point in time GSR is not a parameter that therapists use for migraine-specific biofeedback. This might change in the near future for two reasons. Firstly, the brain area that rules over the generation and control of the 'galvanic skin response' is one that migraine sufferers urgently want to spruce up, the PFC.[1,2,3,4,5] With time and some empowerment from the world wide migraine revolution, a growing number of patients will duly demand more from biofeedback therapists than general relaxation and warm hands.

Secondly, studies from Japan and the Netherlands show amazing results of a GSR-based biofeedback training with epilepsy patients, who were *unresponsive to drug treatment*: After only one month with only twelve half-hour sessions, 60% of those 'problem epileptics' *at least halved* their seizure rate; and the better they learnt to control their GSR, the fewer seizures they had left.[6,7,8,9]

These stunning results with drug-resistant epileptic seizures can only be trumped by the most elegant and direct form of therapy: EEG biofeedback for the brain. On average, of these iffy patients with intractable seizures, unresponsive to any medication, *more than 80%* at least halved their seizure rate with brain biofeedback (neurofeedback).[10,11] That's pretty darn good, I reckon.

Biofeedback therapy pitfalls

Therapists in various fields have been using the biofeedback principle for decades for numerous purposes. Nevertheless, too many migraine sufferers seem to be ill-informed, partly because therapists, on average, are notoriously lousy at beating their own drum, and partly because … (well, what would you say?).

---

[1] Zahn TP et al "Frontal lobe lesions and electrodermal activity: effects of significance" Neuropsychologia 1999;37(11):1227-41
[2] Critchley HD et al "Neural activity relating to generation and representation of galvanic skin conductance responses: a functional magnetic resonance imaging study" J Neurosci 2000;20(8):3033-40
[3] Critchley HD "Electrodermal responses: what happens in the brain" Neuroscientist 2002;8(2):132-42
[4] Nagai Y et al "Activity in ventromedial prefrontal cortex covaries with sympathetic skin conductance level: a physiological account of a "default mode" of brain function" Neuroimage 2004;22(1):243-51
[5] Critchley HD et al "Volitional control of autonomic arousal: a functional magnetic resonance study" Neuroimage 2002;16(4):909-19
[6] Nagai Y et al "Clinical efficacy of galvanic skin response biofeedback training in reducing seizures in adult epilepsy: a preliminary randomized controlled study" Epilepsy Behav 2004;5(2):216-23
[7] Nagai Y et al "Changes in cortical potential associated with modulation of peripheral sympathetic activity in patients with epilepsy" Psychosom Med 2009;71(1):84-92
[8] Spronk D et al "Discrete-trial SCP and GSR Training and the Interrelationship between Central and Peripheral Arousal" J Neurotherapy 2010;14:217-228
[9] Nagai Y et al "Biofeedback and epilepsy" Curr Neurol Neurosci Rep 2011;11(4):443-50
[10] Sterman MB "Basic concepts and clinical findings in the treatment of seizure disorders with EEG operant conditioning" Clin Electroencephalogr 2000;31(1):45-55
[11] Sterman MB "Biofeedback in the treatment of epilepsy" Cleve Clin J Med. 2010;77 Suppl 3:S60-7

While studying medical literature, scientific papers, books for patients, websites, blogs and patient forums, I've found a few errors and misconceptions about biofeedback-based therapies. Let's correct them now, before they spread to a wider audience:

1.) Psychophysiological therapy with biofeedback-based tools and methods is not like a drug for attack abortion. I've found posts on migraine forums that expressed disappointment that **"BIOFEEDBACK DIDN'T STOP MY MIGRAINE HEADACHE"**. Therapy is not symptom treatment. Its goal is to help patients to change into ex-migraineurs. The role that biofeedback-based training plays is *teaching the skill to self-regulate the autonomic nervous system*. In plain words: ANS mastery counteracts 'stress' and its devastating consequences. In difficult and complex migraine cases, that alone may not be enough to reduce the attack rate to zero. In simple and easy cases it might.

2.) Biofeedback therapy is not a passive remedy. It seems that some patients were misled into believing that sitting in front of a laptop with a sensor on a finger is a futuristic 'medical' cure, like an *infusion of bio-information* or a *cybernetic irradiation* that acts like a *virtual vaccination* against the migraine virus. Later they discover that **"IT DIDN'T DO MUCH TO ME"**. Indeed, actually it doesn't *do* anything *to* anyone. Biofeedback tools offer information about the ANS and the question is, what can therapist and client *do with* that knowledge.

3.) 'Biofeedback' is one of three fully evidence-based therapies for migraine.[1,2,3,4,5,6,7] It is therefore inappropriate and misleading to put 'biofeedback' in the category 'alternative', 'complementary' or 'natural' remedies. Psychophysiological therapy ('biofeedback') is a behavioral method that leads more patients to attack cessation than medication can: Drugs and 'biofeedback' can prevent migraine attacks roughly equally well, but after stopping either, only the skills learnt with 'biofeedback' keep working.

---

[1] Nestoriuc Y et al "Efficacy of biofeedback for migraine: a meta-analysis" Pain 2007;128(1-2):111-27
[2] Andrasik F "Biofeedback in headache: an overview of approaches and evidence" Cleve Clin J Med 2010;77 Suppl3:S72-6
[3] Penzien DB et al "Behavioral management of recurrent headache: three decades of experience and empiricism" Appl Psychophysiol Biofeedback 2002;27(2):163-81
[4] Holroyd KA et al "Pharmacological versus non-pharmacological prophylaxis of recurrent migraine headache: a meta-analytic review of clinical trials" Pain 1990;42(1):1-13
[5] Pryse-Phillips WE et al "Guidelines for the nonpharmacologic management of migraine in clinical practice. Canadian Headache Society" CMAJ 1998;159(1):47-54
[6] Campbell K et al "Evidence-Based Guidelines For Migraine Headache: Behavioral and Physical Treatments" US Headache Consortium, available from the American Academy of Neurology, 2000; accessed April 9, 2012
[7] Evers S et al "Acute therapy and prophylaxis of migraine: Guidelines of the German Migraine and Headache Society and of the German Neurological Society" Nervenheilkunde 2008;27:933–949

Therefore, labeling behavioral therapies as 'complementary' to drugs, turns the facts upside down. As much as we value pharmaceutical support to get through an attack, medication for migraine is a lot like a crutch for a knee injury: You need it until the rehabilitation and the healing kick in: It helps you limp, but hinders you walking. And nobody in his right mind would say that the targeted knee rehabilitation is 'complementary' to the crutch.

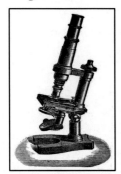

The term 'alternative' therapy is typically used for methods, which aren't validated by scientific studies and whose mechanisms aren't well explained and quantified by our current scientific understanding. In stark contrast, applied psychophysiology is—by the definition of strict science—by far the most 'scientific' therapy of all: It is a constant measurement that puts the autonomic nervous system under the microscope.

As a friendly, respectful and polite person I wouldn't declare medical migraine management to be 'complementary' or list Botox® between Astrology and Chakra Healing; it would deceive patients.

4.) In some cases it may be justified to use biofeedback tools only to teach and monitor relaxation exercises, but when clients assume that the purpose of thermal biofeedback ("handwarming") is to *replace gloves*, it tells me that something went wrong.

5.) In outcome studies 'biofeedback' often gets tested as if it were a *drug*. For instance: On average, vasomotor biofeedback is more effective than thermal biofeedback.[1] But who is average? In clinical practice, good therapists find out what might be most effective for one special person, combine all the required tools and tweak the methods according to the client's progress and needs. Logically, their success rate is *considerably* higher than those of studies. One should also be aware that success rates of therapies reflect the *patients'* characteristics: There are crucial differences between an easy and simple young patient with 3 attacks *per month* compared to a complex and difficult senior sufferer with 3 episodes *per week*, multiple comorbidities and a thirty year history of failed treatments under their belt. Both have "episodic migraine".

---

[1] Nestoriuc Y et al "Biofeedback treatment for headache disorders: a comprehensive efficacy review" Appl Psychophysiol Biofeedback 2008;33(3):125-40

6.) Diabetics use biofeedback training to improve circulation to their feet,[1] which easily can become their Achilles heel (no pun intended).[2] Changes in 'stress' levels due to biofeedback or other life events can influence glucose levels and insulin demands.[3,4] Way cooler is this: Children with insulin-dependent diabetes needed less insulin, after their troubled *parents* did handwarming 'biofeedback' for ten weeks.[5] It goes to show that an improved regulation of the ANS has fast and measurable consequences, even in close others. It would *not* be smart *to underestimate* the potential power of 'biofeedback' or the effect of regular aerobic sport or relaxation training.

Migraine and 'stress'

Stress, in the sense of being distraught, and migraine have a special relationship due to the mutually reinforcing effect: Stress promotes migraine attacks and migraine is distressing by itself.[6]

Everybody's stress resistance and resilience begins to develop in early childhood.[7] We've touched on this topic multiple times.

Later in life, stress contributes to migraine onset[8] (= the beginning of the odyssey). A prospective study in Finland analyzed data from 20,000 employees and identified that *not* high workload, but *emotional* distress leads to the beginning of episodic migraine.[9]

Up to 80% of sufferers report stress as a precipitating factor[10] for an attack. The more stress migraineurs experience in their lives, the more attacks they have to endure,[11] with *a lack of self-efficacy* (= high levels of helplessness) as the main aggravating factor!

Migraine patients were found to be particularly susceptible to stress[12] and to internalize (= 'swallow') their emotional tension.[13] What do you reckon, could that be true?

---

[1] Aikens JE "Thermal biofeedback for claudication in diabetes: a literature review and case study" Altern Med Rev 1999;4(2):104-10
[2] Fiero PL et al "Thermal biofeedback and lower extremity blood flow in adults with diabetes: is neuropathy a limiting factor?" Appl Psychophysiol Biofeedback 2003;28(3):193-203
[3] McGrady A et al "Controlled study of biofeedback-assisted relaxation in type I diabetes" Diabetes Care 1991;14(5):360-5
[4] McGinnis R et al "Biofeedback-assisted relaxation in type 2 diabetes mellitus" Diabetes Care 2005;28:2145–4
[5] Guthrie DW et al "Effects of parental relaxation training on glycosylated hemoglobin of children with diabetes" Patient Educ Couns 1990;16(3):247-53
[6] Holm JE et al "Migraine and stress: a daily examination of temporal relationships in women migraineurs" Headache 1997;37(9):553-8
[7] Tietjen GE et al "Adverse Childhood Experiences Are Associated With Migraine and Vascular Biomarkers" Headache 2012;52(6):920-9
[8] Sauro KM, et al "The stress and migraine interaction" Headache 2009;49(9):1378-86
[9] Mäki K et al "Work stress and new-onset migraine in a female employee population" Cephalalgia 2008;28(1):18-25
[10] Kelman L "The triggers or precipitants of the acute migraine attack" Cephalalgia 2007;27(5):394-402
[11] Marlowe N "Self-efficacy moderates the impact of stressful events on headache" Headache 1998;38(9):662-7
[12] Hedborg K et al "Stress in migraine: personality-dependent vulnerability, life events, and gender are of significance" Ups J Med Sci 2011;116(3):187–199
[13] Gunel MK et al "Are migraineur women really more vulnerable to stress and less able to cope?" BMC Health Serv Res 2008;8:211

Stress is also one of the key ingredients for the transformation of episodic to chronic migraine,[1] which typically occurs after a phase of stressful life events.[2] Especially prone to reaching the dead end of chronic migraine are those episodic migraineurs with PTSD (post-traumatic stress disorder). Who would have thought?

In PTSD the autonomic nervous system can't fully recover from the traumatic stress and remains vulnerable.[3] Even in people, who have not developed PTSD, that vulnerability can be found in the ANS as *'the traces of trauma'*.[4] It looks as if stress *resistance* (= tolerance) and *resilience* (= ability to recover) are central topics for migraineurs. Allow me to summarize this chapter in a limerick:

> As *stress* makes a huge contribution
> to *mig*raine, we need a solution.
> If patients discovered
> biofeedback, they'd love it
> and rise *up* for their own revolution.

Conclusion

Aside from the vital need for adequate symptom treatment during attacks, halting the *process of chronification* must be the number one goal for patients and their doctors. Stress is a major concern for episodic migraine and the looming transformation to chronic migraine. Today is the day that sufferers unleash the power of biofeedback to *terminate the stress terror*, to increase their resistance/resilience by achieving *ANS mastery*, in order to end the unendurable injustice of migraine, to gain their freedom at last.

Contacts

Biofeedback Foundation of Europe (BFE)	**INTERNATIONAL**
Biofeedback Certification International Alliance: www.bcia.org	
Society for Psychophysiological Research: www.sprweb.org	
Association for Applied Psychophysiology and Biofeedback: www.aapb.org	**USA**
North Eastern Regional Biofeedback Society: www.nrbs.org	
Mid-Atlantic Society for Biofeedback and Behavioral Medicine: www.masbbm.org	
(many US states have their own 'Biofeedback' society, e.g. CA: www.biofeedbackcalifornia.org)	
Australian Association for Applied Psychophysiology & Biofeedback: www.ansa.com.au	**AUSTRALIA**

---

[1] Bigal ME et al "Modifiable risk factors for migraine progression" Headache 2006;46(9):1334-43

[2] Scher AI et al "Major life changes before and after the onset of chronic daily headache: a population-based study" Cephalalgia 2008;28(8):868-76

[3] Schore AN "Dysregulation of the right brain: a fundamental mechanism of traumatic attachment and the psychopathogenesis of posttraumatic stress disorder" Aust N Z J Psychiatry 2002;36(1):9-30

[4] Dale LP et al "Abuse history is related to autonomic regulation to mild exercise and psychological wellbeing" Appl Psychophysiol Biofeedback 2009;34(4):299-308

Section Three:
Weapons for the Brain

neuron

"If real is what you can feel, smell, taste and see, then 'real' is simply electrical signals interpreted by your brain.."

Morpheus

Any thought or emotion, idea or perception, whether joyful or horrible, pathetic or grand, comes down to the work of the billions of neurons inside our head, which make up our brain. It would be a truly revolutionary idea to somehow alter the brain of a *migraineur* to the *ex-migraineur* design. Given the mind-boggling progress in neuroscience, perhaps they've come up with something *'brain-boggling'* too? Or is that too far fetched?

Almost like putty

Neuroplasticity refers to the brain's ability to adapt and change throughout its entire life.[1] For instance, you may not recall the Swedish word for "nurse" from page 318, but you might remember the name of the zoo assistant, who sorted the animals after the earthquake (page 153). What about the shampoo with natural Amarula-oil that gently smooths the rough nano-structure of your horrible hair? Any recollection? At least, by now you should know the name of the brain area behind the forehead, which is 'wobbly' in migraineurs. Because I've mentioned it often enough in this book, your brain has built new synapses (= connections) between neurons, so that your knowledge of the PFC is now hard-wired into your brain and accessible to your mind.

That's the essence of *neuroplasticity*. The network of neurons changes constantly under the influence of old and new information. Therefore stroke victims can re-learn to use a 'paralyzed' arm and London taxi drivers can memorize the pubs in Cricklewood. You can see those network alterations in brain scans, for instance as a larger memory area in cabbies.[2] Similar to muscles, brain areas can grow when they're used a lot and their function improves.

---

[1] Pascual-Leone et al "The plastic human brain cortex" Annu Rev Neurosci 2005;28:377-401
[2] Biegler R et al "A larger hippocampus is associated with longer-lasting spatial memory" Proc Natl Acad Sci USA 2001;98(12):6941–6944

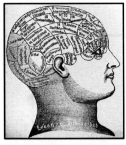
One day, when brain scans can depict every single neuron, we can probably see where your brain has made new connections so that you don't forget the idea of the 'wobbly … '. So far it's not possible to pinpoint the word "sjuksköterska" (= Swedish "nurse") inside someone's brain, but you can already measure that people with a second language use up more oxygen in area 45 than those, who can only speak their mother's tongue.[1]

A mirror for the brain?

Given what we've learnt about *neuroplasticity* and pondering what we already know about the *biofeedback* principle, wouldn't it make sense to expect that both mechanisms should go together very well? When you repeatedly give your brain information about the Crown Inn in Cricklewood, it can learn to drive your cab there. When you repeatedly give your brain information about the autonomic nervous system, it can learn to 'drive' your ANS in a more balanced way. Wouldn't you say that, if you repeatedly give your brain information about itself, it can probably learn to 'drive itself' in a more balanced way?

In front of a mirror you do a better job at putting make-up on or at shaving, right? The mirror shows you, what you are doing, you can correct your actions and so avoid making a mess or hurting yourself. Let's say that your brain is at least as smart as you are. Then your brain should also be able to make use of a biofeedback 'mirror', that shows what it's doing, so it can correct its actions and avoid making a mess and hurting *you*.

Distractible kids and unstable brains

That is the ancient Egyptian hieroglyph for "brain", which goes back 5,000 years to the pharaoh Imhotep, who we all know well from the Hollywood blockbuster "The Mummy".

Though diligent scientists have managed to discover some stuff about the brain and the nervous system over the centuries, neuroscience has only really flourished over the last few decades.

---

[1] Kovelman I et al "Bilingual and monolingual brains compared: a functional magnetic resonance imaging investigation of syntactic processing and a possible "neural signature" of bilingualism" J Cogn Neurosci 2008;20(1):153-69

The reason for that is easy to grasp: It takes sophisticated technology to even begin to understand the function of a network, made of 100 billion nerve cells with thousands of connections each. Brain scanners, EEG amplifiers and fast computers come in handy here. That also explains why so many neuroscientific findings have not made it into the pool of common knowledge yet.

The same thing is true for *applied* neuroscience, which uses this new know-how for therapeutic purposes: Many people haven't heard of it yet. Often patients are surprised to learn that the use of the biofeedback principle on the brain dates back to the 1970's. They also don't know that there are conditions, where neurofeedback (= brain biofeedback) is an evidence-based option. That means that enough good studies were conducted proving its efficacy.

One such condition is *attention deficit disorder* without and with hyperactivity (ADD/ADHD). A meta-analysis in 2009 — based on the many studies since 1976 — concluded that the *highest level of evidence* (Level 5) has now been reached and that neurofeedback training is *specific* and *efficacious* with moderate effect sizes for hyperactivity and *large effect sizes* for inattentiveness.[1]

That is remarkable, because the scientific criteria for these ratings are in brutal favor of drug treatments, hence very difficult to fulfill for *behavioral* therapies. That's on top of the fact that behind applied neuroscience, there is no rich industry, happy to spend millions on studies, in order to earn billions from the results.

Level 5 roughly means: "Many good studies leave no doubt: This works." It doesn't really say how *fabulous* a therapy is; that depends on many factors (e.g. risks, costs, alternatives etc). In chapter 25 I've mentioned another indication, for which neurofeedback therapy is quite established: *intractable seizures*, unresponsive to medication. A meta-analysis confirmed the roughly *80% success* rate of patients, who at least halved their seizure rate.[2] That is *fabulous*, don't you think? Yet, the evidence level rating is only 3, because all the study groups, understandably, were rather small: You can't just round up a few dozen drug-resistant epilepsy patients for a couple of weeks. Perhaps you can, if you have the money.

---

[1] Arns M et al "Efficacy of neurofeedback treatment in ADHD: the effects on inattention, impulsivity and hyperactivity: a meta-analysis" Clin EEG Neurosci 2009;40(3):180-9

[2] Tan G et al "!Meta-analysis of EEG biofeedback in treating epilepsy" Clin EEG Neurosci 2009;40(3):173-9

More interesting is this question: If you were a *seizure* patient and drugs weren't really helping you, would you rather wait until more studies are done and the official rating climbs to level 4 or 5?

My own answer, totally biased and subjective

I certainly would *not* wait and I'll tell you my reasons:

1.) If biofeedback-based brain training (neurofeedback) works well for one brain disorder (e.g. ADD/ADHD), then I can conclude that the principle itself is sound: *Neurofeedback can change the brain for the better.* It is very unlikely that this works exclusively for rowdy kids. It is more likely that it works for many different brain glitches, because that would be logical. I would also assume that neurofeedback training won't help much, when I'm struck down by pneumonia, leukemia, Creutzfeldt-Jakob disease or Ebola virus. But when it's about a brain, that doesn't work the way it should, then I'd be very open to the concept of neurofeedback therapy.

2.) The notion that the studies on intractable seizures were done on *small* groups only, may have an effect on such an official rating, but it wouldn't bother me in the slightest: Drug trials often *need* to be done on large groups in order to make relatively small effects "*statistically* significant". If a study can prove such an effect with a *small* number of participants, it tells me that the *effect* itself was large and, as a patient myself, *that's* what I'm after.

3.) As a cautious and suspicious person, I would ask myself: What is their natural intention? Many neurofeedback therapists are PhD psychologists or psychotherapists. They could make a decent living with talk therapy or trauma resolution, based on an investment in two comfy chairs. Instead, the psycho-professionals spend time and money on neuroscience education, expensive equipment, workshops and conferences, as well as regular computer and software-updates. Why would they do that, if not because they find it more fulfilling and emotionally rewarding? And it can only be satisfying, if neurofeedback indeed is pretty darn successful and makes most of their clients fairly happy.

4.) I would also think of the PEDMIN strategy (see page 103). What is the greater risk? Committing to a logical, neuroscience-based therapy, which has no dangerous side effects, because it's learning and training; or missing out on my only opportunity?

5.) The rather conservative US military uses neurofeedback methods to rehabilitate soldiers with combat-related PTSD while the official evidence level is only 2 for this condition. Obviously they are convinced and are not willing to wait for more studies.

6.) In the US alone more than 200 neurofeedback practices have committed themselves to the program "Homecoming for Veterans": *Free* neurofeedback therapy for soldiers with PTSD. Clinicians in other countries have welcomed the good idea: Australia, Colombia, France, Puerto Rico, UK and Venezuela. I'm a suspicious person, but I've never heard of *'free snake-oil'*.

7.) Of course, one point is a major concern: If it were true that neurofeedback is a valuable tool for the therapy of brain disorders, **"THAT WOULD HAVE BEEN ON PAGE ONE OF EVERY NEWSPAPER"**, right? Could it be a scam, a swindle? Is applied neuroscience a 'rip-off'?

Fortuitously I've found out what really happened: In 2009, when neurofeedback reached *evidence level 5* for ADD/ADHD, all the journalists were very excited. They salivated and wanted to publish that story on the title page of every single newspaper in the whole entire world (Journos are totally into that funky brain stuff and stories about *applied neuroscience* are famous for selling newspapers like hotcakes: The average Joe can't wait to read the latest gossip about the prefrontal cortex). Everything was prepared, but five minutes before the print-run, breaking news came in: The Raiders had beaten the Knickers in the last innings of the playoffs with a historic double-bubble touchdown-homerun for a sudden-death knock-out in the penalty-shootout for the America's Cup. And so, instead of on page one of every single newspaper in the whole entire world, the neurofeedback story ended up in the bin.

Science and neurofeedback-based therapy

We've seen in chapter 25 that a technique like biofeedback, which can tweak the autonomic nervous system (ANS), can be helpful for many disorders, since the ANS is involved in many.

Logically, since neurofeedback training can change the brain's ways, and since the brain is very involved in pretty much every disorder, almost every disorder could potentially benefit from neurofeedback therapies, at least to some degree. 'Neurofeedback' has indeed shown positive results with the following problems:

- Antisocial personality disorder[1]
- Anxiety disorders[2,3,4,5]
- Autism and Asperger's syndrome[6,7,8,9,10]
- Brain injury / concussion[11,12,13,14,15,16,17]
- Cerebral palsy[18,19]
- Chronic fatigue syndrome[20,21]
- Cognitive decline / aging[22,23,24,25,26]
- Complex regional pain syndrome[27]
- Contamination anxiety[28]
- Coma[29]
- Depression[30,31,32]

---

[1] Surmeli T et al "QEEG guided neurofeedback therapy in personality disorders: 13 case studies" Clin EEG Neurosci 2009;40(1):5-10
[2] Vanathy S et al "The efficacy of alpha and theta neurofeedback training in treatment of generalized anxiety disorder" Ind J Clin Psych 1998;25(2):136-43
[3] Moore NC "A review of EEG biofeedback treatment of anxiety disorders" Clin Electroencephalogr 2000;31(1):1-6
[4] Hammond DC "Neurofeedback with anxiety and affective disorders" Child Adolesc Psychiatr Clin N Am 2005;14(1):105-23
[5] Kerson C et al "Alpha suppression and symmetry training for generalized anxiety symptoms" J of Neurother 2009;13(3):146 – 155
[6] Pineda JA "Positive behavioral and electrophysiological changes following neurofeedback training in children with autism" Res Aut Spect Disorders 2008;2:557-581
[7] Kouijzer ME et al "Long-term effects of neurofeedback treatment in autism" Res Aut Spect Disorders 2009;3:496-501
[8] Coben R et al "Neurofeedback for autistic spectrum disorder: a review of the literature" Appl Psychophysiol Biofeedback 2010;35(1):83-105
[9] Coben R et al "The relative efficacy of connectivity guided and symptom based EEG biofeedback for autistic disorders" Appl Psychophysiol Biofeedback 2010;35(1): 13-23
[10] Thompson L et al "Neurofeedback outcomes in clients with Asperger's syndrome" Appl Psychophysiol Biofeedback 2010;35(1):63-81
[11] Ayers ME "Electroencephalic neurofeedback and closed head injury of 250 individuals" Nat Head Inj Found Frontiers 1987:380-392
[12] Thatcher RW "EEG operant conditioning (biofeedback) and traumatic brain injury" Clin Electroenceph 2000;31(1):38-44
[13] Bounias M et al "EEG-neurobiofeedback treatment of patients with brain injury" J Neuroth 2001;5(4):23-44
[14] Walker JE "A neurologist's experience with QEEG-guided neurofeedback following brain injury" in Evans JR "Handbook of Neurofeedback" Haworth Medical Press-Binghamptom, NY 2007:353-361
[15] Thornton KE "Efficacy of traumatic brain injury rehabilitation: Interventions of QEEG-guided biofeedback, computers, strategies, and medications" Appl Psychophysiol Biof 2008;33(2):101-124
[16] Pachalska M et al "Evaluation of differentiated neurotherapy programs for a patient after severe TBI and long term coma using event-related potentials" Med Sci Monit 2011;17(10):CS120-8
[17] Duff J "The usefulness of quantitative EEG (QEEG) and neurotherapy in the assessment and treatment of post-concussion syndrome" Clin EEG Neurosci 2004;35(4):198-209
[18] Ayers ME "Neurofeedback for cerebral palsy" J Neuroth 2004;8(2):93-94
[19] Bachers A "Neurofeedback with cerebral palsy and mental retardation" J Neuroth 2004;8(2):95-96
[20] Hammond DC "Treatment of chronic fatigue with neurofeedback and self-hypnosis" NeuroRehab 2001;16:295-300
[21] James LC et al "EEG biofeedback as a treatment for chronic fatigue syndrome: A controlled case report" Behav Med 1996;22(2):77-81
[22] Albert AO et al ""Theta/beta training for attention, concentration and memory improvement in the geriatric population" Appl Psychophysiol & Biof 1998;23(2):109
[23] Budzynski T et al "Brain brightening: restoring the aging mind" Evans JR "Handbook of Neurofeedback" 2007 Haworth Medical Press, Binghampton, NY: pp. 231-265
[24] Hanslmayer S et al "Increasing individual upper alpha by neurofeedback improves cognitive performance in human subjects" Appl Psychophysiol & Biof 2005;30(1):1-10
[25] Angelakis AE et al "EEG neurofeedback: A brief overview and an example of peak alpha frequency training for cognitive enhancement in the elderly" Clin Neuropsych 2007;21(1):110-129
[26] Vernon D et al "Alpha neurofeedback training for performance enhancement: Reviewing the methodology" J of Neuroth 2009;13(4):214 – 227
[27] Jensen MP "Neurofeedback treatment for pain associated with complex regional pain syndrome" J Neuroth 2007;11(1):45-53
[28] Hampson M et al "Real-time fMRI biofeedback targeting the orbitofrontal cortex for contamination anxiety" J Vis Exp 2012;(59)pii:3535
[29] Ayers ME "EEG neurofeedback to bring individuals out of level 2 coma" Biof Self-Regul 1995:20(3):304-305
[30] Baehr E et al "Clinical use of an alpha asymmetry neurofeedback protocol in the treatment of mood disorders: Follow-up study one to five years post therapy" J Neuroth 2001;4(4):11-18
[31] Hammond DC "Neurofeedback treatment of depression and anxiety" J Adult Develop 2005;12(2/3):131-137
[32] Dias AM et al "A new neurofeedback protocol for depression" Span J Psychol 2011;14(1):374-84

Weapons for the Brain

- Fibromyalgia[1,2,3,4]
- Headache[5,6,7]
- Juvenile criminals[8,9,10]
- Learning disabilities[11,12,13,14]
- Mental retardation[15]
- Obsessive compulsive disorder[16,17,18]
- Pediatric stroke[19]
- Pain[20,21,22,23,24]
- Parkinson's disease[25]
- Schizophrenia[26,27,28]
- Sleep disorders[29,30,31]

But wait, there is more!

---

[1] Donaldson CCS et al "Fibromyalgia: A retrospective study of 252 consecutive referrals" Can J Clin Med 1998;5(6):116-127
[2] Mueller HM et al "Treatment of fibromyalgia incorporating EEG-driven stimulation: A clinical outcomes study" J Clin Psych 2001;57(7):933-952
[3] Kayrian S et al "Neurofeedback in fibromyalgia syndrome" J Turk Soc Algol 2007;19(3):47-53
[4] Kayrian S et al "Neurofeedback intervention in fibromyalgia syndrome; a randomized, controlled, rater blind clinical trial" Appl Psychophysiol Biofeedback 2010;35(4):293-302
[5] McKenzie R et al "The treatment of headache by means of electroencephalographic biofeedback" Headache,1974;13:164-172
[6] Lehmann D et al "Controlled EEG alpha feedback training in normals and headache patients" Archiv Psychiat 1976;221:331-343
[7] Matthew A et al "Alpha feedback in the treatment of tension headache" J Personal Clin Stud 1987;3(1):17-22
[8] Martin G et al "The Boys Totem Town Neurofeedback Project: A pilot study of EEG biofeedback with incarcerated juvenile felons" J Neuroth 2005;9(3):71-86
[9] Quirk DA "Composite biofeedback conditioning and dangerous offenders: III" J Neuroth 19951(2):44-54
[10] Smith PN et al "Neurofeedback with juvenile offenders: A pilot study in the use of QEEG-based and analog-based remedial neurofeedback training" J Neuroth 2005;9(3):87-99
[11] Cunningham MD et al "The effects of bilateral EEG biofeedback on verbal, visual-spatial, and creative skills in learning disabled male adolescents" J Learn Disabil 1981;14(4):204-8
[12] Fernández T et al "EEG and behavioral changes following neurofeedback treatment in learning disabled children" Clin Electroencephalogr 2003;34(3):145-52
[13] Becerra J et al "Follow-up study of learning-disabled children treated with neurofeedback or placebo" Clin EEG Neurosci 2006;37(3):198-203
[14] Breteler MH et al "Improvements in spelling after QEEG-based neurofeedback in dyslexia: a randomized controlled treatment study" Appl Psychophysiol Biofeedback 2010;35(1):5-11
[15] Surmeli T et al "Post WISC-R and TOVA improvement with QEEG guided neurofeedback training in mentally retarded: a clinical case series of behavioral problems" Clin EEG Neurosci 2010;41(1):32-41
[16] Sürmeli T et al "Obsessive compulsive disorder and the efficacy of qEEG-guided neurofeedback treatment: a case series" Clin EEG Neurosci 2011;42(3):195-201
[17] Hammond DC "QEEG-guided neurofeedback in the treatment of obsessive compulsive disorder" J of Neuroth 2003;7(2):25-52
[18] Hammond DC "Treatment of the obsessional subtype of obsessive compulsive disorder with neurofeedback" Biofeedback 2004;32:9-12
[19] Ayers ME "A controlled study of EEG neurofeedback and physical therapy with pediatric stroke, age seven months to age fifteen, occurring prior to birth" Biof Self-Regul 1995;20(3):318
[20] Rosenfeld JP et al "Operantly controlled somatosensory evoked potentials: Specific effects on pain processes" in Rockstroh B et al"Self-Regulation of the Brain and Behavior" Springer-Berlin 1984:164-179
[21] Rosenfeld JP et al "Operant control of human somatosensory evoked potentials alters experimental pain perception" in Fields HL "Advances in Pain Research and Therapy" Raven Press-New York 1985;9:343-349
[22] deCharms RC et al "Control over brain activation and pain learned by using real-time functional MRI" Proc Natl Acad Sci USA 2005;102(51):18626-31
[23] Jensen MP "Neuromodulatory approaches for chronic pain management: Research findings and clinical implications" J Neuroth 2009;13(4):196–213
[24] Chapin H et al "Real-time fMRI applied to pain management" Neurosci Lett 2012;520(2):174-81
[25] Subramanian L et al "Real-time functional magnetic resonance imaging neurofeedback for treatment of Parkinson's disease" J Neurosci 2011;31(45):16309-17
[26] Gruzelier J et al "Learned control of interhemispheric slow potential negativity in schizophrenia" Int J Psychophysiol 1999;34, 341-348
[27] Gruzelier J "Self regulation of electrocortical activity in schizophrenia and schizotypy: a review" Clin Electroencephalogr 2000;31(1):23-9
[28] Bolea, AS "Neurofeedback treatment of chronic inpatient schizophrenia" J of Neuroth 2010;14(1):47-54
[29] Feinstein B. et al "Effects of sensorimotor rhythm training on sleep" Sleep Research 1974;3,134
[30] Bell JS "The use of EEG theta biofeedback in the treatment of a patient with sleep-onset insomnia" Biof Self Reg 1979;4(3):229-236
[31] Hoedlmoser K et al "Instrumental conditioning of human sensorimotor rhythm (12-15 Hz) and its impact on sleep as well as declarative learning" Sleep 2008;31(10): 1401-1408

- Stroke[1,2]
- Tinnitus[3,4,5,6,7]

Already mentioned and referenced:
- ADD/ADHD
- Alcoholism
- Drug-resistant epilepsy
- Performance enhancement
- PTSD
- Substance abuse

... to name but a few.

Migraine and neurofeedback therapy

- Migraine[8,9,10,11,12,13,14,15,16]

Two *excellent* studies have formally investigated the benefits of neurofeedback therapy for persistent severe migraine:

● Carmen (2004)[13] reported the outcome of 100 successive cases of episodic and chronic migraine, previously unresponsive to drug treatments. He found that 95% of those patients who completed at least six sessions of *infrared neurofeedback* eventually reported "*significant improvements*", which meant, the intensity of their migraine headache became *at least* so low that clients could not distinguish it anymore from a mild garden-variety headache, and they weren't troubled by it either. This turned out to be a replicable and reliable outcome criterion, better than pain ratings.

---

[1] Ayers ME "Assessing and treating open head trauma, coma, and stroke using real-time digital EEG neurofeedback" in Evans JR et al "Introduction to QEEG and Neurofeedback" Academic Press-New York 1999:203-222
[2] Doppelmayr M "An attempt to increase cognitive performance after stroke with neurofeedback" Biofeed 2007;35(4):126-130
[3] Gosepath K et al "Neurofeedback training as a therapy for tinnitus" HNO 2001;49(1):29-35
[4] Weiler EW et al "Neurofeedback and quantitative electroencephography" Int J Tinn 2001;8(2):87-93
[5] Schenk S "Neurofeedback-based EEG alpha and EEG beta training. Effectiveness in patients with chronically decompensated tinnitus" HNO 2005;53(1):29-37
[6] Dohrmann K et al "Neurofeedback for treating tinnitus" Langguth G et al "Progress in Brain Research" 2007;166 Elsevier-London:473-486
[7] Busse IM et al "Neurofeedback by neural correlates of auditory selective attention as possible application for tinnitus therapies" IEEE Engin Med Biol Soc 2008:5136-5139
[8] Tansey MA "A neurobiological treatment for migraine: The response of four cases of migraine to EEG biofeedback" Headache Curr Treat Res 1991;90-96
[9] Othmer SO "EEG biofeedback training Megabrain Report" J Mind Technology 1994;2:43-47
[10] Siniatchkin M et al "Self-regulation of slow cortical potentials in children with migraine: an exploratory study" Appl Psychophysiol Biofeedback 2000;25(1):13-32
[11] Walcutt DL "The Efficacy of Neurofeedback on Migrainous Neuralgia" Rosemead School of Psychology, Biola University-La Mirada, CA 2001
[12] Kropp P et al "On the pathophysiology of migraine--links for 'empirically based treatment' with neurofeedback" Appl Psychophysiol Biofeedback 2002;27(3):203-13
[13] Carmen J "Passive Infrared Hemoencephalography: Four Years and 100 Migraines" J Neurotherapy 2004;8(3):23-51
[14] Stokes DA et al "Neurofeedback and biofeedback with 37 migraineurs: a clinical outcome study" Behav Brain Funct 2010;2(6):9
[15] Walker JE et al "QEEG-guided neurofeedback for recurrent migraine headaches" Clin EEG Neurosci 2011;42(1):59-61
[16] Collura TF et al "Clinical benefit to patients suffering from recurrent migraine headaches and who opted to stop medication and take a neurofeedback treatment series" Clin EEG Neurosci 2011;42(2):VIII-IX

Carmen's article describes the *reality* of a therapy practice for migraine: Some so-called simple and easy cases (*of persistent severe frequent episodic migraine, unresponsive to medication!*) were free of any complaints after only six neurofeedback sessions, whereas more complex and difficult clients (e.g. chronic migraine with medication overuse) needed 20 or up to 30 session to reach the aforementioned criterion of "significant improvement". Thermoimaging confirmed the therapy results.

Dr. Carmen, a psychologist in private practice, also analyzed those cases who dropped out before the sixth session (24 of 100) and determined in 75% of the male fall-outs "psychological reasons". Of the females, 63% quit for "allegedly financial" and 32% for "psychological reasons". Surprisingly, "addiction to migraine medication" was responsible for only 17% of the total dropouts.

In summary, 100% of the compliant men and 92% of the compliant women were liberated from debilitating migraine headaches (In regard to the four women, who failed to achieve a "significant improvement": It might be illuminating to have them tested for estrogen dominance; see chapter 17).

● Walker (2011)[1] studied the fate of 71 patients with recurrent migraine headaches, who underwent a QEEG (see page 165) in his neurology practice. 46 patients elected to do neurofeedback based on the abnormalities found in the QEEG, "to remediate their migraine headaches". 25 others chose to continue to rely on drug treatment only and served as a control group.

In comparison to a normative database, Dr. Walker found an excess of so-called "Hibeta" (21-30 Hz) magnitude ('volume') in various electrode locations of his patients' QEEGs. Excess in this frequency range can be characterized as unsettled energy: If the brain were a muscle, you would call it tension.

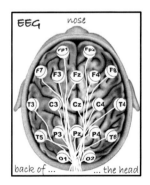

Each partaking migraineur received five 30-minute sessions of 'neurofeedback' to train down the "Hibeta" at each electrode site where it was elevated. The number of sessions ranged from 12 to 32, with an average of 24 sessions.

---

[1] Walker JE et al "QEEG-guided neurofeedback for recurrent migraine headaches" Clin EEG Neurosci 2011;42(1):59-61

The Migraine Revolution

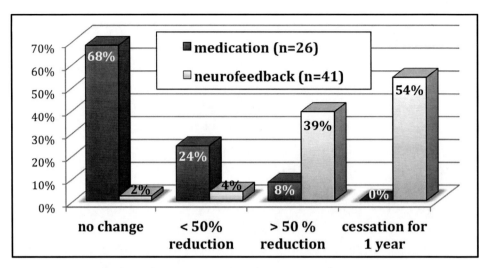

The graph shows the results (five patients dropped out of the neurofeedback group, one of them received medication):

As expected, the control group didn't change much while 93% of the neurofeedback group had *at least* halved the rate of their attacks. In 54% of cases the neurofeedback training led to complete and sustained *liberation* from the migraine tyranny.

This is actually an authentic demonstration of the effects of competent neurofeedback therapy in real life: Of the 71 migraine patients of that neurologist, more than a third didn't even want to try a promising non-drug therapy. Five trainees abandoned the neurofeedback prematurely; perhaps they "TRIED IT ONCE AND THE RESULT WAS HELL" or because the first few sessions "DIDN'T DO MUCH TO THEM" or they hit some other form of difficulty (see chapter 6).

"If the neurofeedback therapy is so good, why didn't they all end up migraine-free?"

We don't know, but if someone forced me to speculate I would say: Some of them could have had a *hormone imbalance* (e.g. estrogen dominance). Some might have been deficient in *magnesium*, *vitamins B2* or *D3* or *omega-3* fatty acids. Some may have been low in CO_2 due to *overbreathing*. Some may still have had an imbalanced *ANS* while in some others the *PFC* still wasn't up to scratch. Some could have been suffering from some *toxicity* issue or some IgG-based *food intolerance* and some may have had a dysfunction in pathways of *dopamine* (= a 'joyful' neurotransmitter, esp. in the prefrontal cortex, PFC).[1]

---

[1] Cannon PR et al "Migraine and restless legs syndrome: is there an association?" J Headache Pain 2011;12(4):405–409

Some possibly had unresolved *trauma* or *schema* issues. Some others perhaps were stuck in a *dysfunctional family* situation,[1,2,3] for which their migraine is a stabilizing element. Some may indeed have been *addicted* to migraine medication, because a specific part of their prefrontal cortex was too compromised.[4] Some others may have had so much *iron dirt* in their brain's "*pain matrix*"[5] that they could have set off the security scanner at the airport. After years and decades of migraine seizures and medication gluttony, some may have been *too brain-damaged*[6] to become pain-free, while some others may have been *too mind-damaged* to change their identity as a suffering migraine victim into a proud and happy ex-migraineur. Of course, all of these are mere speculations.

Considering how many factors can potentially sabotage a good therapy outcome, it is almost puzzling that straight neurofeedback therapy alone *terminated* the migraine terror for more than half of the trainees. On the other hand, this is consistent with the shared clinical experience in the field of neurotherapy.

Those compliant patients, who did *not quite* reach migraine-freedom in Walker's study, should neither be complacent nor feel discouraged. Targeted testing can identify the interfering factors and once they are addressed, a different method of neurofeedback (e.g. infrared neurofeedback) or biofeedback may finish the job.

It is unfortunate that Dr. Walker's article didn't reveal how complex and 'difficult' the study participants were. We do know that he is a neurologist in Texas, which means that primary care physicians usually refer the patients to him. This makes it unlikely that the study group consisted of *walk-in-the-park* cases of *occasional* migrainous headache. It is rather likely that he sees a lot of patients who the family doctors prefer to pass on. We've also learnt that 35% opted to forego the opportunity of neurofeedback therapy and that five trainees gave up early. Either one speaks for complex and 'difficult' migraineurs, stuck in a life-script of suffering.[7]

---

[1] Miksch A et al "What is helpful for kids with headache?--Qualitative analysis of systemic family interviews at the end of a solution and resource oriented group therapy for children and adolescents with primary headache" Prax Kinderpsychol Kinderpsychiatr 2004;53(4):277-87
[2] Kröner-Herwig B et al "Biopsychosocial correlates of headache: what predicts pediatric headache occurrence?" Headache 2008;48(4):529-44
[3] Gaßmann J et al "Risk Factors for Headache in Children" Dtsch Arztebl Int 2009;106(31-32):509–516
[4] Gómez-Beldarrain M et al "Orbitofrontal dysfunction predicts poor prognosis in chronic migraine with medication overuse" J Headache Pain 2011;12(4):459–466
[5] Tepper SJ et al "Iron deposition in pain-regulatory nuclei in episodic migraine and chronic daily headache by MRI" Headache 2012;52(2):236-43
[6] Szabó N et al "White matter microstructural alterations in migraine: a diffusion-weighted MRI study" Pain 2012;153(3):651-6
[7] Steiner C "Scripts People Live: Transactional Analysis of Life Scripts" Grove Press-New York 1994 (reissue ed.)

As human beings, we tend to defend our world-view against disruptive new info (= *"confirmation bias"*, see page 100). A poor attachment in childhood often leads to an *emotional coping style* and *avoidant-dismissive attitudes*. All three together prompt *open hostility:*

> "None of the studies of neurofeedback for migraine were done in a **PROPER**, randomized, double-blind, placebo-controlled study design. **THEREFORE THEY ARE USELESS!**"

The aggressive judgment **"THEY ARE USELESS"** indicates to me that someone has made up their mind and nothing will change it. So let's rephrase: "*... study design. Aren't they useless?*" Neurofeedback therapy is not medication. Drugs need to undergo rigorous drug trials, before they get an official approval. That is reasonable, because very few drugs turn out to be totally free of risks and side effects. Therefore the risk-benefit ratio needs to be determined as precisely as possible. The appropriate study design for that is randomized, double-blind, placebo-controlled in order to guarantee that no confounding factor makes the drug look better than it really is.

Neurofeedback therapy is not a drug and an outcome study is *not a drug trial*. Since behavioral therapies typically don't bear hidden risks of long-term damage, they don't need to be approved by the drug-supervision authority (US: FDA, Oz: TGA). All that *double-blind* stuff doesn't apply, because behavioral therapies *always* depend to some extent on a good relationship between client and therapist. *Randomization* is also quite an idiocy for studies of behavioral therapies, because the client's free choice and motivation are paramount in clinical practice. And that's what it's about, isn't it? The *placebo effect* doesn't apply, because it refers to a mental effect in *medication* treatment. You need to measure it in drug trials, because if it's massive (e.g. Botox®, see page 59), you might as well use a cheaper, more harmless substance. In stark contrast, behavioral therapies are *meant* to elicit empowering mental effects.

Of course, it is interesting to find out whether the observed effects are "*specific*" and we know that already about neurofeedback therapy from ADD/ADHD and epilepsy studies. Sometimes it is also nice to show a *control group*, mainly in disorders that tend to change, like "seasonal affective disorder" (= winter depression), especially if the therapy takes you far into spring. Got it?

In short: Life is not a trial either and what patients need to know about a *therapy*, can be found in *clinical outcome studies*.

Why have I never heard of neurofeedback therapy?

With the theoretical knowledge from chapter 8 and the credible confirmation that it really seems to work well in practice, it has become clear that neurofeedback-based therapy is by far the *most promising* way out of the migraine misery. Carmen's and Walker's outcome studies have verified what has been known amongst therapists for quite some time:

'Neurofeedback' is not a *miracle* cure for every migraineur, but under the *precondition* that ...

- possible *'body blocks'* (ANS, hormones, Mg, VitD3+B2, IgG, CO_2 etc.) as well as
- possible *'mind hurdles'* (unhelpful beliefs, hopelessness, trauma, schema etc.)
  EITHER • do not interfere   OR • can be identified, addressed and overcome,

then even many 'difficult' and complex cases of severe, frequent, drug-resistant migraine *can* achieve complete cessation (or at least a *drastic* reduction) of attacks with neurofeedback therapy.

As part of a *comprehensive rehabilitation* to overcome 'body blocks' and 'mind hurdles', neurotherapy can end the tyranny for many. This is awesome, but inevitably leads to the question in the headline: "If it's that good, why have I never heard of neurotherapy before?"

1.) The thing that is "that good" is the *brain* and its ability to adapt and recover. Neurofeedback therapy (neurotherapy) is just the means by which we take advantage of our amazing brain.

2.) Applied neuroscience is still a *young discipline* and although colorful brain scans in science magazines are fascinating, it's not a topic that people discuss in the cue at the cheese counter.

3.) Doctors don't know much about it either and although more and more MDs are getting engaged in this field, the vast majority of family docs are completely *overwhelmed* already by ever more challenging patients and a sick load of administrative tasks.

4.) Professionals from several different fields have joined the neurofeedback community, but PhD psychologists have been cracking the whip since the beginning. *Psychology* has a long history of internal fights between different schools of thought and so neurofeedback professionals can endlessly bicker amongst themselves—like angry fishwives in winter—about having the best method or the longest cables. That leaves neither time nor energy for educating the public about neurofeedback's therapy potential.

5.) Migraine *books* are mostly authored by doctors and we can't expect them to write: "Okay, I'll tell you a bit about medication, but drugs don't end the tyranny. You should rather read 'The Migraine Revolution', because neurofeedback is the therapy of choice for migraine, especially as part of a comprehensive rehabilitation program. All the best to you. Yours sincerely, Dr. Oliver Bernholz, MD"

6.) Please meet *the tyrant's helpers*. Migraine info on the internet (websites, blogs, forums) is dominated by a handful of professional chronic migraine patients, who unfortunately show all the problematic psycho-behaviors that have made me sound like a broken record since chapter 5: emotional coping style, dismissive-avoidant attitudes, cognitive distortions, unbudging helplessness and strong medical beliefs. In the true spirit of commitment and consistency,[1] they can't help it but guide migraine patients down the same track, which has led *them* into irrevocable *chronification*, based on false info, bad thinking habits and unhelpful beliefs (see chapter 7 for a complete list of "barricade" myths). These omnipresent opinion leaders—beacons of hopelessness—advocate relying on migraine drugs and pain killers, complemented by Crystal Healing. If you *don't* want to end the tyranny, they can truly teach you how to LIVE WITH MIGRAINE DISEASE AND HEADACHES. And if you've ever wondered who came up with the absurd argument "IF IT WERE TRUE, IT WOULD HAVE BEEN ON PAGE ONE OF EVERY NEWSPAPER ...", now you know the answer. I'm afraid not everyone will welcome the migraine revolution. We'll have to fight.

7.) Finally, the correct answer to your question: "Why have I never heard of neurotherapy?" Because I didn't write this book earlier, sorry.

How does neurofeedback therapy work?

You've already learnt that the brain's native language consists of electric potentials, supported by biochemical substances ("ink"). You know that the EEG can listen in on and quantify the brain's busy chatter. You probably remember that scientists discovered the heralds of agony in the QEEG already 72-36 hours before the head pain's arrival.[2] And you also know that LoRETA can even eavesdrop in 3-D. What I haven't told you yet is how the brain can be changed. Well, let's get cracking.

---

[1] Cialdini RB "Commitment and Consistency: Hobglobins of the mind" Chapter 3 in "Influence" Allyn & Bacon 2001:52ff
[2] Bjørk M et al "What initiates a migraine attack? Conclusions from four longitudinal studies of quantitative EEG and steady-state visual-evoked potentials in migraineurs" Acta Neurol Scand Suppl 2011;(191):56-63

Weapons for the Brain

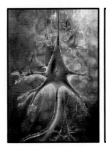
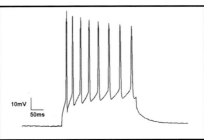
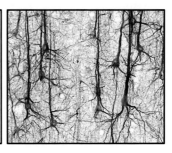

Since you've mastered the crash course Neuroscience 101, you know that neurons (= nerve cells) fire off action potentials at particular *frequencies*. Now I'd like you to imagine that a neuron in the brain is *like* a singer in a choir. Then the firing-frequency of the neuron would be equivalent to the pitch of the note of the singer: Low frequencies are like low notes, more to the left on a piano keyboard. High frequencies are like high notes, more to the right on the piano.

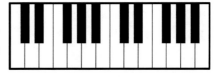

The voices in a choir are now equivalent to the frequency ranges in the brain (as seen in the graph). And the volume of the singers is analogue to the electrical energy in the brain, measured in the EEG at the scalp in microvolt.

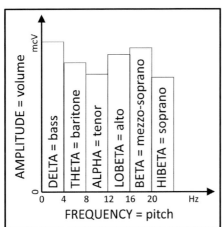

The brain contains 100 billion neurons, so you need to think of the intergalactic solar systems' congregation of super-choirs, each consisting of groups of choirs. I hope that you've booked a concert hall the size of China for them.

Although the venue is spacious, it's not enough to have the singers stand in closely-packed rows, you need to arrange for several levels in order to accommodate them in layers.

It's a smart move to place the groups of conductors at the very pre-front of the hall, facing the choirs, so they can conduct, duh.

Once you've got them all in, you mount 19 microphones to the roof of the building. That will give you a good impression in which area of the hall the choir groups are struggling to perform well.

After a few boring welcome speeches by some smug officials there is an announcement that all the choir groups now form one single super-duper ensemble with the name "brain-choir". As expected, all the delegates and singers are excited: "**Hooorrraaayyy**"

Once they've warmed up their voices, you might want to give them their first song "Sit still, my love, your eyes keep shut" by some contemporary composer. You get the recording equipment ready and off they go. After a while you think "That went well" and you give them a second song "With distant gaze in calm I rest", quite a catchy tune and high in the charts since day one.

After that you quickly clean up the recordings from external noise like the garbos[1] and some idiot with his lawnmower. Then you run the recordings through some expensive software that compares the parameters of the brain-choirs performance with a database of really, really good concerts from previous years.

Let's say that you've found that the sopranos were too loud in 12 of the 19 recorded channels. So you let them sing again and every time the sopranos are too loud in those channels, you shake your head. When the sopranos pull back a bit, you give thumbs up. And since it gets displayed on a huge video wall, the brain choir can see your feedback and the sopranos learn to hold back a bit. They might need a couple of songs to form a new habit, but with your help the brain-choir and its prefrontal conductors can learn to keep the sopranos under control. That wasn't too hard, was it?

Congratulations, you've just replicated Dr. Walker's study about QEEG-guided neurofeedback with migraine patients.

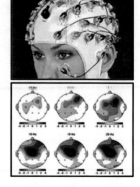

Walker recorded QEEGs with 19 channels, but instead of microphones he used EEG electrodes. Then he cleaned the data from garbage and compared the patient's recording to a database of really, really healthy brains. He found an excess of 'Hibeta' energy, which is somewhat equivalent to shrill soprano voices, overdoing it. This also characterizes the Hibeta excess. You find it in brains that are somehow tense or too intense, e.g. in anxiety, PTSD etc.

---

[1] garbos = Aussie for garbage collectors, trashmen in the US, dustmen or refuse collectors in the UK

During the therapy sessions ('songs') Walker arranged his neurofeedback training software in a way that the brain ('choir') received a *positive* feedback ('thumbs up') whenever the power of the Hibeta ('sopranos') was okay and a *negative* feedback ('shaking your head') when it was too much ('sopranos too loud').

Luckily Dr. Walker didn't need a gigantic video wall; a normal-sized computer screen was sufficient since his patients' heads were nowhere near the size of China.

The absence of negative feedback ('shaking your head') and the appearance of positive feedback ('thumbs up') is *rewarding* for the brain, like a treat for the puppy dog from page 46. The neurofeedback software can give the *reinforcement* (= reward) in many different ways, similar to what you've seen in the biofeedback chapter: numbers, graphs, animations, video clips, DVD films or even video games (which is great if you see kids for therapy).

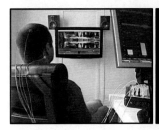 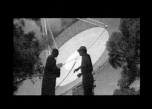 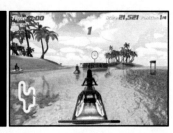

I personally like working with DVDs, because there is a huge selection of top-quality documentaries available with captivating images and rich soundtracks. That way my client's brain is keen to tame the sopranos and so keep the picture large and the sound audible, which a brain easily understands as 'thumbs up'.

Films for feedback are also advantageous in that they keep the client's mind busy and out of the way. In contrast to biofeedback, which is usually done with *conscious* attention, neurofeedback is typically a *subconscious* training. Consciousness is not required for learning by reward (= operant conditioning). Even a sea slug (aplysia californica) can learn with operant conditioning[1] although it doesn't even have a brain and only 20,000 neurons in its entire nervous system. Most migraine patients beat that hands down.

Once the brain has learnt to shut up the sopranos, it knows how to do it. That's why it's neuro*plasticity* and not neuro*elasticity*.

---

[1] Cook DG et al "Operant conditioning of head waving in Aplysia" Proc Natl Acad Sci USA 1986;83(4):1120-4

Neurofeedback versus Biofeedback

Technically speaking, neurofeedback is a form of biofeedback, yet professionals usually use the two words like so. →

Applied Psychophysiology	Applied Neuroscience
Biofeedback (body signals)	Neurofeedback (brain signals)

The photo below shows the setup for an EEG-neurofeedback session (My wife was kind enough to pose as a model):

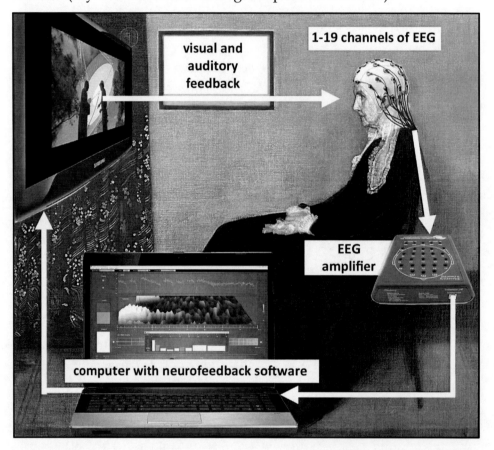

For obvious reasons people say "*neurofeedback session*" and not "*a neurotherapy-session using one of the many neurofeedback-based methods*" This is relevant, as it sometimes happens that a client responds very well to one neurofeedback method, but less so to another one.

If we wanted to be really precise, we would also state which signal gets measured to represent the brain's activity. Jonathan Walker used EEG in his migraine study, whereas Jeff Carmen utilized the PFC's infrared radiation (call it *warmth*, if you will).

Chapter 26

Show Me Some Warmth!

"When life descends into the pit, I must become my own candle; willingly burning my self to light up the darkness around me."

Alice Walker

Infrared neurofeedback

When you 'work up a sweat', it means you're getting hot, because you're active, right? The same applies to the brain: When neurons are active, they generate chemical energy and warmth by burning glucose. Sensibly the amount of warmth accurately represents the amount of activity.[1]

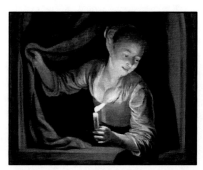

That is the basis for a very elegant technique that tells us with colorful pictures where exactly the PFC is 'wobbly'. You are probably bored beyond belief, because you remember question #3 from the final exam to the home study course "Introduction to brain scanning" on page 169. And so you knew straight away that I'm talking about PFC Thermoimaging,[2,3] am I right? Fantastic.

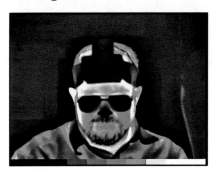

← This is a picture of Dr. Jeff Carmen[4] (the bloke from the study with 100 migraine cases). Since it's a thermal image, his nose and his glasses are very dark (= much cooler). The thingo on his forehead is a sensor for infrared neurofeedback.

Jeff had been working as a psychologist and biofeedback expert mainly with migraine patients for more than 20 years before he developed a system for infrared neurofeedback, which turned out to be highly effective in the rehabilitation of the PFC and migraine.

---

[1] Trübel HK et al "Regional temperature changes in the brain during somatosensory stimulation" J Cereb Blood Flow Metab 2006;26(1):68-78
[2] Shevelev IA et al "Thermoimaging of the brain" J Neurosci Methods 1993;46(1):49-57
[3] R Coben et al "Sensitivity and specificity of long wave infrared imaging for attention-deficit/hyperactivity disorder" J Atten Disord 2009;13(1):56-65
[4] Carmen J "Passive Infrared Hemoencephalography: Four Years and 100 Migraines" J Neurotherapy 2004;8(3):23-51

The grumpy face on the right belongs to the famous author of the bestselling book "The Migraine Revolution" (which also turned out to be highly effective for the rehabilitation of migraine). If you look closely, the area over *his left* eye is a tad darker. That's where grump lives. Other than that, his PFC doesn't seem to have suffered from too many soccer headers.

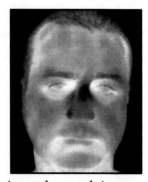

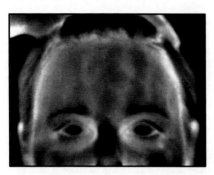

← This too is a thermal image of a *normal* PFC. It's evenly colored and that means that all areas are working. Okay, 'colored' is a weird word when the example is in gray-scale, but you get the picture: When the entire forehead is uniformly gray, that's what we want, okay?

Compare ↑ normal to this one → of a young man who suffered a brain injury in a motorcycle accident, which earned him a month in a coma. Later he had decent difficulties with speech fluency and logical thinking (= PFC).

Can you guess, which part of his helmet-less head hit the tree?

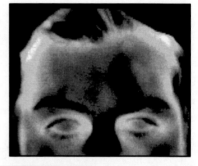

If you've identified "his forehead, above his left eye", because the black fleck represents sluggish PFC areas, then you are correct. Gosh, you are so amazing! We're on the second page of this chapter only and you've already diagnosed a traumatic brain injury.

Let's make it much harder. Which of the two thermo-images below shows the client ⬇ with the paranoid delusions and chronic anxiety? Don't dare to stuff this up or I will get into trouble; the other one is my wife!

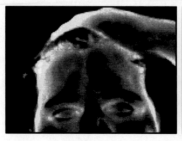 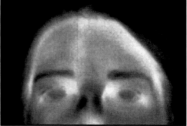

Show Me Some Warmth!

May I assume you saved my ... peace at home and picked the left image with the dark, cold prefrontal cortex as the client with the more severe psychiatric disorder of the two? Thank you.

On the right we see the PFC of a young woman during a migraine attack at the start of the headache phase. The PFC is 'weak', particularly left and center; and the white lines are her temporal arteries with a lot of blood flow. ➡

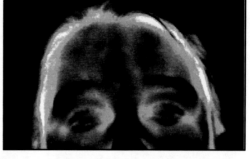

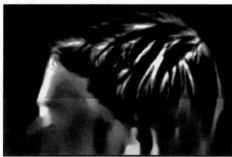

⬅ Here you find the side view of an atypical migraine in an adolescent male. The 'white' scalp under his hair shows that the brain needs to get rid of a lot of thermal waste. Or: During the migraine seizure the brain is working up a sweat.[1]

As awe-inspiring as thermal images are, infrared neurofeedback is even better. The headset on the right has three sensors built in, which measure the warmth of the PFC via the infrared radiation; essentially the same as what the thermal camera does. That's the signal we use for PFC training.

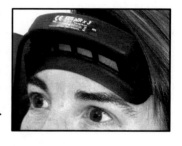

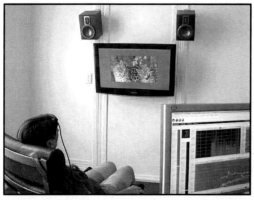

During the session with infrared neurofeedback, we force the PFC to work a bit harder, either by stopping the DVD or by fiddling with the picture. When the PFC lifts its game, we give it thumbs up by running the film or with full picture and sound quality.

---

[1] Dreier JP "Spreading convulsions, spreading depolarization and epileptogenesis in human cerebral cortex" Brain 2012;135(1):259–275

The PFC can only raise the heat radiation by *activating* more neurons and it seems, once they're awake anyway, they might as well do their regular job. That's what we want (If we were just interested in a warm forehead, we could simply put a bonnet on). So what we're aiming for is an evenly active prefrontal cortex. The measurement of the infrared radiation is merely a means to an end.

If all goes well, the sluggish PFC areas become more and more active and the dark flecks lighten up over the course of the therapy. Do you fancy a few cases? Below are the PFC thermoimages of a 20 year-old female with severe obsessive-compulsive disorder (OCD) *before* and *after* successful infrared neurofeedback therapy:

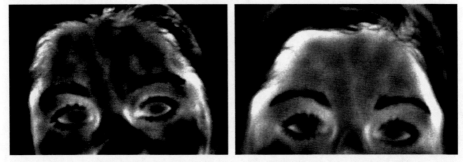

The next case is a 20 year-old man with mild mental retardation, attention and language deficits, hugely improved after IR NFB.

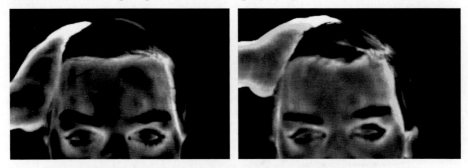

If you're worried about *your* brain injury patient from earlier:

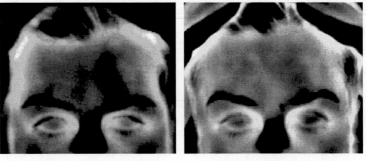

Show Me Some Warmth!

I think the thermal images speak for themselves. In cases of therapy failure, the PFC doesn't change and the inactive areas remain dark in the images. That can happen and we've talked about that earlier. Infrared neurofeedback, like every other therapy, is not a *miracle* cure for every case. It's just an awesome tool.

The next example is a 15 year-old boy with migraine before and after nine sessions. The rate went down from daily attacks to ten a month. The thermal image confirms that he's not finished yet:

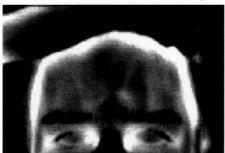 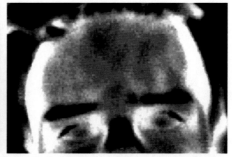

The last case is a 74 year-old lady before the first and before her sixth session. She still has some way to go, but she is already down from 15 severe attacks per month to 1 or 2. That's a start.

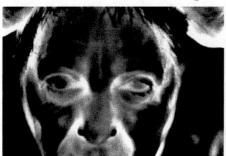 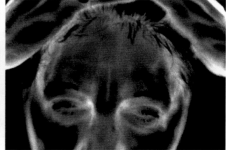

All the case examples and most of the thermal images are from Dr. Jeff Carmen, Manlius, NY (www.stopmymigraine.com). Thanks a lot, Jeff! These pictures were converted from color-coded thermal data to grayscale and are for educational purposes only. Also, the expert name for infrared neurofeedback is *"passive infrared hemoencephalography"* (pIR HEG). If you're looking for a therapist, please visit the directory at www.TheMigraineRevolution.com or ask the usual suspects (Google, Yahoo …).

Please do not attempt to 'cure' your migraine with a hot water bottle on your forehead. The sluggish areas of the prefrontal cortex need to *work up a sweat* in order to end the tyranny. Got it?

Keeping an overview

Neuroscientific research and neurotherapeutic applications are developing rapidly. Here is a brief and incomplete overview:

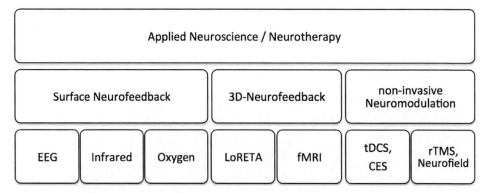

Elucidations along the bottom row from right to left:

- TMS: transcranial magnetic stimulation; more for research[1] than for therapy[2]
- Neurofield: low intensity, pulsed electromagnetic field stimulation (pEMF)[3]
- tDCS: transcranial direct current stimulation; experimental, adjunctive therapy
- CES: cranial electrotherapy stimulation; for insomnia, anxiety, depression[4]
- AVE: audio-visual entrainment; pulsing lights/sounds to boost frequencies[5]
- pRoshi: frequency-variable visual dis-entrainment[6]
- fMRI: spectacular, prohibitively expensive research application[7]
- LoRETA-neurofeedback; wait for chapter 31
- Oxygen: near-infrared Hemoencephalography; for PFC neurofeedback too
- Infrared: Show me some Warmth (chapter 26)
- EEG neurofeedback: see chapters 28 to 32
- surface neurofeedback: measurements from the surface of, through the skull
- Neuromodulation: therapeutic principle that migraineurs don't hear about until they're due for an occipital nerve stimulator, a highly invasive method with a pathetic success rate of 40% responders (= 50% headache reduction)[8]

Let's focus on effective steps to end the migraine tyranny: infrared and EEG surface- and LoRETA 3D-neurofeedback.

---

[1] Brigo F et al "Transcranial magnetic stimulation of visual cortex in migraine patients: a systematic review with meta-analysis" J Headache Pain 2012;13(5):339-49
[2] Brighina et al "rTMS of the prefrontal cortex in the treatment of chronic migraine: a pilot study" J Neurol Sci 2004,227(1):67-71
[3] typically used as an adjunctive therapy to neurofeedback; for more info visit www.neurofield.org
[4] McCrory DC "Cranial electrostimulation for headache: meta-analysis" J Nerv Ment Dis 1997;185(12):766-7
[5] Noton D et al "Migraine and photic stimulation: report on a survey of migraineurs using flickering light therapy" Compl Ther Nurs 2000;6(3):138-42
[6] Anderson DJ "The treatment of migraine with variable frequency photo-stimulation" Headache 1989;29(3):154-5
[7] Zotev V et al "Self-Regulation of Amygdala Activation Using Real-Time fMRI Neurofeedback" PLoS One 2011;6(9):e24522
[8] Saper JR et al " Occipital nerve stimulation for the treatment of intractable chronic migraine headache" Cephalalgia 2011;31(3):271–285

Chapter 27

Listening Through the Wall

"With the gift of listening comes the gift of healing."
Catherine de Hueck

EEG recording technology

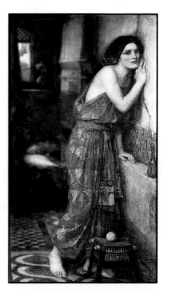

When you want to eavesdrop on your neighbor's matrimonial noise or pre-divorce arguments, you probably have to overcome a sound barrier, e.g. a wall. To make the muffled sound audible, you hold a water glass against the wall and listen through the glass. The air in the glass amplifies the sound volume, enabling you to listen carefully and to collect the necessary material to update the latest gossip.

When we need to listen to the brain-choir to check up on the sopranos or to aid the pre-frontal conductors, we also have to overcome a sound barrier. Providentially,

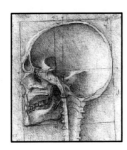

humans don't have to carry their brains in their hands or in a backpack, since our creator had the perspicacity to place our brain inside a protective bony safe: the skull. That's good for scoring goals in soccer with headers, but it makes recordings from the brain, literally, a tiny bit harder.

Although the brain's overall energy intake is in the vicinity of 25 Watts, much of that is lost to sustenance and only 10 Watts are available for singing.[1] This results in a measurable signal on the surface of the brain in the dimension of single-digit millivolts (mV). One millivolt is one thousandth of a Volt; a button cell watch battery has 1-2 Volt.

So the signal is weak-ish on the brain's surface already and then there is the skull as a sound barrier. Now we've hit the wall.

---

[1] Kandel E et al "Principles of Neural Science" Elsevier 1981

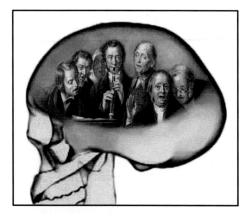

A water glass won't help in our attempt to eavesdrop on the brain and drilling holes into the skull seems fairly impractical for daily diagnostic and neurofeedback with conscious clients.

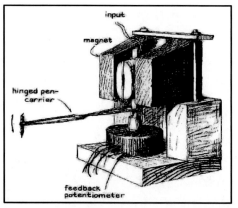

Hans Berger, the chap who recorded the first human EEG in 1924, allegedly did so with a device like this one to the right.[1] ➡ Some coil amplified the weak voltage at the skull and a long lever wiggled a pen over a strip of paper. He pulled the paper strip at a constant speed and so he could see the number of wiggles per second drawn onto the paper.

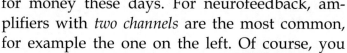

⬆ Berger recognized a waxing and waning rhythm at the back of the brain of his subject and since he was an ace in ancient Greek and familiar with the alphabet, he called that rhythm "*alpha*".

Technology has made leaps and bounds since 1924 and a wide assortment of digital EEG amplifiers is available for money these days. For neurofeedback, amplifiers with *two channels* are the most common, for example the one on the left. Of course, you can also have four channels of EEG or combine neurofeedback and biofeedback with one device like the one on the right, which is the size of a pack of cigarettes.

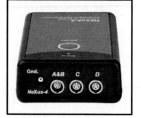

---

[1] Berger H "Über das Elektroenkephalogramm des Menschen" Arch Psychiatr 1929;87:527–570

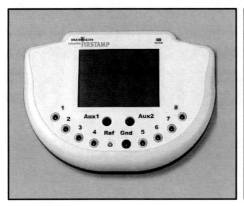 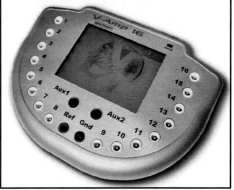

⬆ These two amplifiers[1] with 8 and 16 channels respectively can easily keep students and their professors busy for a semester or two. For QEEG/LoRETA, we need 19 data channels (+ references).

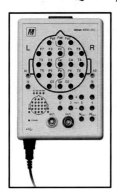 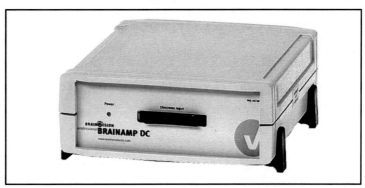

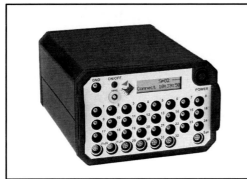 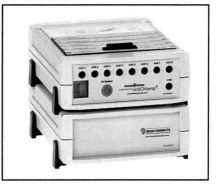

These four beautiful boxes[2,3,4] with 21, 32, 24-32 and up to 160 EEG channels are more than capable of recording QEEGs/LoRETA. Dense array EEGs with 128 or 256 channels are used in research.

[1] FirstAmp and V-Amp (8 or 16 EEG + 2 auxiliary channels, DC, 24 bit), www.brainproducts.com
[2] top left: Mitsar 201 (21 EEG + 4 aux ch, AC, 16 bit) / top right: BrainAmp (32 EEG, DC, 24 bit), www.brainproducts.com
[3] bottom left: Nexus 32 (32 EEG or 24 EEG + 8 aux ch, DC, 24 bit), www.mindmedia.nl
[4] bottom right: actiChamp (32-160 EEG + 8 aux ch, DC, 24 bit), www.brainproducts.com/productdetails.php?id=42

Now that we have a fine digital EEG amplifier—fine enough to make good ol' Hans Berger go green with envy—we only need to connect the brain through the skull to the electronic box. Easy.

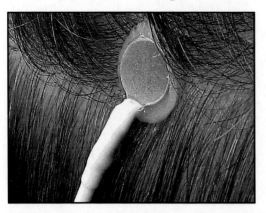

For that connection we first prepare the scalp a bit with a special gel. Then we put a tiny dab of a conductive and sticky paste on the *electrode* and pop it onto the scalp. If we've done a good job and with a bit of luck, the electrode will stay there and transmit the weak brain signal to the dear amplifier.

That's how it is for most types of neurofeedback training where one or two channels with 3 to 5 electrodes can do a lot of good for clients and patients. However, for a full QEEG and LoRETA we would have to prepare at least (19 ch + 2 ref + 1 gnd =) *22 spots* on the scalp and pop 22 single sensors on. This could take a while; especially if you want to make sure that the electrode is in the right place.

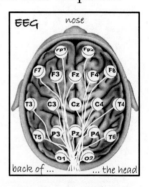

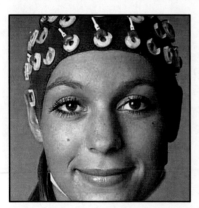

And so it is common practice to use an *EEG cap*, either with built-in electrodes or with ring sockets in the fabric that hold the sensor at its designated location. That not only looks good, but also in about 20-30 minutes all the electrode sites are prepared, the quality of the connections is checked and the recording can start. That is certainly acceptable when it's done once in a blue moon.

These days more and more therapists themselves implement QEEGs and LoRETA into their work and run these tests much more often than once in a blue moon. And now the 20-30 minutes for the preparation become a logistic *nightmare* in a busy practice.

Listening Through the Wall

Of course, there is a solution to this growing problem (otherwise I wouldn't have mentioned it, duh). A novel EEG cap system makes it possible to prepare clients for QEEG and LoRETA in about 5 to 8 minutes. The secret of the actiCAP is a sophisticated, electronic processor—built into the sensor—that guarantees the best possible contact to the scalp *without* the time-consuming skin preparation.

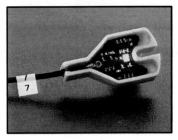

Unless it's the very first time, putting the prepared actiCAP onto the client's head is a matter of seconds since the bonnet is made of a firm, but slightly stretchy material. Let's rather say 'pliable' or 'compliant' instead of 'stretchy', because we need to ensure that the sensors are placed correctly and a flabby, sloppy cap can't do that.

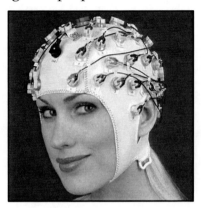

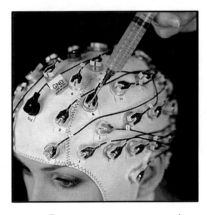

With all the sensors in place, we inject a small amount of highly conductive electro-gel into the socket, next to the contact pin, to bridge the gap to the scalp. And here comes the kicker: As soon as the quality of the electric connection between scalp and sensor[1] has reached the desired level of perfection, a diode lights up *green*.

In case a connection deteriorates, for whatever reason, the electrode diode turns *yellow or red* and it also shows in the control software. That is particularly useful when you see something unexpected in the raw EEG and want a confirmation that you're looking at valid data, before jumping to conclusions. Imagine you diagnose "parasitic aliens" in your client's brain, perform emergency surgery and it turns out that a sensor contact had dried out!   (Just kidding.)

---

[1] Experts know this as the impedance, which is the same as (DC) or analogue (AC) to resistance; low impedance is desirable.

373

On top of all that, the actiCAP also uses *active shielding* technology, which is a bit like the protective force field in Star Trek. While the trekkies' force field works against klingons, the active cable shielding protects the fragile brain signal on its audacious voyage to a place, no man has gone before: into the EEG amplifier.

Once the delicate messages from the brain have made it into the amplifier they're safe, since they'll continue their adventure as a sturdy digital data stream into the computer. The end result is a perfectly *clean* EEG.

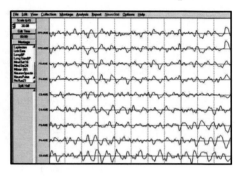

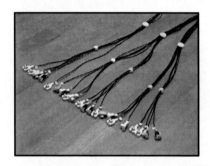

Ordinarily, handling so many cables is infuriating, because they usually behave like mating snakes, deliberately entangling themselves. In order to keep the 'signal-serpents' separated, the actiCAP comes with an ingenious *cable management* system.

The actiCAP[1] was originally designed for *research* and meets the extreme demands of space flights and Himalayan expeditions. This is not the first time that technology, developed for one field, turns out to be even more useful in a different area. Think of Teflon as an example. Whilst researchers certainly benefit from the actiCAP's technology, it might have an even greater impact on the therapeutic applications mentioned here: QEEG/LoRETA, multi-channel neurofeedback and LoRETA-3D-neurofeedback.

Particularly those complex and 'difficult' migraine patients with allodynia, whose scalp is utterly sensitive and tender, will welcome the actiCAP's *skin-prep-skip* feature. It allows us to record clean brain-signals of a strength measured in *micro*volts (= millionth of Volts) without scrubbing the client's irritable scalp.

In other words, modern technology makes it possible to attentively listen to the whispering brain, barely touching its wall.

---

[1] for more detailed information about the actiCAP visit www.brainproducts.com

Chapter 28

Wiping Migraine Off the Map

> "All you need is the plan, the road map, and
> the courage to press on to your destination."
>
> Earl Nightingale

QEEG-guided neurofeedback

Throughout this book I've mentioned QEEG (quantitative ElectroEncephaloGraphy) multiple times. Let me briefly remind you of what you've already learnt and now remember:

- QEEG is a form of brain analysis;
- 19 or more electrodes measure the brain's electro-chatter at the scalp,
- an amplifier converts the weak signals into the digital format that computers understand,
- special software filters the various frequencies ("voices") and their respective power ("volume"), so
- heaps of metrics (=measures) get compared to a database that represents a normal, healthy brain of the same age and gender.

QEEGs are used for different purposes in research and clinical practice; for example to predict the response to a drug or to monitor medical treatments;[1] but for no good reason, it is not the standard tool in the average neurologist's office yet. Any one of the brain scanning techniques from chapter 7 has certain strengths and advantages.

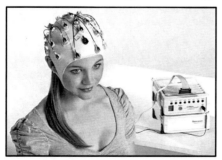

The QEEG is fast enough to keep up with the brain's rapid babble, is readily available, comfortable, economical and it helps you figure out how to get rid of a problem with neurofeedback.

---

[1] Sneddon R et al "QEEG monitoring of Alzheimer's disease treatment: a preliminary report of three case studies" Clin EEG Neurosci 2006;37(1):54-9

In that way the QEEG is for the brain what a blood test is for the body. In order to find the right remedy you want to identify the *disturbing bug*. In the case of a disease of the *body*, the word 'bug' means the disturbing bacterium that causes the pneumonia, for example. In the case of a disorder of the *brain*, 'bug' means the disturbing activity pattern that leads to migraine attacks. The high-tech equivalent is a *computer bug*, which can't be corrected with medication either. That's why drugs can't end the tyranny.

The goal of QEEG-guided neurofeedback therapy is training the brain to behave more like a normal healthy one and thereby to correct the disturbing bug in the operating system. In a seizure disorder like migraine, we wouldn't be too surprised to find a bug in the beta frequency bands (= mezzo-soprano/soprano), because seizures are often connected to fast EEG-patterns and bursts of beta ("beta seizure pattern").[1,2] Let's have a look at a brain of a now ex-migraineur before and after neurofeedback therapy:

Brain maps are typically a *color-coded* view from above. I changed these into *grayscale-coded*: Mid-gray means normal, white indicates scarcity and black shows an excess of the metric at hand.

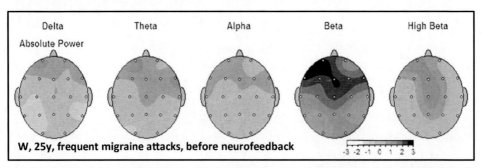

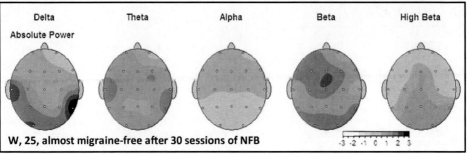

---

[1] Kuruvilla A "Beta band seizure pattern" Neurol India 2001;49(2):217
[2] Wendling F et al "Interictal to Ictal Transition in Human Temporal Lobe Epilepsy: Insights From a Computational Model of Intracerebral EEG" J Clin Neurophysiol 2005 Oct;22(5):343-56

This 25 year-old woman with very frequent migraine attacks went to see a neurologist, but instead of giving her the latest abortive drug, like most doctors do, Dr. Lucas Korbeda[1] did a QEEG on her. 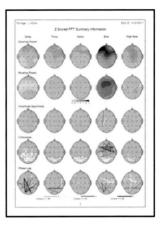 Knowledge and experience allowed him to determine the metrics responsible for this woman's migraine-seizures among the numerous measures that a QEEG calculates. Please note that this is only the report's summary sheet for a brief overview.

We've only looked into how loud the voices of the brain-choir are, which is our way of talking about the power of the frequency bands. Beside that, a QEEG informs about the power of every *single* frequency and much more:

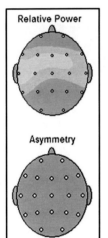

● *Relative Power* tells us how much every voice or frequency contributes to the total choir volume.
● *Asymmetry* is about balance and imbalance between choir groups.
● *Coherence* informs us whether the melody of two choir groups has the right amount of similarity to create an amazing harmony.
● *Phase metrics* are about speed and timing between ensembles.

This is just the very basic stuff and there are lots and lots more meaningful statistics that give trained experts a wealth of information about an individual brain.

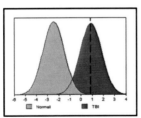

The QEEG-system that Lucas and I use[2] offers the option to analyze whether a brain shows the signs of a *brain injury* (TBI), e.g. after a *concussion*. To be precise, it tells us the likelihood that a brain belongs in the basket of proven injured brains.[3]

---

[1] Dr. J Lucas Korbeda (MD, PhD-TNBC), board-certified neurologist and Assistant Professor of Neurology at The Florida State University-College of Medicine and Director of the Tallahasse NeuroBalance Center, www.tallneurobalance.com
[2] NeuroGuide by Dr. Robert Thatcher, www.appliedneuroscience.com
[3] Thatcher RW et al "EEG discriminant analyses of mild head trauma" Electroencephalogr Clin Neurophysiol 1989;73(2):94-106

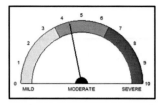

Moreover, the NeuroGuide system can provide an index (with data tables) that represents the *severity* of the traumatic brain injury (= TBI) based on how much the suspected injury has hurt this brain's function.[1]

This is relevant for many migraine sufferers, because a brain injury (e.g. concussion) is *often* the origin of the dysfunction that leads to migraine attacks.[2,3] Headaches are a frequent symptom of TBI, but especially migraine is the *cardinal symptom* when brain injuries occur in war zones.[4,5] Normally a war zone is indeed A HOSTILE PLACE. It is conceivable that the factor that stops TBI-headache episodes from becoming TBI-migraine attacks is something that active combatants certainly don't have: *a feeling of safety* (see p. 107). It might be interesting to measure the oxytocin levels of the many brain-injured war vets who returned from duty as migraineurs.

This also serves as an example that migraine results from a brain dysfunction *and* a lack of feeling safe, or in the words of the cognitively distorted: "MIGRAINE IS NEUROLOGICAL *AND* PSYCHOLOGICAL." Got it?

Given all these features and the painstaking scientific rigor behind the NeuroGuide system, it is no surprise that not only top-notch clinicians and universities worldwide use it, but also the US military in countless bases and VA institutions.[6]

A QEEG is often conducted together with a *neuro-psychological test*, which is like a fitness-test for the brain. To save time and effort, NeuroGuide can give us a calculation of the brain's fitness in the form of a brain *performance index* from the QEEG data.[7]

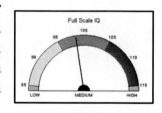

Learning disabilities in children and their severity can be identified in a similar manner by comparing the activity patterns of an individual brain to those of kids who struggle a bit in school.[8]

---

[1] Thatcher RW et al "An EEG severity index of traumatic brain injury" J Neuropsychiatry Clin Neurosci 2001;13(1):77-87
[2] Lucas S et al "Characterization of headache after traumatic brain injury" Cephalalgia 2012;32(8):600-6
[3] Ruff RL et al "Relationships between mild traumatic brain injury sustained in combat and post-traumatic stress disorder" F1000 Med Rep 2010;2:64
[4] Theeler BJ et al "Mild head trauma and chronic headaches in returning US soldiers" Headache 2009;49(4):529-34
[5] Neely ET et al "Clinical review and epidemiology of headache disorders in US service members: with emphasis on post-traumatic headache" Headache 2009;49(7):1089-96
[6] for a list of institutions using NeuroGuide visit http://www.appliedneuroscience.com/Universities.htm
[7] Thatcher RW et al "EEG and intelligence: relations between EEG coherence, EEG phase delay and power" Clin Neurophysiol 2005;116(9):2129-41
[8] Chabot RJ et al "Sensitivity and specificity of QEEG in children with attention deficit or specific developm. learning disorders" Clin EEG 1996;27(1):26-34

Seeing what's readily available, my dear readers will understand that *it sickens me* to read of migraine patients who have *their ovaries cut out*—in sheer despair—after their doctor *assured* them that their migraine-onset after an accident must be a coincidence: "A concussion can't possibly cause migraine attacks since MIGRAINE IS SWELLING AND INFLAMMATION OF BLOOD VESSELS." And caused by the ovaries? This is crazy.

This goes far beyond ignorance/incompetence. There is always the option to say "I don't know" and to send the patient to someone who does know. So it is rather *failure to render assistance, menacing indifference* or simply the current *standard of care*(-lessness).

When will the proletarian migraine masses finally rise up against this unendurable injustice and terminate the terror?

QEEG-guided neurofeedback for migraine

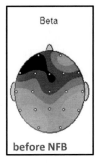
before NFB

After pinpointing the excess left-frontal beta activity as the migraine-driver in his patient's brain, Lucas targeted exactly that in his neurofeedback training sessions with her. Soon her brain choir learnt to attenuate the gung-ho mezzosopranos, which pretty much ended the migraine attacks.

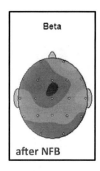
after NFB

As we can see ourselves from the brain-map after the neurofeedback therapy, the very targeted training largely reduced the excess beta and thereby *wiped the migraine off the map*.

It also demonstrates that neurofeedback therapy is neither a *miracle cure* nor a *magic bullet*. After 30 sessions the patient was not completely migraine-free and we can even see that there is still a bit too much beta energy in her brain. In such cases we need to broaden our view and look at driving factors in body and mind. There is no reason to content oneself with rare attacks when the possibility is to eliminate migraine and all its drivers forever.

On the other hand, I assume this 25 year-old woman wasn't too disappointed with the drastic improvements and with the fact that she got away *with* her ovaries intact and *without* getting stuck on the track to chronification that she was definitely on.

Big thank-yous to Dr. Lucas Korbeda (MD, PhD), Assistant Professor of Neurology and Director of the Tallahasse NeuroBalance Center (www.tallneurobalance.com) for the case (Thanks, Lucas!) and one more to Dr. Robert Thatcher, the genius behind NeuroGuide (Thanks, Bob!).

Complementing QEEG-guided neurofeedback

This next case was donated by Dr. Richard Soutar (PhD), a former professor of psychology and sociology as well as a pioneer in the field of applied neuroscience/neurofeedback. I'll present the story of Richard's client in a telegraphic style to keep things zippy:

- Woman in her 30s, works with computers
- migraine-onset as a teenager (= about 20 years of migraine history)
- 3-6 attacks per month, usually sent her home from work, 24 hours long
- premonitory symptoms: heightened sensitivity to light and sound
- triggers: intense emotions, frustration, anger; no food triggers
- family: disconnected relationships, mother: controlling and intrusive
- professional: stressful work environment
- behavior: perfectionistic, controlling, defensive
- physical: premenstrual syndrome (PMS)

With an average of 4.5 attacks per month, she would have lost 54 days per year which adds up to 36 months in 20 years, not funny. ↓ Richard did a QEEG on her and the overview doesn't show much:

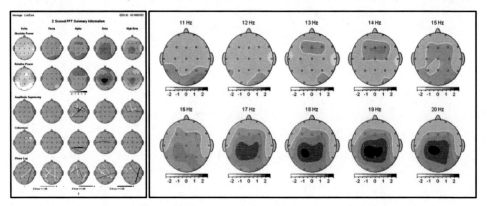

On a closer look at the *single frequencies*, ↑ we can see the excess beta at 17-20Hz (= overeager mezzo-sopranos again). The LoRETA analysis (see ch. 7) reveals the source of the dissonance:

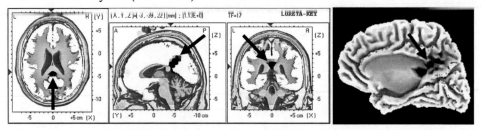

You've probably guessed it, it's the *posterior cingulate cortex*.

Like most, this brain area contributes to many different functions, for example to memory retrieval and pain,[1] but especially to behavioral flexibility and cognitive control.[2] It's a bit as if here the hurts and fears from the past become the dogged determination to control the world with the Self: tense mind protects aching heart.

> "You've told us that the problem in migraine brains is the 'wobbly' PFC and suddenly it's the *'post-area cinema cortex'*, according to Richard. How can that be?"

First, it's the *posterior cingulate* (= Latin for girdle's rear part) and not the *'post-area cinema'*. Second, a QEEG is a snapshot in time, usually done in the morning on a brain at its best. You're right, we can't see any 'weakness' in the PFC in this snapshot. That could be very different *after* a stressful day at work, *after* a frustrating talk to her mother or *during* the client's premenstrual week, when she is cranky and due for an attack. The PFC is supposed to 'keep it all together', but in the presence of intense negative emotions, it can exhaust its limited resources and fail.[3] That's probably why attacks tend to start *after* an emotional turmoil like stress, anger or frustration. Third, we're seeing more than normal 'intensity' in that posterior area and that happens to match the overall picture of a tetchy personality. Isn't that interesting? Finally, we know that *several factors* drive migraine and it's best to address them all.

This was Richard's rehabilitation program with his client:
- 'doping' with magnesium and omega-3 fatty acids
- psychotherapy for the emotionally driven behavioral issues
- re-evaluation of the work environment
- QEEG-guided neurofeedback: training beta down in that 'post-area'

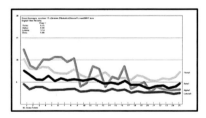

The progress chart indicates that the neurofeedback training went well and that the mezzo-sopranos dialed down their intensity without any drama, but we don't know *when* the client's migraine attacks ceased. After attack cessation, it is wise to continue for a while in order to cement the change; but you can gradually space out the sessions for that.

---

[1] Nielsen FA et al "Mining the posterior cingulate: segregation between memory and pain components" Neuroimage 2005;27(3):520-32
[2] Pearson JM et al "Posterior cingulate cortex: adapting behavior to a changing world" Trends Cogn Sci 2011;15(4):143-51
[3] Heatherton TF et al "Cognitive Neuroscience of Self-Regulation Failure" Trends Cogn Sci 2011;15(3):132–139

After 44 sessions this ex-migraineur was symptom-free and stopped seeing Richard. These are her achievements

- She reviewed and identified childhood issues,
- changed jobs,
- reduced perfectionism,
- learned to handle her emotional triggers with aplomb and
- reclaimed 1.8 months of life per year back from the migraine tyrant.

One year later the client was still migraine-free without any further sessions. Below are the brain-maps for the mezzo-sopranos before and after Richard's *wipe-out* rehabilitation program.

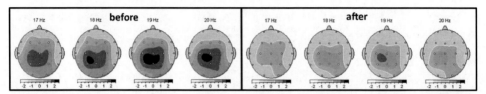

Thank you to Dr. Richard Soutar[1] for this interesting, well documented case (Thanks, Richard!).

Other EEG-based assessments

NeuroGuide is not the only QEEG-system and some specialists take it so far to run the a client's data through more than one of them. That can be helpful to discover the root of a very *specific* dysfunction. In children with dyslexia the QEEG-guided training boosted the kid's *spelling* a lot, but not their *reading*.[2] For that you need to collect the EEG-data *while* they're struggling with reading (= *Activation-QEEG*) to ascertain how their brain creates the struggling and the reading-failure. In contrast, migraine is the consequence of a *global* lack of stability and balance and that's why neurofeedback approaches without QEEG can work just as well.

It is understood that a 'proper' QEEG includes the comparison to a normative database, but there are other EEG-tests. For example, the down-to-earth neurofeedback-coach Peter van Deusen created a very sophisticated assessment that looks at activation patterns via ratios and relationships within the brain itself. Many are perfectly happy with Pete's "TLC" system,[3] which flattens The Learning Curve (= TLC) for the clinician and can also end the tyranny.

---

[1] Dr. Richard and Barbara Soutar in Roswell, Georgia/USA: www.newmindcenter.com
[2] Breteler et al "Improvements in Spelling after QEEG-based Neurofeedback in Dyslexia: A Randomized Controlled Treatment Study" Appl Psychophysiol Biofeedback 2010;35(1):5–11
[3] Peter van Deusen, The Learning Curve Inc., www.brain-trainer.com

Chapter 29

Recipes for the Brain

"This is my invariable advice to people: Learn how to cook- try new recipes, learn from your mistakes, be fearless, and above all have fun!"

Julia Child

Symptom-based neurofeedback therapy

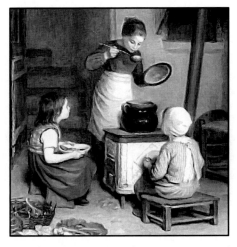

Training the brain towards 'normal' based on an assessment has an amazing face validity and usually works very well. We've seen that in case examples and studies. On the other hand, that doesn't mean QEEGs are the only approach to successfully training the brain. Especially for migraine, using a tried and tested recipe and adjusting it to individual reactions is very common.

The roots of neurofeedback reach back to the late 1960s and are more of a serendipitous discovery than an intentional invention. A sleep researcher at UCLA identified a hitherto unknown EEG waveform, at first in the brains of cats and monkeys, and later in humans too. He called it SMR or *sensory-motor rhythm*, because it showed up in those parts of the cortex that process <u>sensory</u> information (= body sense) or <u>motor</u> commands (= movements).

Then, in an experiment, cats were trained to produce more of that SMR wave with the help of a reward, mixed from milk and chicken broth and it was observed that their sleep improved.

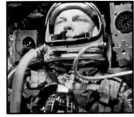

Later the same professor was involved in a completely unrelated investigation of the toxic effects of rocket fuel, which used to give the US air force and NASA quite some grief: The astronauts of the Mercury program claimed that they saw the natives waving at them when their spacecraft flew over the islands in the Pacific.

Even though Pacific islanders are indeed very friendly, it was clear that the astronauts were hallucinating, thanks to the fumes of the rocket fuel. During his tests on cats as guinea pigs, Professor Sterman made a surprising observation. When exposed to the fuel, all 50 cats displayed signs of intolerance like barfing, howling, panting, drooling and finally grand-mal epileptic fits. However, 10 of the 50 cats were *much more resistant* to seizures and it turned out that they were the ones who had participated in the earlier SMR braintraining experiment.

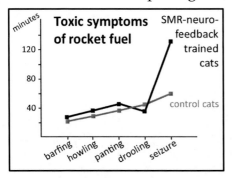

Long story short, SMR neurofeedback training was found to be a viable recipe for intractable seizures in humans (see p. 340). The neurologist Oliver Sacks became aware of this research, and in the 1970 edition of his book "*Migraine*" he speculated that, if this new EEG biofeedback could be helpful for seizures, then perhaps it might one day be helpful for migraine as well. How right he was!

Two of the early pioneers in the field of neurofeedback therapy were the physicist Dr. Siegfried Othmer and his wife Susan Othmer, a neurobiologist. They first discovered neurofeedback as parents of a boy with severe epilepsy and later became clinician and scientist, as well as teachers and activists. Sue Othmer turned out to be a highly gifted therapist and she gradually optimized her methods based on her observations on thousands of patients.

Two of the pioneers' personal friends, who had undergone neurofeedback training for other reasons, reported later that their migraine attacks had ceased, which alerted the Othmers to the possibility that neurofeedback could also help severe migraineurs.

At that time (in the late 1980s) migraine was still considered to be *just a headache* caused by SWELLING AND INFLAMMATION OF BLOOD VESSELS and clinical neurofeedback therapy was in its infancy even for epilepsy and rambunctious kids. Back then popular training protocols were SMR training (= more alto, please!) for the right side and Beta training (= more mezzo-soprano, please!) for the left side of the brain. In either case the other voices were generally admonished to limit their volume to reasonable levels.

For one EEG channel we need *one active* and *one reference* electrode, or "plus" and "minus". The two hemispheres (= halves) of the brain have different tasks and the left half needs to be a smidge faster than the right; so to train the hemispheres separately, plus and minus have to be on the same, trained side.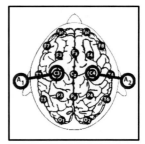

It was also common that Sue Othmer's migraine clients would show up with acute symptoms like headaches. The neurofeedback training on the *hurting* half of the head usually drove the pain over onto the *resting* half. The gifted therapist would then follow by moving the active plus-electrode over to chase the headache there.

One day Sue got tired of the backing-and-forthing and simply placed active and reference electrode on either side of the head. Promptly, the migraine pain vanished, as it didn't have anywhere else to hide. This method of *interhemispheric training* became her favorite method and her trademark in the field. All that thanks to migraine cases.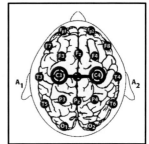

Case examples and skepticism

"One male client had a long history of severe, *chronic* migraine with daily headaches. The client had even been to the Mayo Clinic to little benefit. After ten sessions of interhemispheric neurofeedback he judged himself to have improved by 25%. By session 20, he was experiencing some headache-free days. By session 30, headache frequency and severity were further reduced. By session 40 he was experiencing 5-7 day stretches without any head pain. He rated his improvement overall at 80-90%." In short, he got his life back.

Sue Othmer soon discovered that migraine clients responded faster (with symptom improvements) when she placed the electrodes one notch further out. This recipe has become the workhorse in the Othmer training method, not only for migraine and other seizures, but also as a starting point for the many issues caused by the dysregulation of brain arousal. All that thanks to migraine cases.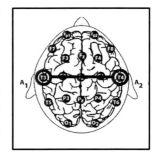

> "Another client had attacks typically lasting for three days. By the tenth session, there were fewer episodes and they lasted only 8-10 hours. By session 20, he declared: 'This is the best my brain has felt for years.' By session 30, his migraine was history. He was sleeping better and felt more calm and focused."

Large collections of positive case examples can be extremely informative, because they tell us what works well with those clients who are eager to change into ex-migraineurs, unspoilt by those who are not. Unfortunately, the ever-present drug propaganda and some sufferers' dismissive-avoidant attitudes have managed to create an atmosphere of *illogical skepticism,* especially towards such a successful and essentially risk-free method, as can be seen in the statement: "IF IT WERE TRUE, IT WOULD HAVE BEEN ON PAGE ONE OF EVERY NEWSPAPER."

Here I'd like to point out how *irrational* it is to be more critical and skeptic of a benign behavioral therapy than of drugs: The pharma giant GlaxoSmithKline (GSK) *pleaded guilty* and paid a $ 3bn fine for various fraudulent actions like bribing doctors and pushing useless and harmful drugs *against better knowledge.*[1] Before anyone starts tearing up about the 'harsh' punishment: $ 3bn (=3,000 million) is merely a fraction of the additional profit that GSK earned from their illegal deeds. So, who deserves our distrust?

No matter how helpful medication often is, migraine patients who delude themselves into naïvely relying on the pharma-medical industry and into dismissing behavioral methods like neurofeedback therapy are also following a recipe, a recipe for disaster.

Over the years Sue and Siegfried Othmer have trained more than 5,000 neurofeedback clinicians from all over the world:

> "One practitioner, a chiropractor in Syracuse, NY, told us of her success with migraine, and sent us a number of case reports. One of her clients had had a history of daily migraine headaches for thirty years, and they had gotten worse over the last twenty. She was taking Imitrex® for the migraine and Zoloft® for depression. After ten sessions of training she judged her depression to have improved by 50%, and her headache incidence by 80%. By twenty sessions, she could report that she hadn't had a migraine attack for two months. By session 30, she no longer considered herself depressed and there had been no headaches to report. By session 40, she was also medication-free."

Evidently, one way to battle migraine is to follow Sue's recipe.[2]

---

[1] news agency Reuters on July 2nd, 2012; www.reuters.com/article/2012/07/02/us-glaxo-settlement-factbox-idUSBRE86116E20120702
[2] http://www.eeginfo.com, in Europe www.eeginfo.ch; as well as www.homecoming4veterans.org

Chapter 30

On the Crest of Slow Waves

"You can't stop the waves, but you can learn to surf."

Jon Kabat Zinn

Infraslow fluctuations neurofeedback therapy

The summit of Mt Everest is 8848m *above sea level*. Without this *reference* there is no altitude, as it is the vertical *distance* to the reference sea level. Clear?

EEG devices too measure a *difference,* the difference in electrical potential between the plus and the minus lead. We call plus "active" and minus "reference",

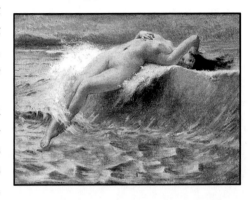

but that's just a convention and doesn't change the amount of difference. You could also say that sea level is 8848m *below* the summit of Mt Everest, if you wanted to; it's the same difference.

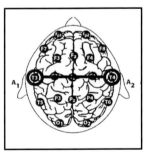

By placing the active and the reference electrode on either side of the head, Sue Othmer changed her method substantially. Not only are both hemispheres now involved, but the signal also embodies the *difference* between those areas and is mainly influenced by the *relative timing* of those choir groups (In chapter 28 we've learnt about timing/phase).

Sue, being a gifted therapist, observed that fine adjustments of the rewarded frequency (= pitch) could have a noticeable impact on the brain and its owner. Also, every client seemed to have special needs regarding the training of their brain's timing; an individual, *optimal frequency*, at which good things happened, when trained with reward. For instance, hyperactive kids would fidget a bit less during the training and there would be a report from mom next week that she noticed a positive change: "He did his homework by himself" or stuff like that. Things change when brain timing shifts.

Again, it was migraine clients who displayed the most convincing reactions and thereby confirmed the concept of an optimal reward frequency (ORF) for every brain. Those who came in with headaches felt immediate relief, when the ORF was hit. Sue reports:

> "A client history from our own office illustrates the optimization procedure. This person had had headaches every day for most of her adult life; in the beginning they used to be PMS-related. The migraine attacks would last for three days and medications would only dull the pain. She came into the second session with a headache, and it vanished within six minutes of training. This vanishing of an ongoing headache is the best indication that the optimum reward frequency has been found. At the third session, she said: *'I feel so good that I am afraid that it will go away.'* Minor headaches were still coming and going. At the fourth session, she declared: *'I think I am in heaven.'* and *'It's hard to remember how I was before neurofeedback, with headaches all the time.'*"

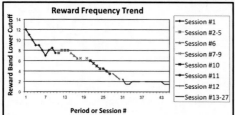

As in this case, especially in migraineurs Sue Othmer often had to lower the reward frequency not only during the neurofeedback session, but also from week to week. As data-driven scientists the Othmers documented this trend thoroughly:

> "The tendency to move the reward toward the lower frequencies became ever more common as more and more intractable migraine cases came our way. Eventually we came to the lowest frequency that our software would allow, 0-3 Hz, and we accepted this limitation for a period of two years, from 2004 to 2006. During that time there were increasing numbers of clients with various brain instabilities, not only migraine, who ended up training at this lowest frequency. It stood to reason that many of these would benefit even more at even lower frequencies, if those were available."

Training the brain at 0.1-1 Hz, below the frequency range of traditional EEG, is not too unusual. German scientists and clinicians have been dealing with these "slow cortical potentials" for years, for instance in migraine research and therapy [1,2,3] (see ch. 8).

---

[1] Kropp P et al "Prediction of migraine attacks using a slow cortical potential, the contingent negative variation" Neurosci Lett 1998;257(2):73-6

[2] Siniatchkin M et al "Self-regulation of slow cortical potentials in children with migraine: an exploratory study" Appl Psychophysiol Biofeedback 2000;25(1):13-32

[3] Kropp P et al "Slow cortical potentials in migraine. Predictive value and possible novel therapeutic strategies to prevent an attack" Funct Neurol 2005;20(4):193-7

Sailing into uncharted waters

During the years 2006-2010 the Othmers observed with every step they took to expand the technically available reward range, that the majority of their clients eventually found their optimal training at the lowest frequency; and also that previously *unresponsive* patients suddenly made progress. Here's a report from a psychiatrist who utilizes neurofeedback in his practice, and who also benefited for his own migraine during this period of transition to the "infra-low frequencies" (ILF):

> "I had an interesting experience the other day that I'd like to share. I get migraine headaches and used to train at 12-14 Hz (at the locations T3-T4). The training was helpful and the severity and frequency of my headaches reduced. However they still occurred from time to time. With the evolution of ILF training I've recently trained at 0.6 Hz as this seemed the most comfortable frequency. Having not had a migraine attack for many months, the other day I began to experience the typical visual aura that I get and knew a headache was on its way. No matter what reward frequencies I had tried in the past, I have never been able to abort an aura, even though I could influence the subsequent headache (often not getting one but sometimes just getting a mild one). For some reason with this aura I decided to be more aggressive and set the T3-T4 reward frequency at 0.01 Hz. The aura was gone within a few minutes and no headache emerged. I was rather astounded and obviously grateful. So I add this story as personal/experiential support for the added benefit of training at the very lowest reward frequencies—at least for those migraine conditions that had only partial benefit at higher reward frequencies."

Gifted therapists also receive a special 'reward'. When they're doing particularly well with certain patients or a condition, their reputation attracts extraordinarily difficult and complex patients.

> "With word spreading of our work, we were starting to attract some of the most unusual and severe cases of migraine, some of whom were coming from great distances, not only traveling under difficult circumstances, but also at great sacrifice of their family resources. And with our earlier methods, sometimes we were not able to help these people either." This was heartbreaking for all involved, because indeed we were seen as the last hope by some of these folks. With the new methods, it was far more likely that we would at least make progress that was worthwhile in the eyes of the family."

Siegfried's term "new methods" means training at 0.01Hz.

Beliefs and reality

In this book I've explained repeatedly the mechanisms that lead some migraineurs into unhelpful attitudes and behaviors, e.g.

- human psychology (from negativity to confirmation bias)
- handicapped minds (from cognitive distortions to hopelessness)
- maladaptive schemas (from unworthiness to vulnerability)
- wobbly PFC (from early life stress to neuroticism)
- misleading myths (incurable genetic disease, inflammation etc.)
- zeitgeist (drugs as quick fix, medicalization of problems etc.)

In short and without ill intentions we can summarize that a few poor souls end up in the deplorable role of "*nutty skeptics*", who believe that the hostile world is after them and that they're doomed to die suffering. While interesting, encouraging and inspiring for all other migraineurs, reading these patient reports of aborting auras and migraine attacks with neurofeedback training must be an unacceptable provocation for the 'nutty skeptics'.

When it comes to infra-low frequency neurofeedback, the poor souls may take comfort from the fact that even amongst the highly educated academics involved in neurofeedback, there are a few who also bitterly complain that *their beliefs* don't match the undeniable success of the Othmers' neurofeedback approach—especially *for migraine* and as a result of their work *with migraine*.

And so, while Sue and the many Othmer-trained clinicians unwaveringly use infra-slow frequency neurofeedback to help the most atrocious migraine cases claim parts of their life back, Siegfried is forced to keep fighting an uphill battle, not only against the considerably larger and stronger natural enemies of behavioral therapies (like doctors, drug firms and self-serving politicians), but also against the persistent animosities from a few righteous and vociferous proponents of a *competing* neurofeedback method, who have their own, selfish agenda and simply don't share the Othmers' vision to improve people's lives with neurofeedback therapy.

The Othmers' envious rivals will probably never comprehend that the agony they themselves had to endure during their own horror-trip as parents of a beautiful boy with horrible epilepsy, gave them an inexhaustible source of unstoppable energy: their *commitment to the mission* to help others—with neurofeedback.

Overcoming inertia

There is an obstacle that not even the most battle-hardened, passionate and committed neurofeedback pioneers can overcome:

> "It is astounding to observe just how many people are willing to live with their occasional migraine attacks, even though these are the very ones that are most readily remediable. We once had a mother suffering through an episode in the waiting room while her son was getting neurofeedback for his ADHD. She obviously believed in the method, and she could afford the fees. And yet she would not avail herself of the remedy that she was making available to her son. 'Oh, it's just once a month...' Still, that's twelve days of misery per year, which is more days than most Americans are allotted for vacation."

One is tempted to think that in this case thoughtlessness and foolishness are behind the mom's silly indifference, but I think the issue lies much deeper in a lack of self-worth, self-care and self-love. Or in psychological lingo, an *unworthiness* schema.

If you asked me, I would say that it's about time for migraine patients to support one another in order to open these invisible cages of their upbringing. If you prefer the colloquial version: You've got to kick each other's butts to end the frickin' tyranny. Being based in California, Siegfried phrases that more politely:

> "In the course of our more than 25 years of work in the field of EEG neurofeedback, migraine has gone from being thought of as essentially intractable to being largely optional. The urgency of the day is for migraineurs themselves to discover the remedies that are now available to them. They should not look to the professionals to lead the way. Neurofeedback is a much more demanding discipline than these professionals are accustomed to. The following case illustrates the problem of professional comfort level:
>
> A 24 year-old female with a 6-year history of progressively worsening migraine, unremitting of late, with two hospitalizations just in 2009 for migraine attacks, has three neurologists and a family physician who have been treating her all this time. They have tried over 40 different medications, and finally referred her for neurofeedback. After six sessions she goes more than a week without a migraine attack. She visits her family physician (who referred her initially), who says: *"I guess our medications finally kicked in."*

This doc's remark seems arrogant, but I think it shows that neurofeedback's proven power is simply beyond his comprehension.

Reality and theory

With their own hardware and software the Othmers finally reached reward frequencies of 0.0001 Hz or 0.1 mHz (= milliHertz). Some traditionalists conclude that this can't be and are appalled. A frequency of 1 Hz means one full oscillatory cycle per second and so the equivalent of 0.1 milliHertz would be more than 2:45 hours. You can't reward an event within a 30 min neurofeedback session if it takes so much longer than the session itself. Ergo, it's all a hoax.

This is a wonderful example of a cognitive distortion amongst professionals (see page 90: *'If I think so, then it is so'*). When the presented reality doesn't fit into the theory with all its assumptions, they conclude that the *reality is wrong!* Of course, that is nonsense and the idea that Sue and Siegfried Othmer would or could apply and teach a method that doesn't work is simply bizarre.

The technically lackadaisical layperson might rightfully think: "So what? Listen, mate, once or twice a week, a devil wakes up in my brain, spills burning lava, maltreats my pain network with a sledgehammer and dances a polka on my nausea nerve. Seriously, I give a **** whether those Othmers use Hertz, milliHertz or picoHertz. If it helps, let them use nanoHertz. Who cares? I certainly don't."

Are you saying that you are not puzzled that these infraslow frequencies of the Othmer method are even below the ranges that were found to influence seizure activity (0.02-0.2 Hz)?[1] Or are you not interested in the finding that especially the *phase* of very slow EEG fluctuations (0.01-0.1 Hz) corresponds with the subjective perception of external stimuli (e.g. light, noise, odor)?[2]

"No, I'm saying, when people don't have migraine attacks anymore, that can't possibly be wrong. If a theory doesn't explain what really happens, then it is no good. Like the old baloney that there is no therapy for migraine; it's obviously wrong. Period."

There is no hoax behind the Othmer method. The error lies in the assumption that so-called *'frequencies'* below 0.1 Hz still represent *'oscillations'*. In thermal biofeedback ('handwarming') we train the ANS with the *slow fluctuations* of the finger's skin temperature. Also, you neither have to drive 50 miles nor for a full hour in order to reach a speed of 50 miles per hour. It's the same for 0.1 mHz!

---

[1] Vanhatalo S et al "Infraslow oscillations modulate excitability and interictal epileptic activity in the human cortex during sleep" Proc Natl Acad Sci USA 2004;101(14):5053-7

[2] Monto S etal "Very slow EEG fluctuations predict the dynamics of stimulus detection and oscillation amplitudes in humans" J Neurosci 2008;28(33):8268-72

The usefulness of ILF/ISF neurofeedback

We can call it *infralow-frequency* (ILF) or *infraslow-fluctuations* (ISF) neurofeedback therapy, but let's have a look at how helpful it is for typical migraine problems; for example for the much discussed issue of migraine 'trigger' factors. Siegfried recounts:

> "We had one case with several decades of migraine history involving a person with a number of well-known triggers—red wine, sleep deprivation, stress, etc. She came for forty training sessions, as had been recommended, but when we reviewed her training history it turns out that she never had another full-blown migraine from the first session on. Further, it turned out that she had gone back to some of her earlier habits of late-night partying, returning to a stressful professional regimen, and re-acquainting herself with red wine...."

No more migraine, no more triggers; is it really that simple? Here is a report from an Othmer-trained clinician:

> "One man, a 60-year-old, who came for fibromyalgia and traumatic brain injury, was completely unable to function with large changes in barometric pressure. He was a truck driver and at times had to pull over and lie on the floor of his truck until the pressure changed because his pain became so severe he couldn't tolerate it while driving. He lost the reaction to barometric changes with neurofeedback training." Siegfried comments: "This case also demonstrates that this neurofeedback method enhances brain stability and function generally, as opposed to targeting migraine attacks specifically."

That doesn't mean that neurofeedback training is a miracle cure that heals every ailment. If I was diagnosed with pneumonia, leukemia, Creutzfeldt-Jakob disease or Ebola virus, I would hope that some medical treatment with drugs, surgery and radiation can safe my life. Neurofeedback certainly can't save lives like doctors can, or can it? Well, this is another report from a therapist:

> "When I first started as a neurofeedback therapist, I had an eleven-year-old boy walk into my office with suicidal intentions because a neurologist had told him to stop playing his favorite sport (baseball), and to come to terms with the likelihood that he might well have untreatable migraine for the rest of his life. After a few sessions, he was 50% migraine-free, and the intensity had also decreased 50%. I no longer treat this boy for migraine attacks because he doesn't get them any more...and he continues to enjoy his favorite sport of baseball. I'll never forget the look on his face when I told him we would likely get rid of his migraine. The very first session, he walked out with no pain."

What a smart move, not to follow through with the suicide idea, don't you think? Luckily, somebody told this this young baseball fan that there is a better solution to end the migraine tyranny than ending his own life. Suicidal thoughts are not uncommon in young migraine patients; migraine with aura drives 23% of them in this dark direction.[1] The likelihood for a suicide attempt is 4.4 times higher in migraine sufferers.[2] It makes me sick to think how many desperate migraine sufferers took their own life, because they had no idea that there is a better option than choosing between suffering and dying: a migraine revolution.

Show me your figures

How about some data? Due to their extensive work with war veterans at six US military bases, Sue and Siegfried have lots of outcome data for clients with PTSD. More than 10% of them also suffer from migraine and so we're looking now at the effect of neurofeedback on 49 migraineurs with PTSD, a decent group size:

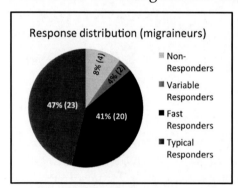
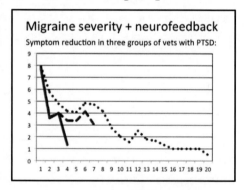

Four ex-soldiers did not benefit and in two cases the outcome couldn't be determined. In 88% of cases the average headache intensity went from 6.6 (out of 10) down to 1.6. Roughly half of these responders needed about 10 sessions, the other half 20-40 sessions of neurofeedback therapy for that. Needless to say that many other symptoms (e.g. depression) resolved in the same manner. Given that many vets receive financial benefits based on their PTSD diagnosis, it is remarkable that only 8-12% didn't make progress.

Further information, videos and the contact info for Othmer-trained therapists world wide can be found at www.eeginfo.com.

---

[1] Wang SJ et al "Migraine and suicidal ideation in adolescents aged 13 to 15 years" Neurology 2009;72(13):1146-52
[2] Breslau N et al "Migraine headaches and suicide attempt" Headache 2012;52(5):723-31

Chapter 31

Overpowering the Migraine Beast

> "The strength and the power of despotism consist wholly in the fear of resistance."
>
> Thomas Paine

Power for speed

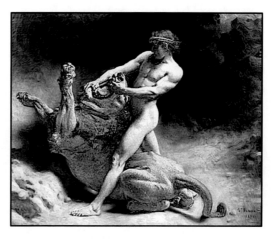

While severely affected migraine patients stockpile triptans in their freezer, therapists discuss *how* they can make the neurofeedback process for attack cessation even shorter. The immense processing power of modern PCs, novel methods of data crunching and developments in neuroscience make very sophisticated and noticeably more efficient neurofeedback approaches possible.

Many complex and 'difficult' migraine sufferers (despite systematic discouragement by the current regime) continue to search for treatment alternatives; be it for true defiant persistence ("I'm not going to give up") or be it to confirm their high levels of experienced helplessness and hopelessness through repeated failures ("... BUT I'LL TRY ANYTHING"). In either case, experience shows that *the more chronic the clients are, the less patient* they will be during their next attempt before concluding: "IT DIDN'T DO MUCH FOR ME." Also, it becomes predictable (and understandable) that for highly reactive and 'difficult' clients any encounter with any form of inconvenience is more likely to lead to a declaration of failure in the spirit of "I TRIED IT ONCE AND THE RESULT WAS HELL". In short: *Harder cases need faster solutions.*

Therefore neurotherapists are under serious pressure to prove to their migraine clients quickly and convincingly that this won't be one of the well-meaning disappointments, fraudulent inadequacies, outright con-schemes and walloping lies they've experienced prior.

Surface Z-score training

One of the innovations in the camp of QEEG-guided neurofeedback is the training of Z-scores instead of the raw values for volume, harmony, speed and timing of the choir-groups. Z-scores express how 'abnormal' a measured value is. For example, if the Z-score for the soprano's volume is 2.1, it means that it is more than twice as loud as the 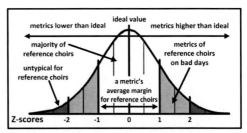 margin for reference choirs. That is too loud and probably worth changing, depending on which microphone-channel recorded it and what the client's most pressing problems are.

We've already seen Z-scores in QEEG brain-maps, because they are the result of the comparison with the database. The true innovation here is the possibility to make that comparison *during* the recording, in real-time, live or "on the fly". If the graphic card is fast too, we can even look at *instantaneous, Z-scored brainmaps*:

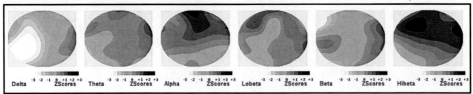

Z-scores allow us to forget about pesky measurement units (like microvolts or milliseconds) and let us calculate the *similarity* between our problem-choir and the reference choir. They make it easy to train several choir groups at the same time and so it's a bit like having an *army of singing teachers* and voice coaches helping.

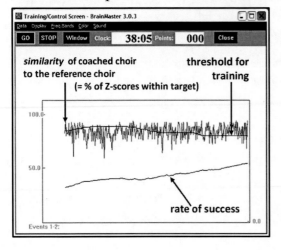

All this might seem like *geek-stuff* to the technically challenged. Yes, it is pretty nerdy, but it indeed serves the purpose of making an already mighty weapon even better.

Z-score neurofeedback can be done as 1- or 2-channel training. Using 4 channels is a popular solution, but the real fun starts with all 19 channels, called "full cap".[1] Once the EEG-cap problem is solved (see chapter 27), *full-cap surface Z-score neurofeedback* seems indeed faster in difficult cases. A seasoned clinician reports:

> "... Z-Score training and ... have resulted in substantial improvement in patients. For example, a stroke victim who after just 3 full-cap 'harmony' sessions regained use of his arm and was able to close his hand as if holding a baseball ... Quite honestly, I have never seen this kind of rapid progress in certain patients with any other training format."[2] (edited for reading ease).

One of the more amazing details is that neurofeedback — even with *hundreds* of metrics — does not require conscious attention. So we can let the mind watch a film, while the brain-choir gets its high-tech singing lessons. The mind's contribution is the wish for a bright picture, when the feedback is set up for that. Easy, ey?

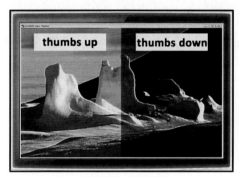
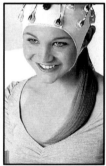

LoRETA neurofeedback training

As a quick refresher, LoRETA is short for *low resolution electromagnetic tomography*, essentially a *3-dimensional EEG*.[3,4] We have already seen several LoRETA images, for example the 3D-image of Richard's patient's overeager mezzo-sopranos in the posterior cingulate cortex (ch. 28) as part of the QEEG analysis; the LoRETA slice-pictures and 3D-images were generated *after* the data-recording.

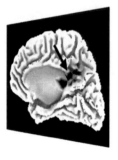

---

[1] Collura TF "Whole-Head Normalization Using Live Z-Scores for Connectivity Training" NeuroConnections 2008;1(4): 12-18
[2] Robert McCarthy, Ph.D. McCarthy Counseling Associates, PA; testimonial on www.appliedneuroscience.com
[3] Béla C "LoRETA: a three-dimensional EEG source localization method" Ideggyogy Sz 2011;64(9-10):306-9
[4] Pascual-Marqui RD et al "Functional imaging with low-resolution brain electromagnetic tomography (LoRETA): a review" Methods Find Exp Clin Pharmacol 2002;24SupplC:91-5

Tomos means *slice*, a tomography creates *pictures of slices* like these from a LoRETA study showing the wobbly PFC in migraine brains.[1] Normally a lack of activity is depicted in blue, so I changed it and here the wobbly areas are seen as white:

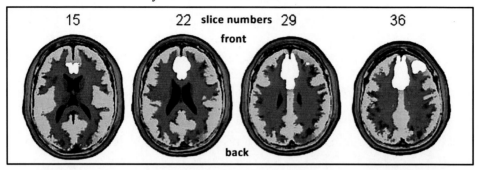

The weakish frequency band is the tenor, a finding which is consistent with the brain's predisposition to create seizure activity.[2] The next three LoRETA slices show the excessive activity *during* a migraine attack as dark and black. Note the silence at the front:

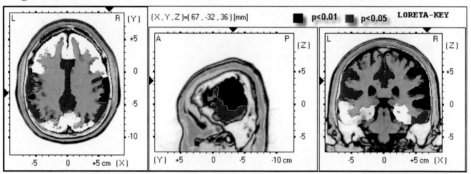

The PFC at the front of the brain is visibly silent, which effectively lets the brainstem loose.[3] The migraine beast is running wild and we can watch it with LoRETA. How cool is that?

However, all of these pictures were calculated from data *after* the recording. For neurofeedback we must inform the singers straight away how they're doing, otherwise they can't learn. So we need to run all the computations that produce the 3-dimensional EGG not after, but *during* the recording. Would it be worth it?

---

[1] Clemens B et al "Three-dimensional localization of abnormal EEG activity in migraine: a low resolution electromagnetic tomography (LoRETA) study of migraine patients in the pain-free interval" Brain Topogr 2008;21(1):36-42

[2] Puskás S et al "Quantitative EEG abnormalities in persons with "pure" epileptic predisposition without epilepsy: a low resolution electromagnetic tomography (LoRETA) study" Epilepsy Res 2010;91(1):94-100

[3] Keeser D et al "Preliminary EEG and Low Resolution Electromagnetic Tomography (LoRETA) measurements results of a migraine patient: An Electrophysiological Evaluation" poster presentation 2011, Technical University Munich

We already know from real-time fMRI neurofeedback that we can expect faster results when the neurofeedback uses *3-dimensional information*.[1] That is like placing the microphones inside the brain-choir to get closer to the singers. FMRI neurofeedback is prohibitively expensive and only a research application, but LoRETA can give us 3D-EEG information on the fly.

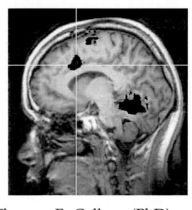

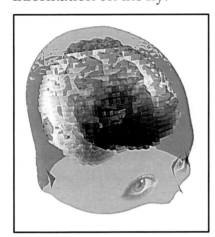

Dr. Thomas F. Collura (PhD), a biomedical engineer, neurophysiologist and boss of BrainMaster Technologies Inc.[2] — known for their innovative energy — was the first to present a *3D-visualization software* for LoRETA. It shows in real-time the activity levels for every frequency band as tiny color-coded cubicles. Trust me, it looks amazing in color. Below we see a training screen for Tom's LoRETA neurofeedback.

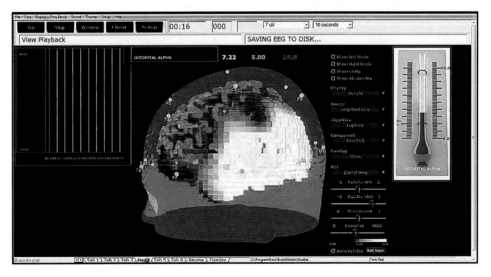

---

[1] deCharms RC et al "Control over brain activation and pain learned by using real-time functional MRI" Proc Natl Acad Sci USA 2005;102(51):18626-31

[2] BrainMaster Technologies, Inc., Bedford, (near Cleveland) OH/USA; www.brainmaster.com

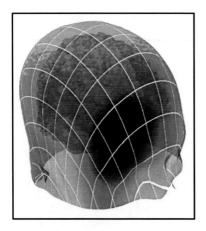

BrainMaster's software also has a cute graphic for the 2-dimensional surface EEG, which looks like a checkered, real-time brainmap-beanie.

"With this system we open the door to an unprecedented level of visualization ..., suited to the needs of the 21st century" says Collura.

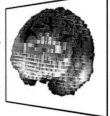

How could anybody contradict that?

LoRETA Z-score neurofeedback

With the vast amount of data that the 3-dimensional LoRETA provides, it would come in handy, if there was something like a quality-controlled, normative database for LoRETA, which could be used to calculate 3-dimensional LoRETA Z-scores. That would make things easier for the clinician, whose first priority should be the client and not the programming of the neurofeedback protocol.

In choir-lingo: It's awesome that we get to move the microphones closer to the singers, but now we need the comparison with the reference-choir more than ever, because we're dealing with even more data. Our focus is the choir, not the recording gear.

Dr. Thatcher, whom we already know from the QEEG chapter, has created such a LoRETA database[1] and a software for LoRETA Z-score neurofeedback. To make things easier for the therapists — who are mostly psychologists, counselors and neurologists and neither brain scientists nor computer programmers — Thatcher created a program that assists with matching the patient's EEG-data with symptoms and complaints, based on published neuroscientific research; a highly appreciated tool.

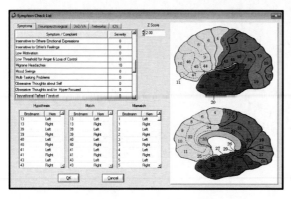

[1] Thatcher RW et al "Evaluation and validity of a LoRETA normative EEG database" Clin EEG Neurosci 2005;36(2):116-22

This is the kind of screen that the neurotherapist watches during a NeuroGuide LoRETA Z-score neurofeedback session:

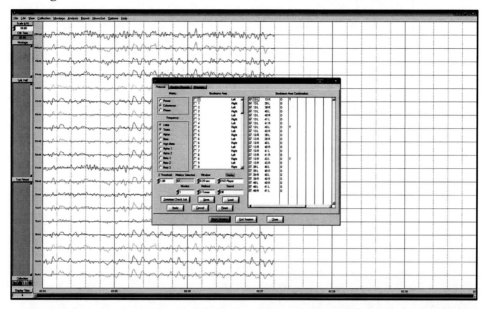

And this could be what the client get's to look at: a nice DVD, this time with the picture size conveying the thumbs up or thumbs down. Who would want to have an *occipital nerve stimulator* implanted, if they knew the alternative is watching 'Planet Earth' with an EEG-cap on your head? What would you prefer, surgery or video?

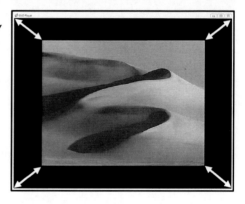

Full-cap neurofeedback and migraine

LoRETA Z-score neurofeedback is *not a new therapy*; it is a systematic refinement of a tried and tested brain training that utilizes the biofeedback principle to take advantage of the brain's neuroplasticity. The new part is where the data come from that are used to guide the brain to better function. So there is no need to re-run all the studies that were done to establish the method itself. Just like a surgeon doesn't have to prove the value of cancer surgery *again*, when he gets a better knife.

"Well, is LoRETA Z-score neurofeedback 'a better knife' for migraine therapy?" Our new friend Lucas, the top-gun neurologist from chapter 28, compared *QEEG-guided 1-channel training* to his pet method: *full-cap Z-score neurofeedback*, alternating surface (2D) and LoRETA (3D):

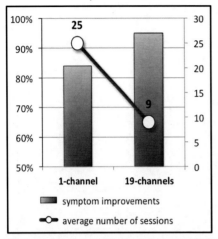

He analyzed 65 mixed cases from his neurology practice who had received neurotherapy. Dr. Korbeda found a slightly better *symptom improvement rate* for full cap training, which doesn't say much between two mixed groups of patients; but the *average number of sessions needed* went down from 25 to 9 (= "nine", with a range of 3-24).

Below we see parts of the initial and final QEEG reports of a

- 58 year-old female, long history of chronic migraine and daily headache;
- the first brain-map showed a marked increase in bass (1) and soprano volume (2), as well as too much baritone (3) and horrible disharmony amongst the soprano groups (4), not uncommon in chronic pain patients.

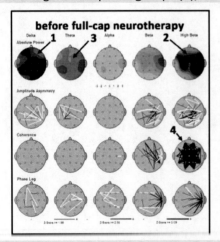
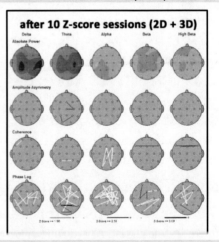

- the brain-map after only 10 sessions is almost flawless (⬆) and so we're not surprised to learn that the woman is migraine-free and headache-less.

Full cap Z score neurotherapy is *not a miracle cure* either, but it's good to know that we have revolutionary weapons like these in our arsenal, that can overpower the migraine beast and set us free.

Thanks again to neurologist Dr. Korbeda, FL (www.tallneurobalance.com): Thanks Lucas!

Chapter 32

The Magic of a Whisper

> "Sometimes a whisper speaks volumes."
> Scott Sheddan

Low energy neurofeedback system (LENS)

As instructed by his king,[1] the Saxon alchemist J. F. Böttger tried to *make gold* and instead discovered that he accidentally created the first European *porcelain*.

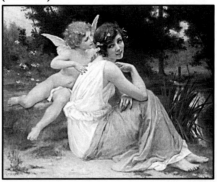

A similar thing happened to the American psychologist and biophysicist Dr. Len Ochs. During the development of an inventive neurotherapy system he discovered that he had accidentally created *low energy neurofeedback*. A fascinating story that he should tell you one day over a beer or a magnesium-rich mineral water.

Before we get caught up in the philosophy and biophysics of the LENS, let's have a look at a case of *migraine resolution*. This one was bestowed upon us by Dr. Gil Winkelman (ND, MA) a naturopathic physician with additional degrees in genetics and counseling, practicing in Portland, OR (www.insightstohealth.net):

- 44 year-old woman, migraine attacks since her teen years, beginning with menarche (= onset of menstruation), corresponding to ovulation and period, oral contraceptives made her episodes more frequent and severe
- TBI: highly likely, several bad falls during horse-riding around age 7
- prodromal symptoms: chocolate and coffee cravings
- attack symptoms: right-sided headache, sensitivity to light/noise/heat, barfing
- genetic disposition: mother and grandmother are/were migraine sufferers
- physical comorbidities: history of endometriosis
- sleep: can sleep from 8.30pm to 7am and still not feel refreshed
- energy: very low; sense of well-being: not good
- mood: irritability, depression, bouts of 'suspicious thoughts'
- medication: Zoloft® (best-selling anti-depressant drug), Imitrex® (triptan)

---

[1] Augustus II the Strong was Elector of Saxony, Imperial Vicar, King of Poland and Grand Duke of Lithuania

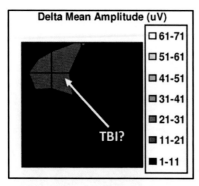

The client saw Dr. Winkelman specifically for LENS therapy for herself and her autistic son. Her first LENS assessment-map revealed high amplitudes of Delta (= loud bass), supporting the suspicion of a traumatic brain injury in the past. It also fits with *depression*, as the left-frontal area of the brain is entrusted with *embracing life*. If it's bruised and limping, it can't really hug the world.[1]

A view for change

Looking at things differently can be very helpful. For example, if you have back pain, you might see a *physiotherapist* and learn that your posture is lousy and that you need shoe inserts to make up for your unevenly long legs. In contrast, if you see a *chirotherapist*, you might be told that you have several blockages in your spine and your posture is the best your movement system can come up with *under the given circumstances* of currently present spine blockages.

In this imperfect analogy a QEEG and the ensuing neurofeedback training is *more like* the physiotherapist who tells you how to sit, stand and walk correctly to make your back pain subside. LENS is *more like* the chirotherapist looking at blocked spine segments:

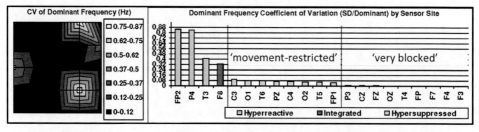

LENS therapists find 'blocked' brain segments by looking at the variability of the brain signal. Areas with too little flexibility are considered as suppressed[2,3] (= 'blocked') and impaired like a boys choir while their voices are breaking. The quantified EEG-patterns are merely the best the brain can do *under the given circumstances*.

---

[1] Braun CM et al "Mania, pseudomania, depression, and pseudodepression resulting from focal unilateral cortical lesions" Neuropsychiatry Neuropsychol Behav Neurol 1999;12(1):35-51
[2] Raffin CN et al "EEG suppression and anoxic depolarization: influences on cerebral oxygenation during ischemia" J Cereb Blood Flow 1991;11(3):407-15
[3] Poh MZ et al "Autonomic changes with seizures correlate with postictal EEG suppression" Neurology 2012;78(23):1868-76

The frequency suppression-map of Gil Winkelman's patient showed a decent number of 'blocked' brain segments. He started weekly LENS treatments, gradually 'unblocking' the impaired sites and thereby restoring her brain's function.

During the 6th session she stated that "her brain is functioning slightly better and she is able to remember things and think things through. She is able to multi-task and is finding it easier to do Jumble and Sudoku."

At the 7th session she reported: "Sleep, mood and headaches are much better. She had no headaches this week. She has more energy; memory and multi-tasking are much better. She is doing very well and didn't realize how bad things were. She still has some aphasia whereby she can't remember certain words."

In the 8th week of LENS treatment Gil wrote: "Mood is very good and energy is much better. She hiked for the first time in a long time. No migraine attacks but had a small headache she related to being tired."

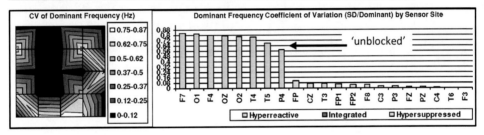

Another frequency-suppression-map showed that four more sites were unblocked, allowing for the better function as reported.

The news at the 9th session: "For the first time in at least 20 years she did not have a migraine attack at the start of her period."

After the 11th session she considered herself done: "Patient had a good week. Headaches were minimal as she had the start of one that went away. She has had the best multi-tasking ability and it continues to improve. Anxiety has decreased as well. She wishes to improve word finding ability although she says it was never good." Other than that "she feels great". She feels great? That sounds a lot like *embracing life* to me, which goes with the restraint at the left front of her 'bass' map (= Delta band). All that in just 11 sessions? How is that even possible?

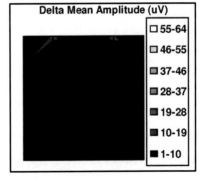

How the LENS works

Dr. Winkelman's client is an example of how even *thirty years of migraine history* with physical and mood issues *don't necessarily* constitute a 'difficult', hard-to-crack case. The woman seemed to be well informed, didn't accuse Gil of abuse or maltreatment when her irritability went up after the 3rd session and was capable of factually reporting her observations of her own level of function. Mind you, she did have her husband's full support; a factor that can make all the difference, especially when it's missing.

The case also demonstrates what the LENS can and can't do. It *restored* the brain's stability and function, possibly to the best it has ever been; but *not* beyond that point: The client's word-finding skill did *not* improve, because it had never been better.

That too is analogue to the chirotherapy for the spine which can't give you stronger back muscles than you've ever had; it only *restores* the movements of the segments to the state before the blockages. It is, however, astounding that in this case (and many others) the restoration of function by a gradual *release of EEG-suppression* was completely sufficient to solve this woman's issues with *migraine, mood, sleep and energy* within eleven treatment sessions. If she now wants to work on her word-finding weakness, she might see a therapist who does QEEG-guided neurofeedback for that.

The truly burning question is: How did the LENS do that? The answer has two parts. Part one is the kind of information that the LENS system feeds back: At any given moment, at any electrode location, one frequency has the greatest power (In our choir analogy that is the loudest note recorded by the microphone). This 'loudest' frequency is called *dominant frequency* (= the main pace).

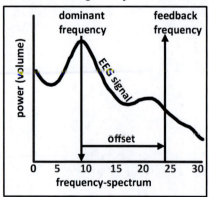

The LENS software receives the brain's *dominant frequency* and — based on that — calculates a *feedback frequency* by adding an offset of 2 to 20 Hertz. For example, when the dominant frequency of the brain is 9Hz and the pre-determined offset is 15Hz, the resulting feedback frequency will be 24Hz.

"Fascinating, but what is that good for?"

The Magic of a Whisper

Imagine you're walking in a park at your own favorite pace. Suddenly you hear a *marching band* play a loud and proud, catchy tune. Before you know it, you've abandoned your prior walking pace and march along to the rhythm of the music. This effect is particularly strong, when the band's pace is close to your own walking rhythm. Then it's nearly impossible *not* to *march along*.

When a bunch of neurons are stuck in a rut (=EEG suppression) and don't function all that well, because they've forgotten how to change pace, then you would want a *marching band* to tempt them to *march along*. That would help the stuck neurons to abandon their prior working pace (= dominant frequency). When the feedback's pace is *close* to the neuron's working rhythm (= low offset), then it's nearly impossible for them *not* to *march along*.

Dr. Len Ochs developed his system as a *marching band for stuck neurons,* originally with light goggles providing the feedback. Later he discovered that a much more effective feedback signal is running from the EEG amplifier *directly* to the brain.

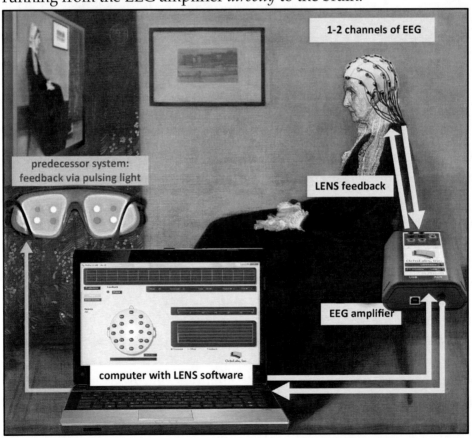

The LENS effect

Every electronic device emanates a tiny amount of electro-magnetic energy. Depending on the device it can be more (e.g. cell phones) or less (e.g. digital watches), but it's never completely absent. Most people don't notice this *low energy* ever, but there are some 'hypersensitive' individuals who react to it, when it gets too much for them. Even EEG-amplifiers emit a minute amount of that low electro-magnetic energy, since they're electronic devices too.

Dr. Ochs later discovered that the software program code, which operated the light goggles of the original system, unintentionally influenced the minuscule low energy emission from the EEG device; the LENS software *wiggles the low energy* emanation in the rhythm of the desired feedback.

The technical term for *wiggling the low energy* is pulse-width modulation (PWM) and it is caused by the timer-chip that puts out a square wave for switching the goggles on and off. Meanwhile the LENS system doesn't use pulsing lights anymore, since the *low energy wiggle* has been found to be the more effective way to tempt the neurons to get out of their rut and march along with the band.

The secret is that the feedback (= the marching band's pace) is derived from the current dominant frequency (= rut rhythm) and by selecting the offset, the therapist can regulate the strength of the unblocking effect, according to the client's resistance and resilience. That means that client and therapist need to cooperate well to adjust the offset as well as the number and duration of the feedback messages to the predicted reaction. This keeps the therapy process itself pleasant and gives the neurons the opportunity to get comfortable with their regained freedom and their restored function.

The 'kindalike'-analogy would be the chirotherapist who also can't treat all the spinal blockages of a lifetime in a single session. If he did try, your nervous system would probably end up pretty fired up or completely exhausted; either wired or tired, the typical signs that it was a bit too much change for one session.

Sometimes technically inept people mistake the LENS for either a *magnetic* stimulation like TMS or *electric* brain treatment like tDCS or CES (see page 368). Neither one is true; the LENS feedback is merely *a faint breath* riding on the low energy's very gentle hum. That the neurons *listen*, that's the *magic of the whisper*.

Less is more

The wiggle of the low energy is an absurdly weak signal of 0.000,000,000,001 Watts only, which completely flies in the face of the popular idea that *severe problems* require radical and invasive solutions. Although the analogy with chirotherapy is useful as an introduction, here it ends abruptly, since spinal manipulations aren't usually done with such an amusingly feather-light touch.

It is indeed astounding that the *shifted frequency information,* which the LENS returns to the brain, can have such a profound effect. Here is an example of a 2 year-old kid with ALPS, a blood disease treated with prednisone[1]. As a result the child had many developmental delays. The QEEG report shows how his brain normalized within only 9 (in words: nine) LENS sessions:[2]

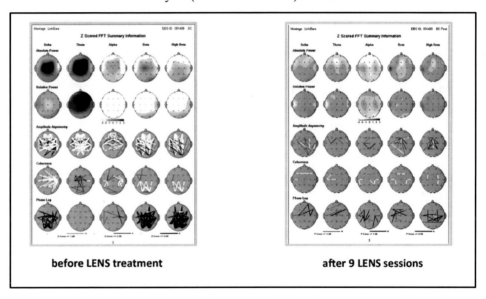

before LENS treatment   **after 9 LENS sessions**

Even laypeople without your QEEG knowledge can see that the brain-maps on the left contain a lot of 'bad' and the ones one the right look almost 'clean'. This is his father's original report:

> "Before the treatments David could not walk, crawl, feed himself, talk or think for himself. During the treatments David started crawling and talking. Then he started feeding himself, stacking blocks and coloring by himself. Shortly after he began walking by himself. David now has a vocabulary of 250 words, he can take 20 steps by himself. He is now a normal boy."

---

[1] Prednisone is a gluco-corticosteroid medication, an artificial version of the body's hormone cortisone/hydrocortisone
[2] The case example was submitted by Dr. Nicholas Dogris (PhD), Psychologist and Neurotherapist in Bishop, CA

Coming out

This outcome study[1] presents the real-life results of 100 unselected patients, treated with LENS at the Stone Mountain Center in New Paltz, NY. The 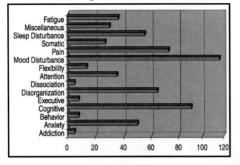 graph shows the variety of complaints that brought patients of all ages to the LENS treatment. Almost 25% were 51-60 years old, an age when symptoms tend to add up. Still, the LENS treatment managed to cut through:

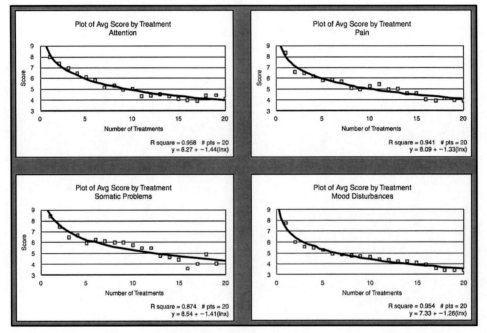

The statistical parameters and the analysis of the EEG data leave no doubt that the reduction of complaints was caused by the LENS treatment: The change in symptoms shows a very high correlation with the change in the EEG marker.

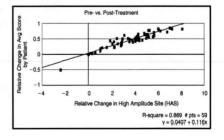

---

[1] Larsen S et al "The LENS (Low Energy Neurofeedback System): A Clinical Outcomes Study on One Hundred Patients at Stone Mountain Center, New York, Journal of Neurotherapy, 2006;10(2-3):69-78 / www.stonemountaincenter.com

The results of Dr. Larsen's outcome study are remarkable, also considering that those patients were treated between 2001 and 2005, based on the technology and methodology from around the *halfway* mark of the system's 20 year development phase. Today, therapists can resort to an abundance of sophisticated LENS tools, consisting of different carrier waves, duty cycle saturation-levels and other such incomprehensible technical variations that make this unique instrument even more efficient.

Of course, the US army has adopted the LENS to help soldiers, for example at the Brooke Army Medical Center in San Antonio, the largest of its kind in the US.

LENS for migraine

The last three migraine case examples stem from the well-known therapist Ann Marie Brown, located in Port Jervis, NY. She is an LMHC, NCC, BCN, FLC and SME, which means that she is a Licensed Mental Health Counselor, National Certified Counselor, Board-Certified Neurotherapist, Fabulous LENS Clinician and also a Splendid Migraine Eraser. Let's have a look at her first client:

- case #1: Charlotte, 53 years, migraine with aura for 12 years
- suspected origin: early life stress, lifelong family-dynamic issues
- onset: mother died 2 years prior, family issues
- physical comorbidities: allergies, sinus problems
- tried medical treatments, chirotherapy, acupuncture, neurologist, ENT-doc
- LENS: 12 x 1 session/week + 1 session/2 weeks + 1 session /month

before LENS treatment	after 14 LENS sessions
3 migraine attacks per week	occasional mild headaches
daily Topamax® (anti-seizure drug)	weaned off
daily Xanax® (anti-anxiety drug)	weaned off
when needed Zomig® (triptan)	not needed
comorbid anxiety	emotional control, articulates concerns
flat affect	energetic, animated, funny
problems handling stress	handles stress with ease
high level of hopelessness	"LENS has helped in more ways than just with the migraine attacks"
overall symptom-score: 191	overall symptom-score: 53

Once the attacks had ceased, Charlotte started to space out the sessions and now sees Ann Marie once per month (= maintenance).

Ann Marie's second migraine case is quite different

- case #2: Tina, 44 years, migraine with aura for 2 years
- suspected origin: hormonal imbalances
- LENS: 9 x 1 session/week + 4 sessions/2 weeks + 1 session /6 weeks

before LENS treatment	after 14 LENS sessions
5-7 severe attacks per month	none
OTC pain medication during attacks	none
overall symptom-score: 195	overall symptom-score: 22

Charlotte (case #1) appeared rather 'difficult' with high levels of hopelessness whereas Tina's story (case #2) almost reads like a car repair report, doesn't it? — The last client is different too:

- case #3: Robert, 27 years, migraine without aura for 1 year
- suspected origin and onset after: traumatic brain injury
- LENS: assessment + 8 treatment sessions + final assessment

before LENS treatment	after 9 LENS sessions
daily attacks upon awakening	none
head pain intensity: 10 out of 10	zero
medication: Excedrin® (with caffeine!)	none
problems with sleep and focus	both improved
overall symptom-score: 192	overall symptom-score: 16

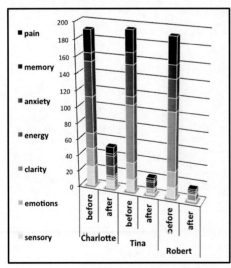

Robert's head injury was recent, he was high-functioning before; both factors made this case comparably fast. It demonstrates that the *severity* of the symptoms, usually the patient's biggest concern, doesn't make the treatment long or difficult.

LENS is *not a miracle cure* for every ailment and problem including tooth decay, low salary and global warming, but many migraine patients do well with it.

Like porcelain-maker J.F. Böttger, Dr. Ochs is also a great *alchemist*, because Len's system enables LENS therapists to turn a *mere whisper* into *a golden opportunity* to end the migraine tyranny. A list of adept LENS providers can be found at www.ochslabs.com.

Huge thank yous to my mates Ann Marie, Gil, Nick, Stephen and Len for their contributions!

Chapter 33

The Side Effects of Change

> "Any change, even a change for the better,
> is always accompanied by drawbacks and discomfort."
> Arnold Bennet

Risks and side effects

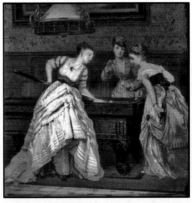

The expression "risks and side effects" is typically used in the context of medication, because drugs deliberately interfere with the body's usual, natural affairs. For example, nowadays lots of migraine patients who previously enjoyed the blessings of triptans get put on anti-seizure medication once they have frequent attacks. That is surprising for two reasons:

1.) Seizures (e.g. epilepsy) are a *contraindication* for the prescription of triptans.[1] That's not a problem, as long as migraine is SWELLING AND INFLAMMATION OF BLOOD VESSELS AROUND YOUR HEAD.

2.) If it were indeed true that MIGRAINE IS SWELLING AND INFLAMMATION OF BLOOD VESSELS AROUND YOUR HEAD, how then is *anti-seizure medication* supposed to deal with all that swelling and inflammation? This is neither logical nor plausible, but *profitable* and that's what counts.

Anti-seizure medication is supposed to tone down the jumpy neurons' agitated chatter by tinkering with their ion channels (see page 161). The desired result is a reduction of the seizure rate[2] and therefore you call that the main effect, if it works.

The downside of *toning down the neurons' chatter* is that other brain functions also get attenuated, for instance in the prefrontal cortex (= a very important brain area controlling the rest of the brain; the seat of the mind and the Self; responsible for thinking, planning, short-term memory, mood regulation, language, pain inhibition and much more; often 'wobbly' in migraine patients).

A side effect is merely the unwanted part of the main effect.

---

[1] http://www.accessdata.fda.gov/drugsatfda_docs/label/2012/020132s024s026lbl.pdf
[2] Bromfield EB "An Introduction to Epilepsy" American Epilepsy Society; West Hartford (CT); 2006

For anti-seizure drugs that means in plain language, they tend to make people stupid, forgetful and grumpy.[1,2] On the other hand, severe uncontrolled epilepsy is statistically more dangerous than the elevated suicide risk on anti-seizure meds.[3,4,5] Drug therapy is a constant trade-off between main effects and side effects. You could also say, that the side effects are the *price* that patients have to pay.

A real-world example from migraine land:

> A secretary, who was worried about losing her job due to her frequent migraine attacks, went on anti-seizure drugs. Predictably, her boss had to sack her, because on the meds she wasn't functioning very well, was forgetful and 'cognitively challenged'. In colloquial language: On migraine drugs she was simply too stupid for the job.

Two thirds of patients with epilepsy take anti-seizure medication and many say: "The side effects are worse than the seizures."[6]

The term *risk* usually refers to the probability of permanent damage, for instance the *risk* for suicide on anti-seizure drugs[7] as a result of the mood-depressing side effect. Or the *risk*[8] of life-threatening damage to the liver or the pancreas, or the *risk*[9] of birth defects caused by mom's anti-seizure medication during the pregnancy. Everything comes at a *price*.

Risks and side effects of behavioral therapies

Behavioral therapies are not drugs; for example they don't tinker with the ion channels of nerve cells. Therefore it is deceptive to talk about *side effects*, since this term is tainted by its association with medication. "Sounds like splitting hair to me." A funny quotation says "Life is a sexually transmitted disease and the mortality rate is 100%" expressing that you can use medical slang for everything. That's witty and not always a problem. Yet, when you're dealing with clients of unusual *sensitivity* and *reactivity* and low *resistance* then you do need to look at the nano-structure of every single hair.

---

[1] Hessen E et al "Influence of major antiepileptic drugs on attention, reaction time, and speed of information processing: results from a randomized, double-blind, placebo-controlled withdrawal study of seizure-free epilepsy patients receiving monotherapy" Epilepsia 2006;47(12):2038-45

[2] Mula M et al "Negative effects of antiepileptic drugs on mood in patients with epilepsy" Drug Saf 2007;30(7):555-67

[3] Kalinin VV "Suicidality and antiepileptic drugs: is there a link?" Drug Saf 2007;30(2):123-42

[4] Bell GS et al "Suicidality in people taking antiepileptic drugs: What is the evidence?" CNS Drugs 2009;23(4):281-92

[5] Bagary M "Epilepsy, antiepileptic drugs and suicidality" Curr Opin Neurol 2011;24(2):177-82

[6] Karceski SC "Seizure medications and their side effects" Neurology 2007;69(22):E27-9

[7] Hecimovic H et al "Depression but not seizure factors or quality of life predicts suicidality in epilepsy" Epilepsy Behav 2012;24(4):426-9

[8] Medline Plus "Valproic Acid" A service of the US National Library of Medicine, National Institutes of Health; June 2012

[9] Panigrahi I et al "Anti-epileptic drug therapy: an overview of foetal effects" J Indian Med Assoc 2011;109(2):108-10

We've seen that in drugs the main effect and the side effect are typically caused by the same mechanism, which makes it normal that they both occur together as long as the patient continues to take that medication.

Behavioral therapies can also lead to discomfort, adverse reactions and unwanted results, but these are 1.) usually temporary and abate soon and 2.) characteristic for the client's reactions to the *challenge of change*.

For example, when people start exercising after years of indolence, languor and atony,[1] they may develop sore muscles over the next days. That is unwanted and painful, but otherwise a completely normal and healthy repair mechanism to challenged muscle fibers; not quite comparable to alterations in the visual system due to anti-seizure medication.[2] You're with me?

After a productive psychotherapy session, a client may be sad about something that was emotionally hurtful in the past. That also is completely normal and a healthy process of emotional healing.

After a neurofeedback session, a client's brain can be a bit too agitated leading to irritability and restless sleep. Big deal. All that is unproblematic and nobody in his right mind would make a fuss about sore muscles, a couple of tears and a sleepless night, right?

Matching the challenge

When people's resistance and resilience is compromised, then things are slightly different. A standard first workout in a gym can easily cause excruciating pain in a patient with fibromyalgia (FM). That is a complex chronic pain condition where the processing of normal signals from the body leads to the activation of the brain's pain network, made possible by problems with the PFC.[3,4,5] Like migraine, FM (fibromyalgia) is connected to early life stress[6] and brain injury[7] leading to diminished resistance and resilience.[8]

---

[1] = fancy words for laziness, here in the sense of not enough physical activity, predominantly sedentary lifestyle, couchpotato
[2] López L et al "Assessment of colour vision in epileptic patients exposed to single-drug therapy" Eur Neurol 1999;41(4):201-5
[3] Williams DA et al "Biology and therapy of fibromyalgia. Functional magnetic resonance imaging findings in fibromyalgia" Arthritis Res Ther 2006;8(6):224
[4] Valle A et al "Efficacy of anodal transcranial direct current stimulation (tDCS) for the treatment of fibromyalgia: results of a randomized, sham-controlled longitudinal clinical trial" J Pain Manag 2009;2(3):353–361
[5] Narasimhan M et al "A tale of two comorbidities: Understanding the neurobiology of depression and pain" Indian J Psychiatry 2010;52(2):127–130
[6] Low LA et al "Early Life Adversity as a Risk Factor for Fibromyalgia in Later Life" Pain Res Treat 2012;2012:140832
[7] Napadow V et al "Intrinsic Brain Connectivity in Fibromyalgia is Associated with Chronic Pain Intensity" Arthritis Rheum 2010;62(8):2545–2555
[8] Schweinhardt P et al "Fibromyalgia as a Disorder Related to Distress and its Therapeutic Implications" Pain Res Treat 2012;2012:950602

If this wasn't a serious, scientific book, one could simply say: The fibromyalgia brain takes incoming body signals *too personally*, because the limbic system is constantly in a state of emotional hurt and the PFC is not mature enough or too weak to take the lead.[1]

Exercise therapy can be enormously beneficial for FM patients and if this wasn't a serious, scientific book, one could say: Exercise therapy that strengthens the body's resistance and resilience can help FM patients to *harden up* a little, improve mood and sleep.[2]

Yet, there is a difficulty that FM patients might have to deal with. As we've said, healthy couchpotatos get sore muscles after their first workout. FM brains declare normal muscles as "hurtful" already. Can you imagine the drama that an FM patient's brain creates from normal muscle soreness? Excruciating, debilitating, blinding pain can easily be the experience and nobody wants that.

Logically, the qualified exercise therapist wouldn't treat the FM patient like a regular couch-potato, but would reduce the intensity and the duration of the workout, would adjust the *challenge* adequately to *match* the FM patient's lower resistance. That normally does the trick to avoid unnecessary suffering, more medication and emotional aggravation in the spirit of the well-known exclamation: **"I'VE TRIED IT ONCE, BUT THE RESULT WAS HELL."**

The many and the few

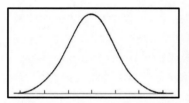

Few adults are dwarfs, most are roughly average size and above that you can find some very talented basketball players. When things come in variations, the majority is usually huddling around the average, whilst only small minorities are "very" either way. For example, if we understand *exercise capacity* in the context of resistance, then one minority—elite athletes—can do hours of hard training; a large group of fitness-conscious lawyers, bakers and candlestick-makers goes through all the machines at their gym or 90 min of Spinning; another large group of couchpotatoes struggles with 30 minutes in front of a Zumba-DVD and the small group of fibromyalgia patients is spent after 5-10 min of brisk walking.

---

[1] Pujol J et al "Mapping Brain Response to Pain in Fibromyalgia Patients Using Temporal Analysis of fMRI" PLoS ONE 2009;4(4):e5224
[2] Jones KD et al "A comprehensive review of 46 exercise treatment studies in fibromyalgia (1988–2005)" Health Qual Life Outcomes 2006;4:67

Understandably, after years of chronic pain and the avoidance of any strenuous activity, FM patients are usually extremely untrained, weak and frail. But that alone wouldn't be a problem.

Challenged balls

When you play billiards,[1] you want to make sure that cue, table and balls are of a standard quality and according to the usual specifications. Also, you would want that the table is level. If all the boxes are ticked, then 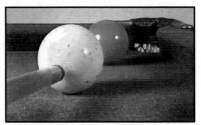 billiards is fun because it is truly up to you and your cue, to give the white ball exactly the right *impact* or *challenge* to push the red ball into the corner pocket. If there is no wind in the parlor and nothing else interferes, the balls will react in a very predictable way and precisely follow the laws of physics.

In that regard, people are very different from billiard balls. Even if they look according to the usual specifications, their *reactions to a challenge* are often not of a standard quality and barely follow the laws of physics. The majority of couchpotatoes will react in a predictable way to a first workout with sore muscles for a few days. In contrast, a minority of fibromyalgia patients can react quite unpredictably, even to the adjusted little wander as a first 'workout'.

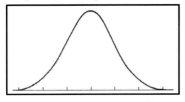 The reason is that inside the group of FM patients, we have another roughly normal distribution: The vast majority of FM-hikers can cope with the slight discomfort after the first cautious walk. A minority will react better than average and report that their pain has even improved after the stroll. Another small group, however, will show certain *adverse reactions* to the brief snappy march with increased pain and higher emotional arousal.

Of these, a few will follow their usual pattern and cry out loud: **"I'VE TRIED IT ONCE, BUT THE RESULT WAS HELL."** The reason is very simple: That's who they are, that's what they do. Their brain hasn't learnt to cope with a challenge without feeling attacked and without raising the pain alarm; and their mind hasn't learnt that either.

---

[1] Original picture by MichaelMaggs, adapted and converted to grayscale

Responses to reactions

Let's recapitulate: Even to the adjusted workout in form of a short brisk walk, which is adequate for most FM patients, a small minority will show an adverse reaction, because their brain is truly hyper-reactive to *any* form of challenge. It is likely that those brains react similarly to other challenges like moving house or an overseas trip. It is also likely that their mind will follow a certain, well established habit which matches their *maladaptive schema* ("life-trap") and their usual schema *compensation* pattern (see chapter 22):

If their dominant, maladaptive schema is "*vulnerability to harm and illness*", they might interpret their brain's exaggerated reaction as evidence that they will never be able to overcome *their special vulnerability*, because **"THE WORLD IS A HOSTILE PLACE FOR FIBROMYALGIA PATIENTS"** and they will probably—once again—withdraw from the challenge of an exercise therapy and avoid physical activity in their daily life as much as possible. That's understandable, but not helpful.

If their schema is "*abandonment*", they will probably be very disappointed that the exercise therapist too has let them down—like so many before—and they will try to find consolation from their doctor, the only reliable person in their life, who is 'compassionate' enough to prescribe more *short-acting opioid* medication (see chapter 3). This too is understandable, but not helpful.

If a hyper-reactive FM patient experiences her brain's exaggerated reaction to the brisk walk according to her maladaptive schemas "*abuse/mistrust*" and "*punitiveness*", then it might happen that she suddenly finds unexpected energy and stamina *to take revenge* by reporting the therapist—the **"ABUSIVE CHARLATAN"**—to a medical board or by writing something defamatory on the internet.

Patients who *play* this form of *game* usually present themselves as particularly *innocent* and *incompetent* to therapists, only to finally *switch* their *role* from "*helpless victim*" to "*merciless persecutor*". We've seen such a case in chapter 6: The hyper-reactive, seemingly 'innocent' Erica indulged in 15 unfamiliar substances, experienced nausea and concluded: **"I'VE TRIED IT ONCE, BUT THE RESULT WAS HELL."** Since **"IT ALSO DIDN'T DO MUCH"** for her migraine, she quit hormone balancing therapy after one week and retaliated by publishing a devastating book report on amazon, advising others to stay away. In short, she paid a high price for a moment of *power* and *revenge*.

All these understandable, yet unhelpful behaviors are made possible by imposing medical beliefs onto patients with functional disorders; by cloaking disorders as diseases (e.g. **"MIGRAINE DISEASE"**[1]) in order to "retain ownership" of the ailment;[2] by prescribing endless symptom treatments[3] although rehabilitation and therapy are required;[4] by hastily labeling *experiences* as "medical symptoms"[5] and by spreading disempowering misinformation to lure patients into dependence on drugs. Patients often willingly resign responsibility to the expert who promises relief and thereby lose their autonomy.[6] Good behavioral therapists inform their clients first up that their *role* is now changing from *passive consumer* to *active collaborator*.

Fibromyalgia, irritable bowel syndrome, migraine and a few more "medically unexplained" disorders, are comorbid to one another and to depression.[7] They are complex and complicated variations of essentially the same basic mechanisms. If this wasn't a serious, scientific book, one could say that they're all disorders of stress and trauma, of glitches in the prefrontal cortex, and of diminished resistance and resilience; aggravated and made truly 'difficult' by misleading medical myths that deprive the affected patients of the opportunity to develop active and constructive coping behaviors and to terminate those various terrors in their own body, mind and brain that medicine alone can neither explain nor 'cure'.

The recent developments in the *comprehensive rehabilitation* of FM are promising, so a FM revolution may not be necessary.[8,9]

Traditionally fibromyalgia is under the care of *rheumatologists* and used to be called "fibrositis" or "soft tissue rheumatism".[10,11] If this wasn't such a serious, scientific book, one could simply say that in the past fibromyalgia patients were also told that **"FIBROMYALGIA DISEASE IS SWELLING AND INFLAMMATION OF THE MUSCLES IN YOUR BODY"**.

---

[1] Young WB et al "Naming migraine and those who have it" Headache 2012;52(2):283-91
[2] Ghazan-Shahi S et al "Should rheumatologists retain ownership of fibromyalgia? A survey of Ontario rheumatologists" Clin Rheumatol 2012;31(8):1177-81
[3] [No authors listed] "Fibromyalgia: poorly understood; treatments are disappointing" Prescrire Int 2009;18(102):169-73
[4] Imamura M at al "Fibromyalgia: From treatment to rehabilitation" Eur J Pain 2009;3(2):117–122
[5] Page LA et al "Medically unexplained symptoms: Exacerbating factors in the doctor-patient encounter" J R Soc Med 2003;96:223–7
[6] Merckelbach H et al "Misinformation increases symptom reporting: a test–retest study" JRSM Short Rep 2011;2(10):75
[7] Cole JA et al "Migraine, fibromyalgia, and depression among people with IBS: a prevalence study BMC Gastroenterology 2006;6:26
[8] Casanueva-Fernández B et al "Efficacy of a multidisciplinary treatment program in patients with severe fibromyalgia" Rheumatol Int 2012;32(8):2497-502
[9] Kayiran S et al "Neurofeedback in fibromyalgia syndrome" Agri 2007;19(3):47-53
[10] Wein AB "Treatment of fibrositis and other inflammatory musculoskeletal disorders with local dexamethasone 21-phosphate injections" Med Ann Dist Columbia 1966;35(8):426-9
[11] Bennett RM "Fibrositis: Misnomer for a Common Rheumatic Disorder" West J Med 1981;134(5):405–413

Sensitivity and reactivity in migraine

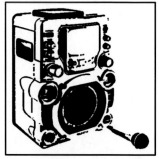

Imagine someone dear gave you a top-notch, first-rate, awe-inspiring karaoke machine as a birthday present. Not only does it have Auto-tune (a merciful software that tweaks your missed notes into the pitch of the right key), but it also offers numerous options to adjust the behavior of that box to your needs and circumstances.

For example, when young and shy children have a particularly tender voice with a low volume, you can adjust the *sensitivity* of the microphone accordingly, so that grandma in the back row can be still be moved to tears by the whispered performance of "Silent Night". You mustn't forget to dial the sensitivity of the microphone *down*, when you take the karaoke box to the pub for the annual end-of-season drinking bout of your sports team, where a few badly intoxicated mates want to bawl the club anthem. Since the pub is very noisy, you might have to dial up the *volume* control of the *amplifier* instead, to make sure that every patron dares to sing along as soon as they can't hear their own crooked voice anymore.

If the sensitivity of the microphone were still in the Christmas setting, the roaring voices of your mates would sound *distorted* due an effect called "overdrive". And whilst powerful rock guitars actually sound better with a bit of overdrive, your sloshed mates surely can't afford any further deterioration of their howled tune.

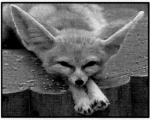

You could have guessed it; the fennec fox in this picture has ultra-sensitive hearing, which allows it to locate insects in the ground and dig in the right spot for a bite to eat. It probably wouldn't have much fun at your season-end festivity.

People can also be ultra-sensitive. For example, sommeliers are wine experts who can taste the subtle differences between separate batches of the same wine, because they've trained their taste-sense for wine by paying a lot of *attention* to even miniscule variations. In contrast, your team-buddies are meanwhile completely trashed und wouldn't even notice the difference between a cask red wine and a beer. I would say, they are rather *insensitive*.

EEG amplifiers also have to be *sensitive* enough to perceive the weak traces of the brain's electrical ramblings through the bony skull, not too dissimilar to the fennec fox, who can hear ants fart deep in the ground of the desert.

So, *sensitivity* is the ability to perceive very weak signals and subtle differences, like the sommelier (the professional wine taster). Similar to the meaning of *sensitivity* is the concept of *perceptiveness*, but you would use the expression "she is so perceptive" to describe someone who pays close attention to social cues and other people's subtle behaviors; whereas sensitivity refers to the sensory system and the reception of stimuli like sound, taste, touch and such.

People with migraine are said to be very *sensitive*. Is that true? Does that mean the *light*-sensitive ones can see in the dark like my cat? Can *sound*-sensitive migraineurs rival the fennec fox and hear insects in the ground? Do *taste*-sensitive migraine patients work as wine tasters? And does every radio station employ a *weather*-sensitive migraineur for the forecast after the news? I don't think so.

We already know that many migraine sufferers are known for alexithymia (see page 87). Allegedly they have a rather below-average *perceptiveness* for their own subtle cues, and so it can happen that alexithymic migraineurs forget to eat, because they don't feel hungry until a hunger headache sets in (see ch. 4 and 13).

We've also seen that only a small minority of so-called *weather-sensitive* migraineurs actually show a reliable over-reaction to certain weather-phenomena and we've explained that with *sensitization*, the escalation of the brain's electrical *reactions* (see p. 194).

Unfortunately and adding to the confusion, the mechanism of *sensitization* explains a cascade of escalating *reactions*. For example, light-sensitive epileptics might react with a fit from the flickering disco-light in a nightclub; but—like everybody else—they can't read the list of overpriced, adulterated cocktails at the dimly lit bar, because their vision is *not sensitive enough* for that.

And those smell-sensitive subjects whose migraine attacks were provoked with intense rose odor in one study? They showed an unusual *reaction* which we explained with the mechanism of *kindling* via *sensitized* pathways (p. 195). Yet, those subjects do not work in the perfume industry as covert cologne spies, decoding the secret recipe of the competition's costly concoction with their nose.

Not even those people with migraine who are allegedly very sensitive to scents and odors can crack the Chanel code, because their sense of smell is *not sensitive enough* for that; otherwise they could earn a fortune as undercover aroma agents.

It seems that the so-called 'well-known fact' that the majority of migraine patients are ultra-sensitive and therefore particularly 'vulnerable' to the harsh environment and to the world's hostility, turns out to be another myth. The occurrence of alexithymia proves that there is rather a tendency in migraineurs to be *insensitive*.

That doesn't mean that migraineurs can't taste the difference between red wine and beer, like your booze buddies, but it shows that it's *not sensitivity* that promotes occasional over-reactions.

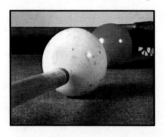

Billiards professionals have to be sensitive to the properties of the table at which they're playing for the championship and like every elite athlete, they have certain preferences in regards to altitude of the location, temperature, air humidity; factors that have a very subtle influence.

It is interesting that the cue's impact challenges the white ball; but it is the white ball's *reaction* that determines, how much it will impact on the *red* ball (here gray, of course). If you wanted to confuse your grandma, you could say: "Granny, look at this: The red ball reacts to the white ball's reaction."

Your gran might not understand what you're trying to say, because she is still in Christmas mood and so you would clarify: "Nana, it's not the push of the *cue* that challenges the red ball, but it's the impact of the *white* ball that makes the *red* ball roll. Did you get it?" And suddenly she would lift her head and with her eyes wide open she would say: "Yeah, now I get it. The red ball doesn't react to the challenge of the push at all. It *reacts* to the white ball's *reaction*." And you would fall into each others arms, hug for a while and then sing "The hills are alive" from the musical "The Sound of Music" and dance through her room in excitement until the cabin neighbors in the nursing home complain and a cranky nurse rips open the door and yells: "What is going on here?" Naïve as you are, you would try to share your excitement and say: "The balls *react* to their *own reaction*", but the nurse seems rather unimpressed by that.

The experience of reactions

In a minority of hyper-reactive patients, anything that has an *impact* or constitutes a *challenge* can lead to a reaction that is stronger than in average patients, even if the impact or 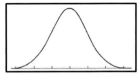 challenge is perfectly adjusted to the reduced capacity, resistance and resilience which is typical or 'normal' for that particular condition. The example that made that clear was the hyper-reactive fibromyalgia patient who over-reacts even to the briefest stroll. The reason is, that the *habituation* ("get used to it", p. 193) to body signals is faulty in FM brains[1] and the ensuing escalating brain reaction is strongly influenced by mood and emotions.[2]

Therefore fibromyalgia sufferers need to understand that their experiences are the *reaction* to their *own brain's over-reaction*. It's a bit as if the dial for volume on the karaoke box is still in the max position and even the kid's whispered voice gets distorted and brutally amplified to levels that cause ear pain and lets wine glasses shatter. And the last thing FM sufferers need is more emotional tension as a reaction to the myth **"THE WORLD IS A HOSTILE PLACE FOR FIBROMYALGIA PATIENTS."**

Instead FM patients need to be informed that not their muscles hurt but their brain creates an overdrive, a distorted reaction. That is perfectly normal in FM brains and no reason for additional aggravation. Rather, it's the reason why they can't dance for half an hour in front of a Zumba-DVD yet and why they need a bit more time until they can do 90 minutes of Spinning or all the machines at the gym. And sure, the experience of pain is quite an *uncomfortable reaction*, but it will pass, like every experience of a reaction passes, be it to moving house or to an overseas trip.

I imagine it can be quite a relief for patients to understand that neither **"THE WORLD IS A HOSTILE PLACE"** nor are they overly *sensitive* or particularly *vulnerable*. They certainly don't crave for additional drama. Their experience is a reaction to their brain's own reaction. So it would be smart to teach the mind to take a back seat and be a neutral and well-meaning observer of that brain's reactions.

---

[1] Montoya P et al "Reduced brain habituation to somatosensory stimulation in patients with fibromyalgia" Arthritis Rheum 2006;54(6):1995-2003
[2] Montoya P et al "Abnormal affective modulation of somatosensory brain processing among patients with fibromyalgia" Psychosom Med 2005;67(6):957-63

Adverse experiences in therapy

For a few patients the greatest challenge is the experience of their reactions to *change*; perhaps due to a general concern about life in the spirit of "You never know what's gonna happen." which assumes that the future will inevitably bring more suffering. That is plausible when the mind holds the idea that "MIGRAINE IS AN INCURABLE, PROGRESSIVE BRAIN DISEASE". Incurable, progressive brain diseases are the devastating *early-onset Alzheimer's* disease[1] or *glioblastoma*, an evil and aggressive brain tumor with an average survival expectancy of 15 months.[2] With such an idea in one's mind about *migraine*, being concerned is understandable, but *not helpful*. Instead, it might be a better idea to remind oneself that whatever it is that is going to happen—"Silent night" or club anthem, moving house or overseas trip, pleasant or less pleasant—it too will pass.

And so it can be a smart move to pay more attention to the present moment and savor experiences for what they are: reactions of one's own brain. Patients with high levels of anxiety sometimes feel *uncomfortable* with the *unfamiliar* experience of *lower* anxiety levels after a neurofeedback session. That is completely normal and clients quickly learn to *get used to it*. Isn't that interesting?

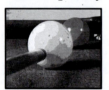

In a small minority of hyper-reactive migraine cases it can happen that a challenge leads to an *uncomfortable* experience. It's a bit as if the billiard balls look like standard quality with the usual specifications, but turn out to be *rubber* balls; the impact of the adjusted push can lead to an *distorted reaction* of the white ball, driving the red ball off the table. That's when the mind has to make a decision: A small minority will interpret their own reaction as proof that "THE WORLD IS A HOSTILE PLACE" and that "THE THERAPIST IS AN ABUSIVE CHARLATAN" so that they can whine: "I'VE TRIED IT ONCE, BUT THE RESULT WAS HELL". They are not suited for behavioral therapies. The vast majority will pick up the rubber ball and say: "Isn't that interesting? Let's try that again." If this wasn't a serious, scientific book one could say: *Change* can prompt the occasionally uncomfortable experience of one's own brain's *reaction* to change. Everything comes at a price.

---

[1] Natale B et al "Early onset Alzheimer's disease - diagnosis, therapy and management" Fortschr Neurol Psychiatr 2011;79(3):144-51
[2] Perry J "Novel Therapies in Glioblastoma" Neurol Res Int 2012;2012:428565

Chapter 34

Guide to Victory

"Your movement is carried internally by so strong a truth and necessity that victory in one form or another cannot elude you for long."

Hjalmar Schacht

Making sense

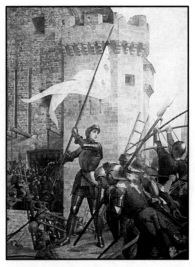

It has become common practice that authors of scientific articles merely summarize the findings of previous studies, present the facts of their own investigation and leave it to the readers *to make sense of it*. That way nobody can criticize their subjective analysis. Since this is not only a serious, scientific book, but also a patient guide, I'm going to offer my interpretation, experience and biased opinion, trusting that readers, who've digested what I've cooked up on more than 400 pages, won't mind burping with me. This is how I see it.

Knowing what we now know, it is completely *obvious* that neurofeedback-based therapies are the most striking weapon in our arsenal and why: Migraine is the product of a slight dysfunction of the brain,[1] resulting in a lack of stability and eventuating in episodic brainstem seizures.[2,3] The ensuing dilation of blood vessels is the logical consequence of neurons running wild, burning energy and demanding sustenance;[4] no mystery remains unsolved.

It is *logical* and *plausible* that neurofeedback therapy, which restores normal brain function, can terminate the migraine terror. We've seen enough credible evidence for that; nobody in his right mind can deny that neurotherapy can end the migraine tyranny.

---

[1] Maizels M et al "Beyond Neurovascular: Migraine as a Dysfunctional Neurolimbic Pain Network" 2012 Jul 3 [Epub ahead of print]
[2] Tajti J et al "Where does a migraine attack originate? In the brainstem" J Neural Transm 2012;119(5):557-68
[3] Rogawski MA "Migraine and Epilepsy—Shared Mechanisms within the Family of Episodic Disorders" in "Jasper's Basic Mechanisms of the Epilepsies" 4th edition, National Center for Biotechnology Information, 2012
[4] Baumgartner C et al "Preictal SPECT in temporal lobe epilepsy: regional cerebral blood flow is increased prior to electroencephalography-seizure onset" J Nucl Med 1998;39(6):978-82

Of course, the current regime will continue to present "migraines" as "primary headaches" and explain this GENETIC DISEASE with neurotransmitter imbalances, inflammation and other biochemical 'stuffs' that seemingly necessitate the continuous purchase of drugs and other medical treatments, and call it migraine "management". Just like in other areas of life, the financial interests of an industry defeat people's needs and rights. That's why we need a revolution.

The best migraine therapy

Many treatments and therapies lead to complete cessation *for some* and to a reduction of attack frequency for *some others*. Thanks to the huge placebo effect in migraine brains, lots of *utter nonsense* can also be helpful *for some*. Even the amputation of face muscles, Botox® injections, PFO closure or the implantation of occipital nerve stimulators *can* result in freedom from migraine *for some*. That doesn't justify endorsing *utter nonsense* as the therapy of choice; especially not, when there is a powerful, logical, plausible, successful and risk-free therapy available. That would be unethical and — more important — really stupid.

What makes neurofeedback-based methods different from the many other useful therapies is: They help not only *some*, but *very many*. That was predictable for the so-called *simple and easy* cases (of frequent severe migraine attacks!). It can also be expected for all the migraine cases due to traumatic brain injury, mood issues and PTSD, given that neurotherapy is traditionally strong with these. Surprisingly, even so-called hormone-related migraine seems to vanish just fine with straight neurofeedback training in many cases.

However, ...

Nevertheless, especially in so-called complex and 'difficult' cases it would be foolish to load excessive weight onto a single therapy's back and risk another "IT DIDN'T DO MUCH TO ME". I cannot warn vigorously enough to *not even think about* neurotherapy as the desired *magic bullet*, the long-awaited *savior* from the evil, the *miracle cure* that makes the blind men walk and the lame ones see.

The question is not "Magnesium or massage or medication or neurotherapy?" It is: "Which of the therapeutic options 1. *do I need to* and 2. *can I afford to* combine to guarantee the best possible outcome for myself *under the given circumstances*?"

Considering options

Let's have a look at this list of all the migraine therapies that we've discussed in this book.

Self-help and lifestyle
- establishing a regular aerobic exercise routine and sticking to it
- learning and practicing slow abdominal breathing, stopping overbreathing
- learning and practicing progressive muscle relaxation
- learning and practicing autogenic training
- establishing stable sleep habits; if indicated, blue-light blocking glasses
- reading about positive psychology
- limiting coffee intake to a minimum, no 'energy' drinks
- following a healthy diet (no fast food, no aspartame,[1] no MSG[2] etc.)
- drinking sufficient amounts of clean water[3] (> 2.5 liters = 85 oz. = 0.66 gal)

Biochemistry (helped by a naturopath, nutritionist, functional medicine expert, ...)
- magnesium—testing and supplementation, if indicated
- omega-3 fatty acids—testing and supplementation, if indicated
- vitamin D—testing and supplementation, if indicated
- zinc—testing and supplementation, if indicated
- coenzyme Q10—testing and supplementation, if indicated
- homocysteine—testing/supplementation: vit B6, B12, folic acid, if indicated
- B-vitamins—testing and supplementation, if indicated
- vitamin B2 (riboflavin)
- Petadolex® (butterbur)
- melatonin—testing and supplementation, if indicated
- IgG-testing and adequate food elimination, if indicated
- considering a gluten-free diet, if indicated
- hair mineral analysis for toxicity issues and mineral imbalances
- Organix (organic acids) analysis, if indicated
- essential amino acids—testing and supplementation, if indicated

Hormones (helped by a doctor who does BHRT)
- estrogen, progesterone, testosterone, SHBG, (pregnenolone, prolactin)
- ACTH, cortisol, DHEA-S, (aldosterone, vasopressin), albumin
- thyroid panel: TSH, FT3, FT4, (RT3, TBG)
- iron status: serum iron, ferritin
- IGF-1, IGF-BP, GHIH (somatostatin), if comorbid with fibromyalgia[4]

---

[1] Briffa J "Aspartame and its effects on health: independently funded studies have found potential for adverse effects" BMJ 2005;330(7486):309-10
[2] Yang WH et al "The monosodium glutamate symptom complex: assessment in a double-blind, placebo-controlled, randomized study" J Allergy Clin Immunol 1997;99(6P 1):757-62
[3] Spigt M et al "A randomized trial on the effects of regular water intake in patients with recurrent headaches" Fam Pract 2011;29(4):370-5
[4] Cuatrecasas G et al "High prevalence of growth hormone deficiency in severe fibromyalgia syndromes" J Clin Endocrinol Metab 2010;95(9):4331-7

Mind therapies (helped by a psychological coach, counselor, psychotherapist ...)
- cognitive-behavioral therapy (CBT)
- acceptance and commitment therapy (ACT)
- schema therapy
- (psychological coaching, solution-focused therapy, positive psychology ...)
- trauma therapy (e.g. EMDR, EFT, TFT, BSFF, hypnotherapy etc.)
- alpha-theta neurofeedback trance
- applied psychophysiology, psychophysiological stress profile (PSP)
- biofeedback-based therapy, e.g. HRV-, vasomotor or thermal biofeedback

Complementary treatments (helped by the respective professional)
- muscular trigger points: assessment and treatment, if indicated
- manual massage (consider lomi-lomi and similar enjoyable techniques)
- chirotherapy, if indicated
- oxytocin supplementation

neurotherapy / applied neuroscience (helped by a neurotherapist)
- infrared neurofeedback (PFC)
- QEEG-guided neurofeedback
- symptom-based neurofeedback
- infra-low frequency neurofeedback
- surface and LoRETA Z-score neurofeedback
- LENS—low energy neurofeedback system

Obviously, there is no shortage of tools from which to build an individual rehabilitation program that is adequate to the case; but what is the case?

Determining the needs

It could be a good idea to start with a factually *written* case description. There are plenty of case examples in chapters 28 to 32 that can serve as a model. Once you have a written summary of your migraine story and with the help of the table on page 208, you should be able to ascertain the levels of *complexity* and *difficulty*. Give yourself a *score* between 1 and 3 for complexity and another one for difficulty (1= low, 2= medium, 3= high).

To make things a bit more complicated, let's add a *third score* in the same manner, a score for the number of *failed attempts*. It's quite a difference if a client has already "tried everything" to little avail.

By multiplying the three scores, you get an overall tally between 1 and 27. For example: "1" in *complexity* times "2" in *difficulty* times "3" in *failed attempts* equals 6 out of 27. Not too bad.

Please note that this is not a standardized, calibrated, adjusted or rectified evaluation tool. I've made it up to help you think about your case from a bit of a distance in the spirit of: "If you were an independent migraine expert and rehabilitation-manager, how would you see this case?" Seeing it written on paper is crucial.

By now you should have a rough idea what the nature of your migraine problem is and an *overarching topic* might emerge, e.g. *trauma, vulnerability, stress/fight, injury, loss/failure, deprivation* ... Whatever the unmet needs are that you are starting to see, chances are that neither drugs nor surgery can give you what you need. What is it that you really need? What is it that you want?

Allocating resources

Resources are usually the factors that limit the achievable success. When it comes to health issues, many people rely solely on public supply (depending on the country): doctor, pharmacy, health insurance; a system perfected for the needs of the industry, not for the needs of the patients. Nevertheless, some people insist on being cared for *inside* that public system, at any cost. And so they celebrate a pyrrhic victory when their health insurance finally gives in and pays for Botox® treatments, only to find out that the soreness after the injections is *just as bad* as the chronic daily headache. As always, the winners are the drug company and the doctor.

Other people may have sufficient funds and access to brilliant therapists, but don't take the time to show up for regular appointments, because their ambitions occupy every minute that's left after the migraine took its fair share of days every month.

In short, there is an abundance of options for self-sabotage and failure. Most of these are based on *unhelpful beliefs* about oneself and the world, deeply ingrained into the subconscious mind and emerging as habits and rules. They can be exposed with the question "Why am I doing this?" as there is no *reasonable* answer, rather an *odd justification*, contradicting wishes, needs and goals:

Therapist: "You cancelled our appointment last week?" - Client: "Yeah, I had a migraine attack on the weekend and I needed the time for a project that my boss gave me." - "A project that you accepted, right?" - "It was important." - "More important than your project to free yourself from the migraine attacks, that steal most of your weekends?" - "I wouldn't say it like that." - "But you acted like that." - "Right. Why did I do that?"

Getting priorities right

Professionally and privately I am of the opinion that people have the right to make their choices as it pleases them; especially after they have been *truthfully informed* about the likely and unlikely consequences of their decisions. As a therapist I don't see it as my duty to persuade people to make those choices that I consider to be better or smarter.

I do, however, see it as my obligation to honestly inform them about what I believe I know and then everybody can make up their mind and do what they want, based on their values and priorities.

I have consulted with chronic pain patients for whom I would have been *the last hope*, but they had already spent their money on an expensive holiday-trip and couldn't afford my fees anymore. On the other side there is Lena, the 16 year-old apprentice cook with headaches every second day, who managed to pay for my services *despite* her measly apprenticeship wages without any other support.

It all comes down to priorities and if someone makes the conscious decision for a holiday-trip, a bigger plasma TV or a new car, I'm perfectly okay with that; but was it *a conscious decision*? Did they really sit down, weigh up the pros and cons and conclude "I'd rather spend my money on a holiday than investing it in a therapy for my chronic pain"?

Or is it rather an *immature behavior*? Like that of a child who spends the bus-money on ice cream, can't get home anymore and sobs until some grown-up have mercy and solves the brat's problem by paying for the ticket? Unfortunately, that doesn't always work for adults. The point here is the urgent advice is to take full *responsibility* for one's own destiny and not to rely on the idea that some grown-up will have mercy and solve our problem.

In this context, it's about the responsibility of *making choices*, of *setting priorities* and about doing what needs to be done in order to reach one's goals. People do have the right to decide to **LIVE WELL WITH MIGRAINE DISEASE AND HEADACHES**, if it pleases them. I'm not sure they have the right to spend their bus-money on ice cream and then exploit others' mercy; to burden others with the effects of their choices; or to lure others into making the same wrong decisions. Remember: Responsible is he who carries the consequences.

"What happened to Lena, the apprentice cook?" After 8 sessions of LENS and psychological coaching she was symptom-free and happy.

Concrete advice

Psychotherapists are usually trained to guide their clients into *figuring it out for themselves*, because the process makes the client grow and heal, whereas advice is disempowering and creates new dependence. In contrast, in my experience clients often make leaps and bounds in therapy, when I start them off with a piece of wisdom. If it was ~~crap~~ bad advice, they'll *figure it out* very quickly.

Therefore, I wouldn't have a problem to give my readers more concrete advice about to how to tackle their migraine problem. Alas, I don't know enough about you and your situation to be more specific than I was so far. Yet, I can share my thoughts about more concrete questions.

Fighting migraine without money

By reading this book thoroughly you've gained a valuable resource: knowledge. For some it may be possible to rid themselves of migraine attacks with changes to their lifestyle and some self-help activities. A client of mine, an elderly gentleman, saw me for daily headaches plus two migraine episodes per week. After the first session he took his homework assignment seriously, diligently practiced slow abdominal breathing and never had another migraine attack again. His remaining headaches were gone after 5 sessions with different biofeedback tools, for example one with EMG to teach him how to relax his jaw muscles. Since he took in everything without arguing, it was a *walk in the park* with a highly chronic patient. This case demonstrates how easy things *can be*, when trust is possible and the commitment is strong.

Slow abdominal breathing, regular aerobic exercises, autogenic training and the other steps in the first part of the list of options can go a surprisingly long way even if the symptoms are fierce. On the other hand, it takes a fair amount of time, energy and dedication to see this strategy through. If you're a career man or woman with family, you may struggle to divert sufficient time and energy to have a decent crack at it. For a student at the start of a migraine career, breathing, running and meditating may well do the trick. If not, it is a good foundation to stepwise introduce some cheap doping (see ch. 15). Though I wonder how many of my readers fall into the category of *freshmen of migraine*, ready to run.

Fighting migraine with money

Patients usually start reading books about their disorder, when the publicly advertised solution (medication) doesn't really cut it. Disappointed by their *own doctor* they decide to gather more knowledge and purchase a book, written by *another doctor* (So much for the plan to gain autonomy by reading a book!).

And so I can assume that many of my readers have already tried to heal their headaches multiple times with easy-to-follow diet tips and the logically appealing tactic of trigger avoidance.

Apart from the rare exception of the concerned mother of a migraine kid or teenager, most readers probably fall into the category of advanced and experienced sufferers, to put it mildly.

Let's cut to it. If migraine is a severe problem and it has been a part of someone's life for several years, any of the listed methods *can* still work, for example the right combination of magnesium, B-vitamins and acupuncture. However, chances are pretty high that after years and years of regular episodes, minor adjustments to the body's biochemistry and to the circulation of the chi may reduce the attack rate, but won't do the full trick anymore of putting a complete stop to migraine. In blunt words: Where is the change?

In order to see a *real change*, patients need to change their mind and their brain. For economical reasons, it is probably better to improve brain function first, before spending resources on mind therapies. In other cases it might be necessary to soften cognitive distortions first, before the patient can accept that it's easier to train a brain for more *stability* than to adjust the ghastly *weather* to their special *vulnerability* and to end the world's overall *hostility*.

Of course, I cannot recommend to make neurotherapy the central tool of a complete migraine rehabilitation program, because the *nutty skeptics* will take that as their cue and yell: "I KNEW IT, HE'S ONLY TRYING TO PROMOTE HIS OWN SNAKE-OIL, THE ALLEGED MIRACLE CURE; BUT MIGRAINE DISEASE CAN'T BE CURED, IT'S GENETIC!" A second reason is that I don't know where you are located and whether there is a neurotherapist in the area. That may sound odd to the citizens of New York, Sydney or London, but there may be a dearth of neurotherapists in Yukon, Wagga Wagga or Stratford-upon-Avon. A third reason is the knowledge that there are many migraine patients with so much *cumulative disadvantage* that they possibly can't afford it.

First choice: weapons for the brain

On the other hand, not everybody is a nutty skeptic, there are quite a few migraine patients in New York, Sydney and London and I know that "migraine management" with medication and other treatments doesn't always come for free either. So let's be audacious for a minute and pretend that your goal is clear and you're willing to do what needs to be done to end the migraine tyranny. Let's also assume that you haven't come to the conclusion that I want to steal your drugs (out of malice), that I want to trick you into a neuro-hoax (out of greed), that I'm trying to talk you out of Botox® (out of envy) or that I'm constantly bluffing you with unsubstantiated lies and impenetrable expert jargon (out of fun).

Let's say, that you were seriously concerned about your migraine, quite desperate and somewhat hopeless before you read this book. Now, after studying the subject under my guidance, you have a pretty clear view and want to start your own as well as the world's migraine revolution. Here are some pointers, in case you see neurotherapy as the most promising direction and want to make it the main building block of your program.

The presented neurofeedback methods work for the majority of migraineurs; the ones that don't work well are not in the book. Don't choose a method, find a therapist. In case there are several neurotherapists at your disposal, pick the one who is best suited for your case or the one you trust or the one who's read this book.

Finding a neurotherapist

- Internet search engines like Google, Yahoo, Bing and the like: "neurofeedback Gold Coast" or "neurofeedback Queensland" or "neurotherapy Gold Coast" or "neurotherapy Queensland". In case you neither reside in Gold Coast nor in Queensland, consider typing the name of your village, county, state instead.
- Links to neurotherapy providers world wide can be found on the rebels' marketplace at www.TheMigraineRevolution.com
- In case there is no neurotherapy provider near your dwelling, you might want to consider neurotherapy during a holiday in Tallahassee-FL, Roswell-GA, Woodland Hills-CA, Portland-OR, Pt. Jervis-NY, Manlius-NY, Dallas-TX, Rutland-VT or Gold Coast-Queensland: Locations with an expert from this book.

- Othmer-trained worldwide: www.eeginfo.com
- LENS clinicians worldwide: www.ochslabs.com

Success with neurotherapy

The reason that I'm suggesting to start the battle with neurotherapy is the overall high success rate and the fast results even in the (suspected) presence of estrogen dominance or other 'body'-blocks. In the vast majority of cases the first changes should be observable after the first 3 or 5 or 7 sessions, depending on the individual case. If nothing changes, additional steps can be initiated to find out, what stalls the expected progress.

One option is engaging in a bit of detective work with a few tests; be it a hair mineral analysis, a hormone panel, a QEEG or any other assessment that you and your therapist deem appropriate under the given circumstances.

A second option is to change the neurofeedback approach. Many neuro-clinicians have more than one tool anyway and would respond appropriately, when nothing changes. Though, not every neurofeedback clinician is a genius and there may come the time to move on. Important in such cases is not to throw the baby out with bathwater: "I TRIED NEUROTHERAPY, BUT IT DIDN'T DO MUCH TO ME." Even with brain therapies, disappointment is *possible*. That's one more reason to be very factual about the whole process and look at it as if it was a math task: Some are easy, some are difficult and some are incredibly complicated and complex. It is amazing enough that for migraine the solution is *often* fast and comparably easy although migraine is allegedly AN INCURABLE, GENETIC DISEASE. However, some cases turn out to be awfully complicated and complex and for their resolution client and therapist need to be very smart and rational.

So instead of venting despair it would be more helpful to state "After 5 sessions of _____-neurofeedback, my therapist suggested a hair mineral analysis and a hormone panel" or "... changed to the _____-approach" or whatever is sensible and goal-oriented in a particular case. Nobody has ever won a battle by complaining how nasty the other army is.

Frankly, I am quite concerned that some utterly 'difficult' migraine patients will once again discourage ill-informed others with undifferentiated failure reports: "I TRIED THAT NEURO-STUFF AND THE RESULT WAS HELL." That "neuro-stuff" may have been Neurontin®, a drug.

Now you might believe that I'm exaggerating, but think about it. For example, how would an average patient know, whether the neurologist collects data for an analog, clinical EEG or for a QEEG. They get a cap on and are told to sit still. How easy is it then to whine: **"YEAH, THEY MESSED UP MY HAIRDO WITH THAT CAP-THINGO. DIDN'T DO MUCH TO ME."** *You* know that a QEEG is different to a clinical EEG, but others haven't got a clue. So let's not get cocky, but rather tell them.

Sure, many 'accomplished' migraineurs are deeply frustrated, emotionally mutilated, spectacularly misinformed and highly suspicious when they come across a book-title that says "We can end the tyranny". Of course they cringe when I tell them that I've specialized in migraine, because I'm too lazy to deal with the difficult conditions that many neurotherapists face every day. Fact is, that with all those exquisite neurotherapy tools most migraine cases are not that hard to crack, irrespective of the severity of the symptoms.

What's hard to crack is the nasty mind-concrete, the paralyzing compound of negativity, confirmation-bias, victim-attitude, expressive hopelessness, emotion-focused coping and dismissive-avoidant attitudes, hardened by the impertinent misinformation by the current regime (Have I talked about that already?).

Again, neurofeedback therapy is not a drug that you try once or twice and then throw in the bin, if it doesn't work as wished for. Do you remember Irene, the volleyball-player (ch. 9)? It may well happen during her rehabilitation process that one day she tries one-legged jumps off a step, but it turns out that her balance isn't good enough for that yet. Then Irene would improve her balance first and then come back to the jumps later, right? She may have been disappointed after the unsuccessful jump-attempt, but she wouldn't be peeved and blame the exercise or even the step.

In case something like that happens in neuro-rehabilitation, you may have to improve your hormonal or mineral balance first and then come back to the neurofeedback training later. You may have been disappointed, but being peeved and blaming the neuro-therapy wouldn't get you anywhere, true?

If you manage to escape the *psycho terror in migraine land* and you *know your tyrant* and you keep *dealing with difficulties* and you stay *on top of the barricades* and you *think about strategy*, then victory in one form or another cannot elude you for long.

First choice: weapons for the body

Another path to victory is addressing the body issues first. That makes sense, for instance when a grave biochemical glitch is suspected which might interfere with brain-therapies anyway. That may be a hormonal or mineral imbalance, a problem with the zinc[1] or iron metabolism[2] (especially in 'menstrual' migraine), a hiccup in the production of some neuro-chemical[3] or an undetected toxin (e.g. lead or copper). So, instead of wasting time, energy and money on untargeted attempts to find a miraculous drug, it can be a good idea to throw out a wide net and fish for gross irregularities in the body's biochemistry. If something is far off normal, then it is dubious and worth correcting, even if authoritative experts assert: "... has no part in the causation of migraine." Well, prove that to me!

Fact is, that even bright people can't know everything and so it's smart to keep an open mind to the possibility that sometimes the unlikely is true. If you ask medical experts, whether copper poisoning can be a cause of migraine, they'll probably laugh at your stupid question, you moron! And yet, we've already seen a case ("copper-boy", p 262) where that was true. So who is the real moron?

The *logically* correct answer to your question would have been: "Based on our current knowledge, copper poisoning is *not generally* the cause of migraine attacks. It is however conceivable in individual cases." Any other answer is just logically wrong and stupid. Can you see that?

The downside of fiddling with the body's biochemistry is that it can turn out to be an endless, expensive and effectless endeavor, especially if the responsible clinician is more of a supplement dealer than a bio-detective. While I wouldn't hesitate to follow Dr. Gil Winkelman's and Dr. Sharrie Hanley's advice to the letter, my B.S.-meter rings the alarm bells, when practitioners "prescribe" products that they conveniently sell themselves at inflated prices.

It would be a tragic fallacy to apply the medical disease model to this field of body-therapies: This isn't about finding the tonic that kills the migraine bug. Rather it's about nourishing, nurturing, supporting and promoting balance. *Care* is the opposite of tyranny.

---

[1] Baker NC et al "Mining connections between chemicals, proteins, and diseases extracted from Medline annotations" J Biomed Inform 2010;43(4):510-9

[2] Vuković-Cvetković V et al "Is iron deficiency anemia related to menstrual migraine? Post hoc analysis of an observational study evaluating clinical characteristics of patients with menstrual migraine" Acta Clin Croat 2010;49(4):389-94

[3] D'Andrea G et al "Pathogenesis of Migraine-Role of Neuromodulators" Headache 2012;52(7):1155-1163

First choice: weapons for the mind

The average Joe's knowledge about psychology makes the *mind* field a *mine*field. What can one say, when those sufferers with the heaviest emotional load angrily insist that =="MIGRAINE IS NEUROLOGICAL, NOT PSYCHOLOGICAL"==? How do you explain to those patients that mind therapies are *not for crazy people* who've *lost* their mind? Would it help to point out that *the smarter* you are the more you will benefit from any mind method? Dumb ones just can't dig it.

Let's say that the esteemed readers of this book have understood that psychological coaching is instead about helping a person to sense their feelings, to honor their emotions, to come to logical conclusions and to make smart decisions that lead to successful actions. The world is so complicated and complex that there is no reason to assume that *anybody* is *so* well equipped by their upbringing that they can't benefit from mind support at all.

If you ask me, it should be the most *normal* step for *every* sufferer of any kind to seek mind-care, as it should be for anybody who is *not* suffering at all; a sign for *presence* of mind, not absence.

The first group of migraine patients who will want to make mind therapies the center piece of their rehabilitation are the ones who wish to do so; the ones who long for affective support, because they are emotionally depleted after years and years as lab-rats, testing pills, potions and concoctions, tortured with syringes and finally threatened with scalpels and implants.

The second group are the ones who notice that they're sabotaging themselves, because parts of their subconscious mind aren't willing to let go of the role as suffering victim. There is even a test for that. First, close your eyes (not yet!) and imagine that you are an eagle, flying over the mountains, through steep valleys, across an open plain, along a river, over a dense green forest to a quiet lake. Feel the fresh air streaming through the feathers of your wings, smell the flowers on the meadow by the lake and hear the insects and the jumping trout. Did you enjoy your voyage?

Second, close your eyes once more (not yet!) and imagine yourself in your future as an ex-migraineur, how your head feels light and clear; see yourself as a relaxed and happy person, visiting a busy Chinese restaurant, drinking red wine, enjoying the waitresses strong perfume, asking her to turn up the traditional music.

Imagine yourself doing things that would have given you headaches in the past when you were still a migraine patient; things that you can do now, since you've terminated the terror.

If you can imagine flying like an eagle, but you *cannot imagine* being an ex-migraineur, then you know that parts of your mind are willing to pay a very high price for something they get from your plight. That may be attention, that may be revenge or that may be the idea that suffering is what you deserve. Unless your conscious mind agrees with that, these parts can be identified and heal.

A third group of migraine patients who might consider making mind therapies their first choice are those whose *defense mechanisms* against emotional pain interfere with successful rehabilitation. One example is the grumpy rejecter whose dismissive-avoidant attitudes give him *a feeling of safety* by anticipating failure and refusing to entertain any thought of success and joy. This strategy is a form of emotional suicide to pre-empt further pain to an already badly hurt and injured soul.

A variation of the grumpy rejecter is the arrogant demander, a narcissistic facade enveloping itself in a protective shield, created from disdain, dismay and dissatisfaction; enjoys himself in the role of the hard-to-please customer and expects to be treated like a king in exchange for the privilege of his presence; formulates questions and criticism without substance by referencing to his assumed position as the ultimate judge: **"... DIDN'T MEET MY EXPECTATIONS."** If you are into friendly human exchanges in the spirit of "I'm okay, you're okay"[1], then the arrogant demander will exploit your wish for basic respect and approval by tempting you to attempt to please him. He is best dealt with by an even more arrogant and authoritative professor of medicine (if there was such a person).

The arrogant demander is typically male. The female counterpart is the noble lady who flags how special and entitled she is with small, subtle gestures. As a therapy client she would ring several times, first to ask about the appointment that she had made and forgotten, then to move it short-notice (preferably to a time outside regular hours) and then to re book. Finally she would show up late or not at all, but refuse to pay for her booking.

---

[1] "I'm okay, you're okay" = title of a popular book about transactional analysis, a breakdown of human interactions

For her, treatments and therapies are opportunities to inform others how special she is. That's probably the over-compensation of an unworthiness schema and a serious obstacle to change.

A last example in this group is the control-freak, an often quite well-informed, intelligent and educated person who tries to limit his high anxiety levels by running an infinite skeptical investigation against the world around him, based on the paranoid assumption that he is under constant threat. Since every piece of gathered information naturally raises more questions than it answers, the control-freak *increases* his own anxiety with his behavior and spirals *out of control* instead. In contrast to the arrogant demander or the noble lady, the control-freak is easy to handle, because of his high intelligence and sense of humor.

It is important to understand that all these behaviors intend to serve a purpose, but fail to lead to an overall healthy emotional equilibrium including satisfying and enriching social contacts.

The fourth group of migraine patients, who could possibly benefit from mind therapies as their first choice, are all those whose personal development left them extremely susceptible to the current regime's propaganda and whose heavy emotional load makes a clear separation between thoughts and emotions an impossible task. Their cognitively distorted view of migraine as an **INCURABLE GENETIC DISEASE** is not just the result of misinformation, but also a form of protest against the unendurable injustice that they have experienced in their role as victims. Their angry assertions can be understood as an accusation against life itself for leaving them immature and defenseless in a world that constantly bullies them (**"THE WORLD IS A HOSTILE PLACE FOR MIGRAINEURS"**). As is often the case, the bullied ones become bullies themselves; the ones who were abused in their past, become abusers themselves; the ones who suffered under someone's ruthless rules, turn into ruthless rulers themselves.

In the internet-era migraine bullies can reach huge audiences and so abuse and manipulate massive numbers of other vulnerable victims, especially when supported by the current regime. And so they seem to be commanding an army of *migraine zombies*. For example, one author of a migraine book wrote: **"IF A BOOK PROMISES A 'CURE' FOR MIGRAINE DISEASE OR SAYS MIGRAINE IS PSYCHOLOGICAL IN ORIGIN, MAKE A NOTE OF THE AUTHOR AND DON'T WASTE YOUR TIME READING ANYTHING BY THAT PERSON."**

Why would anybody give out such an order? As a severely affected migraine patient herself, why would she not write: "I truly hope that other migraine sufferers don't have to live through the same torturous horror-trip that my migraine journey was (and still is). I pray that one day a book gets published that leads migraine patients away from the path that I took; a book that can change things for the better; a book that starts a migraine revolution." Why not?

First choice: body mind & brain

In some cases it might be necessary to combine every tool available to have any positive impact at all. I'm thinking of those with a wicked combination of *multiple functional disorders*, like fibromyalgia, severe irritable bowel syndrome *and* chronic migraine. In an ideal world, we would have rehabilitation centers where several professionals cooperate in a collegial manner to turn such complicated and complex cases around, against all odds. We also wouldn't have global warming, TV-ads or tooth decay.

Another group of migraine patients who might want to tackle the tyrant on all three levels simultaneously are the ones who've decided that this battle has a *very high priority* in their life and so they are willing to mobilize the necessary resources for such a comprehensive approach. Time can be of the essence for some and so they'd rather pay for a few more tests (which are comparatively cheap anyway), speed up the process and increase their chance of rapid success to the highest level possible.

In such cases I'd suggest to find a *neurotherapist* who also acts as a *biochemical consultant* (e.g. a naturopathic doctor, nutritionist, functional medicine practitioner) and who can initiate a hair mineral analysis, the recommended blood tests as well as additional assays to detect or rule out relevant deficiencies or irregularities. If that person is also trained as a *psychological coach* (e.g. counselor, psychologist, psychotherapist), all three bases are covered. Richard Soutar and Gil Winkelmann are two more examples of therapists who can address body, mind *and* brain.

The alternative is to consult with two, three or more therapists at the same time and ask them to cooperate. That is not always easy, but not impossible either. The message should be that they are *not* competing in "Which of you can cure my migraine?" but to consider the conquest of the migraine as a *team* effort.

In case you end up heading a multi-professional team, you cannot ascribe results and reactions to one team-member only. "The program appears to be working" should be the sentence of choice. While it may be entertaining to play the clinicians off against each other, it's not helpful to tell the naturopath that your progress is the sole result of the chiropractor's hands. That's not the right *team spirit*.

Team spirit is also the reason why I haven't included a doctor of medicine in the lineup. Although it would be desirable to also have access to a doctor's expertise and resources, in reality I would consider it already a success, if the family doctor didn't interfere. On average, doctors are *not* known as great team players. With that being said, a rising number of MDs are becoming neurotherapists, some of them are at the top of the field, for example Lucas Koberda, the neurologist who contributed two case examples to this book. Others engage in integrative medicine, naturopathy, bio-identical hormone replacement or other 'dissident' methods and cop the flak from the pharma-regime. So, it is possible and preferable to find a collaborative doc, but not absolutely crucial in the majority of cases.

Guiding principles

Different people have different beliefs. Throughout this book I've used *unhelpful* beliefs as a springboard to present more helpful ones. For example, "MIGRAINE IS GENETIC" is a statement that leads to the belief "I am helpless against migraine". Being helpless is not really helpful.

In contrast, knowing that migraine requires a genetic talent is *helpful*, because it leaves the option open to develop this talent in the direction of *not* having migraine attacks. Therefore, the first guiding principle that arises is the question: "How is this helpful?"

For example, on internet migraine forums you can find posts like: "My doctor recommended yubyub-therapy for migraine. Did anybody have any success with it?" How is this helpful? What does the poster expect?

Since it's a *migraine* forum, chances are high that someone replies "I TRIED IT ONCE AND THE RESULT WAS HELL" or "IT DIDN'T DO MUCH TO ME", either answer is discouraging. How is this helpful? Sure, theoretically it could happen that someone answers: "Ten years ago yubyub-therapy put an end to my migraine, I never had another attack. Since then I'm a member of this migraine forum waiting for people like you to ask this question." or "... end to my migraine, but I dropped it, because I want to be with my mates on this migraine forum."

Unsurprisingly, the members of migraine forums are people *with* migraine. What can they possibly say about yubyub-therapy? Such a question would make sense on the *yubyub-forum*, where yubyub-therapists discuss their cases; or on the forum for *yubyub-patients*; or on the *forum for ex-migraineurs*, if there were one.

The phrase **"MIGRAINE IS GENETIC"** leads to a second principle: "What exactly does this mean?" When migraine is a serious issue, three-word throwaway phrases are not helpful. If people can't be bothered to be sufficiently precise, it's best not to listen. Another example for that is: **"I tried biofeedback, but it hasn't helped my migraines."** Biofeedback is not a method. We have no idea what that person tried. Also, **"migraines"** makes me assume that this person calls the attack "a migraine" and may have tried to use a biofeedback method like an abortive drug for that. That's not too smart.

The third guiding principle is logic and reason expressed in the question: "Does this make sense?" For example, the amputation of face muscles *doesn't make sense*, because the story of nerve-pinching muscles doesn't explain the symptoms of migraine. We can easily apply this principle to the suggested yubyub-therapy and ask "What's the underlying idea? How does it make sense? Is it logical and reasonable?"

- How is this helpful? = orientation towards the goal
- What exactly does this mean? = sufficient precision
- Does this make sense? = logic and reason

May these three principles guide you through the maze of misinformation, confusion, disempowering feelings and passive attitudes. I've tried my very best to give you heaps of useful information, clarification, encouraging thoughts and occasional humor. Now it is up to you to overcome your fear and start the revolution.

I don't know whether anybody believes that God is a shareholder of a drug-company, he burdened mankind with the **INCURABLE GENETIC MIGRAINE DISEASE** to boost his holy profit and is now muttering:

"They're exaggerating. It's just a headache. They'll have to live with it."

I think, if he knew what's going on in migraine land, God would say:

"Stand not idle by whilst your brethren get slowly slaughtered by the diabolic migraine tyrant and hith current nasty regime. Go forth and start thy migraine revolution! Thou can end the tyranny."

Section Four:

Join the Migraine Revolution!

> "All that is necessary for the triumph of evil is that good men do nothing."
> Edmund Burke

> "The revolution is not an apple that falls when it is ripe. You have to make it fall."
> Che Guevara

Today is the day ...

Let's assume you've read the book, understood everything (or at least the gist of it) and you have a hunch that migraine is not "... AN INCURABLE GENETIC BRAIN DISEASE THAT CAN ONLY BE ALLEVIATED BY MEDICATION ". Let's also assume that you believe that *everybody* has the right to live without migraine. You may even be so audacious to conclude: "Freedom-loving migraineurs should support one another during their personal migraine revolution" and "Every migraine sufferer should know about this."

Let's also accept the realities of the world: This book will not be put on the list of required reading for students of medicine. It is also unlikely that pharmaceutical companies will provide a free copy of this book with every purchase of abortive migraine drugs; and I'd be rather surprised if the maker of Botox® decided to invite migraine-freedom-loving rebels on a 5-star cruise to Bora Bora.

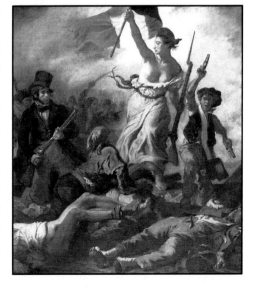

Given that the current regime will certainly not accept *responsibility* to let all migraine sufferers know about this, who do you think should step up to the plate? Who could possibly rise to this challenge? Who will pull out all the stops, lift their game and serve the migraine community? Who will pick up hayfork, scythe or spanner and fight the migraine revolution?

If you have the *vision* to beat migraine and you have the gumption to make that your *mission*, then you might also want to consider to make it a *team effort* to defeat the current regime and to give others the opportunity to find their way out of the misery, to terminate their terror and to end their migraine tyranny too.

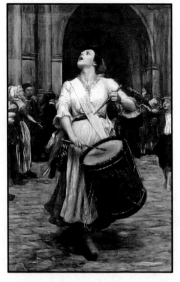

Drumming up strong support for the global rebellion at the same time increases the needed resources for every sufferer's own liberation. And the larger the overall movement becomes, the more tortured souls can be saved.

Today is the day for the people with migraine to raise their shy voices and to unleash their wrath. Let the whole world know that we're ready to fight. Call the suffering masses! Do your part to invite every desperate patient to topple the tyrant and to spread our proud battle cry: Join the migraine revolution!

"What can I do?"

I was about to ask you that same question: What can you do? Let's say you're the secretary-general of the United Nations. Then you could address all the world's lands in the general assembly, call a meeting of the security council and force every country to incorporate The Migraine Revolution into their constitution or face sanctions, embargos and war. That would be an okay first step.

If you're not the UN secretary-general then you need to have a think, how you could create a similar impact with *your resources*. Of course, having complete control over newspapers, radio and TV stations in your country could come in handy here. Let's say you own one measly international network only, then you could replace the hourly news (which are full of crime and disaster anyway) with an encouraging program for migraine sufferers under the title and in the spirit of "The Migraine Revolution". Once that is established you would want to lift your game and persuade all your mates in the playground for network owners to do something similar: daily revolution soap opera or dumping sportscasts for migraine lectures.

Joking aside, that could actually be a strategy: first, use your talents, skills and connections to further the cause, to spread the message and to reach as many migraineurs as possible; and then lift your game and convince your mates, colleagues and peers to do the same. What do you reckon?

In the disappointing case that you're neither the UN secretary-general nor the owner of a single international TV network, you'll find some other way to eventually ask all the 700 million migraine sufferers in the world to join our migraine revolution. Let's start small and with passion, and conquer the world step by step. Okay?

Contributions with love

Let's say you are a bit of an *activist*-type and you love getting involved in your community, your church, your council, your school, your neighborhood or stuff like that. Well, you could become a *Migraine Revolution activist* in your community, church, school or stuff like that and *spread the word by doing what you love doing* anyway. And then you lift your game and motivate other "activists" to join our effort to *free migraineurs* (like Willy).

Let's say you're a *mom of a migraine kid* and reading this book has given you a deep understanding of migraine, then you probably think that *every mom with a migraine kid* should read this book and gain a deep understanding too. I'm confident you'll come up with an idea to reach many, if not *all other migraine moms*. And then you lift your game, because you think that *every teacher* in this country should have a deep understanding for migraine, since they play an important role in a kid's life and around 4% of the brats already have migraine attacks and many more are migraineurs in the making. You've got the moms and the teachers covered?

Let's say you're a bit of a *journalist*-type and you have a blog on the internet. Can you think of a way to reach many, many people and to win them for the *uprising of the sufferers*? I bet you can and you'll also have an idea how to take it one step further. Perhaps win other journalists and bloggers for the good cause?

This might be the opportunity you've been waiting for to *start a video blog* and keep others informed and inspired with your own progress and with the *progress of the world campaign* against the oppression and unendurable injustice of migraine.

And once you've become a *Migraine Revolution video blogger*, you teach others how to videoblog and invite them to join our ranks. Doesn't this sound exciting?

Let's say you are a bit of a *critic*-type and you love to examine things and inform others what's good and what's less good: Well, you could use your critical talent for something great and constructive by scrutinizing the current regime's loyal sources of migraine misinformation and publish your findings.

Let's say you are a fervent *networker*-type and you're good at connecting to people, at linking, relating, involving and uniting. I'm sure you've got all your systems in place to *let our revolution go viral*. Start a Mexican Wave on your networking site to help wash away the chaos of myths that has migraineurs in a headlock. And then lift your game, join forces with others and expand to all other networks and media and reach out to all those who need help.

Let's say you're more of an *observer*-type who likes to watch the world and think about it. Well, this could be an opportunity to get a tiny bit involved and to connect to other observers and think about ways to support the rebellion. For instance by watching the video blogs of liberation and by reading rebellious reports; and by leaving your mark in the form of good comments; to show your appreciation of their efforts and thereby give moral support.

Let's say you typically don't do anything and you can't be moved to change that now. Well, perhaps you could consider to do what everybody can do without putting much effort in:

- visit the website of TheMigraineRevolution.com ○
- subscribe to the YouTube-channel of the Migraine Revolution and give the videos thumbs up by clicking the "Like"-button ○
- visit The Migraine Revolution page on Facebook and "Like" it ○
- join the Yahoo forum for The Migraine Revolution for access to news, updates and relevant, constructive exchanges ○
- write an encouraging book review on Amazon.com ○

We need to be realistic: Some people will scorn The Migraine Revolution ("IT DIDN'T DO MUCH TO ME") and drop discouraging remarks as "*book reviews*" *on amazon.com*. That's exactly what Erica did (ch. 6 + 33). So it would be helpful to stack up many *inspiring* reviews that endorse our Migraine Revolution at its roots: this book.

Gathering in the marketplace

The Latin word for marketplace is forum. Migraine rebels who want to make their own ascent to liberty a team effort and to combine their resources need a meeting point. The marketplace for The Migraine Revolution is the Yahoo group/listserve/forum with the same name. As a reader of this book you not only qualify, but you are urgently invited to join us.

The Migraine Revolution forum is intended for everybody who supports migraineurs' efforts to transform into ex-migraineurs in the spirit of this book. You don't have to *be* a migraineur to be a member and you don't have to *stay* a migraineur either.

The prerequisites for participating in our rebellious forum are:

- reading or having read the book The Migraine Revolution
- willingness to support the struggle for freedom from migraine
- refraining from behaviors that discourage others
- focussing on constructive and helpful exchanges
- kindness, respect and compassion for oneself and others

There are several migraine discussion forums on the internet. The ones I know are dominated by the current regime and by a disempowering, discouraging, disenfranchising and drug-dependent doctrine of migraine as an "INCURABLE GENETIC NEUROLOGICAL DISEASE OF SWOLLEN INFLAMED BLOOD VESSELS THAT CAN ONLY BE ALLEVIATED BY MEDICATION " and "THE WORLD IS A HOSTILE PLACE FOR MIGRAINEURS". This reconfirms the already difficult, subjective experience of feeling helpless and hopeless, strengthens victim-attitudes and maladaptive schemas and reinforces passive-avoidant coping and understandable, yet unhelpful emotional behaviors that lead patients towards chronification.

The Migraine Revolution yahoo forum is meant to be a strong alternative *in the spirit of this book* and with the declared objective to support migraine sufferers to act smart and decisively to end their migraine tyranny. Discussions about medications are permitted, if conducted with an understanding of their use as a temporary crutch or when things have gone wrong.

The forum is moderated, but participants are responsible to moderate themselves and one another. Therapists of all kinds and other experts are welcome until explicit and implicit self-promotion exceed the common purpose: to end the migraine tyranny.

Cast of Characters

> "God writes a lot of comedy... the trouble is, he's stuck with so many bad actors who don't know how to play funny."
> Garrison Keillor

I'd like to express my heartfelt gratitude to the characters who played important roles in my attempt to inform *and* entertain my readers. Revolutions are so much more fun when you don't have to fight them all by yourself.

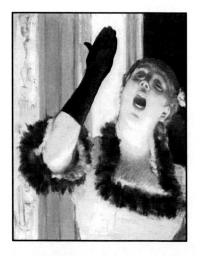

The following characters coincidentally appearing in this work are fictitious. Any resemblance to real persons, living or dead, is purely intentional. More important: No animals were harmed in the making of this book.

- **Tomasso di Andrea da Pontedera**: the famous Italian architect who charged a fortune for stating the obvious problem instead of coming up with a solution
- **Joe**: the patient with the imaginary trembling disorder
- **Dr. Henk van Haaren**: the Dutch eye-doctor who recognized that—although logically appealing—the avoidance of triggers for trembling attacks is not a solution, rather makes it worse
- **Bintje van Haaren**: Henk's wife who helped design a rehab program for trembling disorder, President of the made-up International Society for Foveal Alignment Training (ISFAT)
- **Clare**: the girl who didn't suffer but quit migraine after one attack by doing what needed to be done
- **Daisy**: the worrying and catastrophizing migraine-newbie who showed great promise to become a 'difficult' chronic sufferer
- **Bertrand**: the courageous school-teacher who lost his head for attempting to rouse a rebellion which was destined to fail
- **Fred**: the hard-hitting money-maker with high blood pressure who benefited from his doctor's constructive critical thinking
- **George**: the fine young man who managed to sort the animals after the earthquake thanks to a certain narrowness in thinking

Cast of Characters

- **Kevin**: the over-protected twin with migraine who was never officially diagnosed with triptan- or Botox®-deficiency
- **Larry**: the twin without migraine who received encouragement and support: "Give it a crack, Larry!"
- **Irene**: The temporarily injured world-class volleyball player who didn't succumb to "knee-wobble disease" but instead went through her rehabilitation program like a pro
- **Jenny**: the girl who put her valuable inheritance at risk by clinging to the hope for a magic mold-spray that makes her problems simply go away although a renovation was due
- **Grandma**: the sweet elderly lady who was moved to tears by Christmas carols and who shared your excitement about your insights into the reactions of challenged balls
- **God**: he was playing himself (one of the nicest blokes on the set, one hell of a guy; you should see his trailer!)

Let's not forget the supporting actors with the bit parts—Caroline, Mandy, Neil, Owen and Paula—as well as the technical staff, costume designers, make-up artists, drivers, first aid nurses and the catering service; thanks to all of you guys.

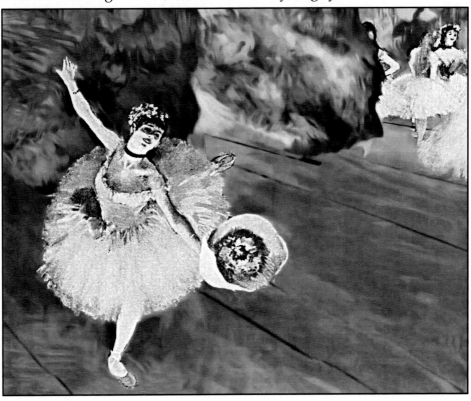

List of Paintings

Page no. *title of the painting* by name of the artist (year of birth/death)

2   *Liberty leading the People* by Eugene Delacroix (1798-1863)
4   *Biblis* by William-Adolphe Bouguereau (1825-1905)
9   *The difficult Lesson* by William-Adolphe Bouguereau (1825-1905)
10 *Young Girl reading* by Jean-Honoré Fragonard (1732-1806)
14 *Lady Jane Grey's Execution* by Paul Delaroche (1797-1856)
16 *The Seven-Headed Hydra Seen at Venezia in 1530* by Conrad Gesner (1516-1565)
28 *Sisyphus* by Tiziano Vecelli "Titian" (1488-1576)
36 *Anatomia del Corazon* by Enrique Simonet Lombardo (1864-1927)
74 *The Star (Dancer on Stage)* by Edgar Degas (1834-1917)
83 *Puberty* by Edvard Munch (1863-1940)
107 *Madonna and Child* by Pompeo Batoni (1708-1787)
118 *Joan of Arc with her Banner* by Harold H. Piffard (1867-1938)
120 Frontispiece from *The Face in the Pool* by J. Allen St. John, pub. 1905 © expired
121 *The Third of May 1808* by Francisco Goya (1746-1828)
122 *Prise de la Bastille* by Jean-Pierre Houël (1735-1813)
135 *Battle at Soufflot Barricades at Rue Soufflot* by Horace Vernet (1789-1863)
156 *The Anatomy Lesson of Dr Nicholas Tulp* by Rembrandt van Rijn (1606-1669)
171 *The Mirror* by Jules Marie Auguste Leroux (1871-1925)
203 *A Game of Chess* Jose Gallego y Arnosa (1857-1917)
214 Weapons of War by Alexander Pope (1849-1924)
215 In the old House by Childe Hassam (1859-1935)
221 *Vitruvian Man* by Leonardo da Vinci (1452-1519)
223 *The skating Minister* by Henry Raeburn (1756-1823)
230 Twins (Grace and Kate Hoare) by John Everett Millais (1829-1896)
231 *Buddhist Monk* Detail from Bezeklik Thousand Buddah Caves in China (9th Century)
232 *The Birth of Venus* by Alexandre Cabanel (1823-1889)
234 *Supper at Emmaus* by Michelangelo Merisi da Caravaggio (1571-1610)
235 *The Gardener* Giuseppe Arcimboldo (1527-1593)
243 *The Love Philtre* by John William Waterhouse (1849-1917)
254 *Still-Life of Fish and Cat* by Clara Peeters (1594-1657)
263 *Sleeping Venus* by Francois Boucher (1703-1770)
265 *Sleeping Venus* by Simon Vouet (1590-1649)
268 *The Awakening of Psyche* by Guillaume Seignac (1870-1924)
269 *The Tightropewalker* Jean-Louis Forain (1852-1931)

List of Paintings

280 *The Archer* by Charles Edward Hallé (1846-1914)
284 *Girl defending herself against Eros* by William-Adolphe Bouguereau (1825-1905)
288 *Pandora* by John William Waterhouse (1849-1917)
290 *The Soul of the Rose* by John William Waterhouse (1849-1917)
294 *American Gothic* by GrantDe Volson Wood (1891-1942)
296 *The Bookworm* by Carl Spitzweg (1808-1885)
304 *Girl with her Pet Bird* by William-Adolphe Bouguereau (1825-1905)
305 *Psyche and Cupid* by William-Adolphe Bouguereau (1825-1905)
308 *Susanna and the Elders* by Artemisia Gentileschi (1593-1656)
309 *The Scream* by Edvard Munch (1863-1940)
312 *Sleeping Girl (Girl with a Cat)* by Pierre-Auguste Renoir (1841-1919)
314 *Ophelia* by John William Waterhouse (1849-1917)
315 The Dreamer by Jean Baptists Greuze (1725-1805)
317 An Interior With a Young Lady at her Toilet Combing her Hair Before a Mirror by Johann Anton de Peters (1725-1795)
362 *Whistler's Mother doing Neurofeedback* based on the painting *Whistler's Mother* by James Abbott McNeill Whistler (1834-1903)
363 *Young Woman With A Lighted Candle At A Window* by Gerrit Dou (1613-1675)
369 *Thisbe* John William Waterhouse (1849-1917)
370 *Choir in the Skull* from *The Village Choir* by Thomas Webster (1800-1886)
375 *The Geographers* José Gallgos y Arnosa (1857-1917)
383 *The Young Cook* by Pierre Edouard Frère (1819–1886)
387 *La Vague* by Guillaume Seignac (1870-1924)
395 *Samson's Youth* by Léon Joseph Florentin Bonnat (1833-1922)
403 *Cupid and Psyche* by Guillaume Seignac (1870-1924)
407 *Whistler's Mother doing LENS* based on the painting *Whistler's Mother* by James Abbott McNeill Whistler (1834-1903)
413 *An elegant Billiards Player* by Charles Edouard Boutibonne (1816-1897)
425 *Joan of Arc at the Siege of Orléans* by Jules Eugène Lenepveu (1819-1898)
443 *Liberty leading the People* by Eugene Delacroix (1798-1863)
444 *La Revolution* by Valentine Cameron Prinsep (1838-1904)
448 *Singer with a Glove* by Edgar Degas (1834-1917)
449 *Dancer taking a Bow* by Edgar Degas (1834-1917)
457 *The Painter's Triumph* by William Sidney Mount (1807-1868)
462 *The Curtsey* by William-Adolphe Bouguereau (1825-1905)

All these paintings are in the public domain and still, I do apologize for taking the liberty of grayscaling, cropping, adapting or otherwise photoshopping them. Not in all cases did my effort lead to true improvements of the original artwork; I'm sorry.

Picture Credits

Foreword — Are you ready for the Migraine Revolution?

Bomb: adapted from a stockphoto (shutterstock 63039805).

Explosion: adapted from File:Operation Upshot-Knothole-Badger 001.jpg This work is in the public domain in the U.S. because it is prepared by an officer or employee of the U.S. Government as part of that person's official duties under the terms of Title 17, Chapter 1, Section 105 of the US Code

Introduction — The Tyranny: Suffering from Migraine

Agony: © Martin Brink

Chapter 1 — The Many Faces of Migraine

PFC: © Martin Brink

Chapter 2 — The Impact and Burden of Migraine

All 8 graphs created with MS Excel, based on data from the referenced study, ⊜

Chapter 3 — Medical Treatments for Migraine Symptoms

All 12 graphs showing statistics created with MS Excel, based on data from the referenced study, ⊜

Human Heart: adapted from a file by Eric Pierce (wapcaplet88), licensed under the Creative Commons Attribution-Share Alike 3.0 Unported license. If you alter, transform, or build upon this work, you may distribute the resulting work only under the same or similar license to this one.

Clostridium Botulinum: adapted from a picture from the Centers for Disease Control and Prevention, part of the U.S. Department of Health and Human Services. As a work of the U.S. federal government, the image is in the public domain.

Injecting Botox: © Martin Brink

Chapter 4 — Avoid Life and You'll be Right

The leaning tower of Pisa © Martin Brink

Chapter 5 — Psycho Terror in Migraine Land

Caveman and Sabretooth: created by the author based on a file by wallace63, licensed under the Creative Commons Attribution-Share Alike 3.0 Unported license. If you alter, transform, or build upon this work, you may distribute the resulting work only under the same or similar license to this one.

Chapter 6 — Dealing with Difficulties

Steeplechase © Martin Brink

Tenzing on Mt Everest adapted from a famous photo © Royal Geographical Society (U.K.); this is a prime example for 'fair use' for these reasons: 1. it is for an educational purpose, not a commercial reproduction (e.g. on T-Shirts) 2. the text refers to the event, not to the work itself 3. it is a famous documentary photo of a significant historic event of public interest (and not a private 'work of art'), the 'artistic' value is limited, Edmund Hillary (who took the photo) was a mountaineer, not a photographer and the photo is merely a visual recording of this historic event 4. the use in this book has no impact upon the market or value of the photo 5. it has been reproduced many times since 1953 (for example on currently more than 1.200 websites) 6. its use as part of an analogy for the difficulties migraine sufferers may encounter, has a 'transformative' character and 7. it is not an 'unfair' use. The Copyrightholder didn't reject these arguments (emails 10.09.2012)

Everest Camps created by the author using a public domain picture file from NASA

Chapter 7 — On Top of the Barricades

DNA and **Twin Concordance** © Martin Brink

Migraine Prevalence shown twice, from the referenced study, ⊜

Horrible Hair and **Shiny Hair** © Martin Brink

IBS Brain Activation adapted from the referenced study, ⊜

Picture Credits

Fear of God's Anger adapted from the referenced study, an open-access article distributed under the terms of the Creative Commons Public Domain declaration, ⚘

PFC created by the author based on a picture from BodyParts3D, © The Database Center for Life Science licensed under CC Attribution-Share Alike 2.1 Japan. If you alter, transform, or build upon this work, you may distribute the resulting work only under the same or similar license to this one.

Bach Scoresheet by Johann Sebastian Bach (1685-1750) Public Domain

Neurotransmission adapted from a picture by the US National Institutes of Health, National Institute on Aging. This work is in the public domain in the United States because it is a work prepared by an officer or employee of the United States Government as part of that person's official duties under the terms of Title 17, Chapter 1, Section 105 of the US Code.

Excitatory Ion-Channel and *Inhibitory Ion-Channel* © Martin Brink

AA Battery adapted from a photo taken by the author

Neuronal Potentials 4 graphs © Martin Brink

Firing Frequency © Martin Brink

EEG Cap adapted from a photo submitted by Brain Products GmbH

EEG 10/20 system © Martin Brink

EEG traces © Martin Brink

EEG FFT created from a screen capture of Neuroguide software with permission from Dr. Thatcher

EEG Frequency Bands © Martin Brink

Brainmaps created from a screen capture of Neuroguide software with permission from Dr. Thatcher

28Hz activity adapted from a data recording, ⚘

QEEG Overview created from a screen capture of Neuroguide software with permission from Dr. Thatcher

MEG machine adapted from an image provided the U.S. Department of Health and Human Services (http://infocenter.nimh.nih.gov/il/public_il/image_details.cfm?id=80), taken or made during the course of an employee's official duties. As a work of the U.S. federal government, the image is in the public domain.

MEG Imaging adapted from a data recording, ⚘

LoRETA Sample adapted from a data recording, ⚘

PET Imaging adapted from a data recording, ⚘

fMRI Imaging adapted from a data recording, ⚘

PFC Thermoimaging adapted with permission from a thermal image provided by Dr. Jeffrey Carmen

DTI Tractography adapted from an image created by Thomas Schulz, licensed under the Creative Commons Attribution-Share Alike 3.0 Unported license. If you alter, transform, or build upon this work, you may distribute the resulting work only under the same or similar license to this one.

Chapter 8 — Know Your Tyrant

Brainstem created by the author from an MRI data recording, ⚘

Cortex created by the author from an MRI data recording, ⚘

Mexcian Wave © Martin Brink

Cortical Spreading Depression (CSD) created by the author from an MRI data recording, ⚘

Brain Scan of the Placebo Effect adapted from the referenced study, depiction of data, ⚘

Evolution created by the author using a picture from TeeKay (Tkgd2007), licensed under the Creative Commons Attribution-Share Alike 3.0 Unported license. If you alter, transform, or build upon this work, you may distribute the resulting work only under the same or similar license to this one.

Triune Brain © Martin Brink *Triunity I* © Martin Brink *Triunity II* © Martin Brink

Chapter 9 — Thinking about Strategy

Volleyball © Martin Brink

Rehab Exercises © Martin Brink

Complexity and Difficulty © Martin Brink

| Chapter 11 | Let's get Physical |

Ergometer © Martin Brink

| Chapter 12 | Passing Gas |

Thoracic Breathing and **Abdominal Breathing** © Martin Brink

| Chapter 15 | Doping for Migraine |

Magnesium Book fair use
HTMA Report display of data, **Organix Report** display of data,
Copper Boy's HTMA and **Copper Boy's Graph of change** display of data,
TIME cover "Early Puberty" fair use because 1. it is for an educational purpose 2. the text refers to the event of TIME Magazin's article about Xenoestrogens 3. it is evidence for the statements of the paragraph 4. the use in this book has no impact upon the market or value of the photo 5. it is merely a transformed grayscale depiction of a color magazin title in the character of a 'thumbnail' picture of a it is not an 'unfair' use
migraine during pregnancy created with MS Excel, based on data from the referenced study,
progesterone during pregnancy created with MS Excel, based on data from the referenced study,
Triunity III © Martin Brink

| Chapter 17 | Balancing Your Urges |

Hormone Solution Book and **Hormone Handbook** fair use

| Chapter 18 | Points of Pain |

Trigger Points and Headaches, adapted from a picture submitted by MindMedia, NL
Stress and EMG Activity created with MSExcel, based on data from the referenced study,
Trigger Points and Depression created with MS Excel, based on data from the referenced study,
Photonic Stimulator adapted from a photo submitted by Ochs Labs Inc.
Medi-Taping on the neck © Martin Brink

| Chapter 19 | Pricks with Benefits |

Migraine Days during Acupuncture created with MS Excel, data from the referenced study
Acupuncture versus Topiramate created with MS Excel, based on data from the referenced study
Acupucture and Migraine Pain created with MS Excel, based on data from the referenced study
Acupuncture versus Sumatriptan created with MS Excel, based on data from the referenced study

| Chapter 20 | Pandora's Treasure Chest |

Acupressure for Nausea adapted from www.homebackpainacupressure.com/acupressure-for-sea-sickness.html with permission: Discover safe and effective acupressure techniques that help you to get drug-free back pain relief at http://www.HomeBackPainAcupressure.com. Virpi Tervonen reveals the most effective acupressure points that relieve lower back and hip pain, sciatica, and stiff shoulders and neck in her new acupressure guide. These safe and simple techniques are demonstrated step-by-step in numerous descriptive photos and video clips. Visit www.HomeBackPainAcupressure.com for more information.
Lidocaine Nasal Spray created with MS Excel, based on data from the referenced study
Nasal Spray © Martin Brink
Massage versus Drug created with MS Excel, based on data from the referenced study
Massage for Attack created with MS Excel, based on data from the referenced study

| Section Two | Weapons for the Mind |

Taxi Drivers adapted from a data-chart from the referenced study
Medial Prefrontal Cortex adapted from a data-chart from the referenced study
fMRI Activation 3D adapted from a figure showing recorded data from the referenced study
Severity of Depression created with MS Excel, based on data from the referenced study

| Chapter 23 | Healing Shocks |

Brain in Trance © Martin Brink
Alpha-Theta Session Graph © submitted by Dr. Siegfried Othmer

Picture Credits

Chapter 24 Feeling Heavy and Warm
Meditation © Martin Brink

Chapter 25 When the Mind Sees what the Body Does
Sonography of Abdominal Muscles © Martin Brink
Knee EMG © Martin Brink ©
EMG Vaginal Sensor submitted by MindMedia, NL
Tongue Display Unit fair use, adapted from the referenced study
Autonomic Nervous System created by the author using parts of a file from Ruth Lawson (sunshineconnelly), licensed under the Creative Commons Attribution 3.0 Unported license. If you alter, transform, or build upon this work, you may distribute the resulting work only under the same or similar license to this one.
When Fear is near figure from the referenced article "The threatened brain" by Stephen Maren, licensed from "Science" via Rightslink, License Date: Sep 10, 2012, License Number: 29*********90. The photo of the "distant" wolf is from Daniel Mott, licensed under the Creative Commons Attribution-Share Alike 2.0 Generic license. If you alter, transform, or build upon this work, you may distribute the resulting work only under the same or similar license to this one. The photo of the "close" wolf is in the public domain (www.wolf-pictures.net)
Tschudi-Madsen-Graph adapted from referenced study, data 🕮
Checking the ANS adapted from Gray's Anatomy (1918), © expired = Public Domain
Psychophysiology submitted by ©-holder MindMedia, NL
Nexus-10 submitted by ©-holder MindMedia, NL
Breathing Belts © Martin Brink ***Low Back EMG*** © Martin Brink ***Neck EMG*** © Martin Brink
Masseter EMG and ***EOG*** submitted by ©-holder MindMedia, NL
Masseter EMG submitted by ©-holder MindMedia, NL
Screenshot RSA by the author with permission from MindMedia, NL
Screenshot HRV and Breathing by the author with permission from MindMedia, NL
Interbeat Interval by the author with permission from MindMedia, NL
HRV Power Spectrum by the author with permission from MindMedia, NL
HRV Display GOOD by the author with permission from MindMedia, NL
BVP Head Sensor and ***Girl with BVP Sensor*** submitted by ©-holder MindMedia, NL
Screenshot Vasoconstriction Training by the author with permission from MindMedia, NL
BVP Finger Sensor (2 photos) submitted by ©-holder MindMedia, NL
Screenshot Vasoconstriction Training by the author with permission from MindMedia, NL
Digital Biofeedback Thermometer © Martin Brink
Finger Temp Sensor submitted by ©-holder MindMedia, NL
2 Screenshots Flower Display by the author with permission from MindMedia, NL
GSR/EDA Sensor submitted by ©-holder MindMedia, NL
2 Screenshots Biofeedback Displays by the author with permission from MindMedia, NL
Microscope adapted from a photo by Dr. Timo Mappes (www.musoptin.com), released into Public Domain (see http://commons.wikimedia.org/wiki/File:Microscope_Zeiss_1879.jpg)

Section Three Weapons for the Brain
Neuron © Martin Brink
Almost like Putty adapted from Nicholas Henri Jacob (1782-1871), Public Domain
Phrenology adapted from Friedrich Eduard Bilz (1842–1922), Public Domain
Brain Hieroglyph Public Domain
Walker Study Results created with MS Excel, based on data from the referenced study, 🕮
Neurons created by the author based on a Public Domain Image
Action Potentials created by the author based on a Public Domain Image

Pyramidal Neurons adapted from Brainmaps.org, licensed under the Creative Commons Attribution 3.0 License. If you alter, transform, or build upon this work, you may distribute the resulting work only under the same or similar license to this one.
Keyboard and ***Frequency Bands=Choir Voices*** by the author
EEG-Cap submitted by Brain Products GmbH
BrainMaps page 360 by the author
Neurofeedback Session © Martin Brink
2 ***Screenshots Biofeedback Displays*** by the author
Whistler's Mother doing Neurofeedback © Martin Brink

Chapter 26   Show Me Some Warmth!
Thermal Selfportrait Jeff Carmen submitted by Dr. Jeff Carmen
Thermal Selfportrait Martin Brink © Martin Brink, ***Thermal Image My Wife*** © Martin Brink
all other **15 thermal images** submitted by Dr. Jeffrey Carmen
Photo ***IR Sensor*** and Photo ***IR Neurofeedback*** Session © Martin Brink

Chapter 27   Listening Through the Wall
Skull adapted from Leonardo da Vinci (1452-1519), Public Domain
Choir in the Skull by the author based on a painting by Thomas Webster (1800-1886), Public Domain
Pengalvanometer by Renato Sabbatini, licensed under This file is licensed under the Creative Commons Attribution 3.0 Unported license. If you alter, transform, or build upon this work, you may distribute the resulting work only under the same or similar license to this one.
8 photos of ***EEG amplifiers*** submitted by the manufacturer (MindMedia, Brain Products) or fair use
Photo ***Single Electrode*** © Martin Brink, Graph ***10/20 Electrodes*** © Martin Brink
4 photos ***EEG-cap / actiElectrode / actiCAP / Injecting Gel*** submitted by Brain Products GmbH
Screenshot ***EEG traces*** by the author, Foto ***Cable Management*** © Martin Brink

Chapter 28   Wiping Migraine off the Map
Foto ***actiCAP and Amplifier*** submitted by Brain Products GmbH
all ***Brainmaps of W, 25*** submitted by Dr. Lucas Korbeda, Tallahassee
Screenshots TBI-Index and Brain Performance Index by the author with permission Dr. R. Thatcher
all graphs of ***Woman in her 30's*** submitted by Dr. Richard Soutar

Chapter 29   Recipes for the Brain
Photo ***Astronaut John Glenn*** by NASA, Public Domain
Toxic Symptoms of Rocket Fuel created with MS Excel, based on data from the referenced study, ☻
3 graphs ***Electrode Placements*** by the author based on graphs submitted by Dr. Siegfried Othmer

Chapter 30   On the Crest of Slow Waves
all graphs submitted by Dr. Siegfried Othmer, adapted by the author

Chapter 31   Overpowering the Migraine Beast
Z-Scores © Martin Brink and ***Brightness feedback*** © Martin Brink
Instantaneous, Z-scored Brainmaps adapted screenshot of personal data
Fun with actiCAP submitted by Brainproducts GmbH, adapted by the author
LoRETA posterior cingulate submitted by Dr. Richard Soutar, adapted by the author
LoRETA in migraine brains adapted from the referenced study
LoRETA of a migraine attack adapted from the references poster presentation
fMRI neurofeedback adapted from the referenced study
4 screenshots of ***Brianmaster Software*** by the author with permission of Brainmaster Technologies
2 screenshots of ***Neuroguide Software*** with permission from Dr. Rober Thatcher
DVD Size Feedback by the author
1-channel versus 19-channels created with MS Excel from data by Dr. Lucas Korbeda
2 QEEG reports ***58 year-old female*** submitted by Dr. Lucas Korbeda

Picture Credits

Chapter 32	The Magic of a Whisper

4 LENS brainmaps **44 year-old woman** submitted by Dr. Gil Winkelman, adapted by the author
LENS feedback frequency © Martin Brink
Whistler's Mother doing LENS © Martin Brink, based on a famous painting, Public Domain
2 QEEG reports **David** submitted by Dr. Nicholas Dogris, adapted by the author
6 outcome graphs **Stone Mountain Center** from the referenced study, ⚖
Brooke Army Medical Center As a work of the U.S. federal government, the image is in the public domain
Graph **Charlotte, Tina & Robert** created with MS Excel based on Ann Marie Brown's data, ⚖

Chapter 33	The Side Effects of Change

Normal Distribution by the author
Photo **Billiards** by Michael Maggs, licensed under the Creative Commons Attribution 3.0 license. If you alter, transform, or build upon this work, you may distribute the resulting work only under the same or similar license to this one.
Karaoke Machine © Martin Brink
Photo **Fennec Fox** by Yvonne N. from Willowick USA, licensed under the Creative Commons Attribution 2.0 Generic license.

⚖ = Copyright does not apply to facts, data, statistics or recordings of natural phenomena.

Thanks a lot to the Wikimedia Foundation / Wikimedia Commons (http://commons.wikimedia.org) and its contributors for providing freely reusable media files such as some of the images used in this book.

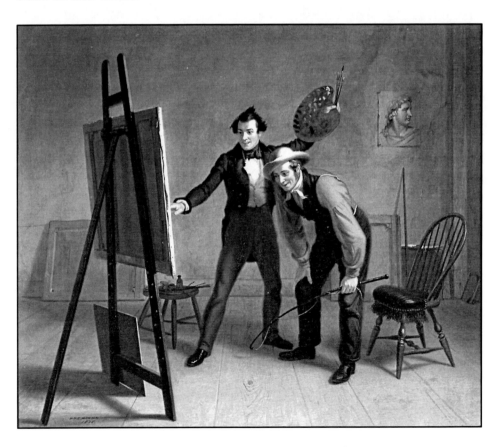

Index

A

Abuse (see Childhood maltreatment)
Acceptance and Commitment Therapy (ACT) 304, 428
Acetaminophen 47, 290
actiCAP 373-374
Action potential 162-163, 359
Acupressure 289
Acupuncture 285-287
ADD/ADHD 25, 190, 347
Agony 13, 96-97, 192, 358
Alcohol 68, 76, 196
Alexithymia 87, 188, 232, 321, 329, 421-422
Alice-in-Wonderland syndrome 18
Allodynia 19, 190, 374
Amygdala 95, 185-187, 190, 309, 322-323
Anxiety 22, 84, 86-87, 90, 111, 115-116, 195, 210, 225, 232, 294, 299, 310, 333, 335, 350, 368
Applied Neuroscience 110, 210, 321, 347, 349, 357
Applied Psychophysiology 317, 327, 342
Aromatherapy 289-290
Aspirin 47, 128, 226
Asthma 25, 27, 137, 232, 236, 333
Attachment Style 106-108
Aura 18, 23-24, 41, 49, 54-57, 68, 151, 172-173, 179-182, 258, 295, 389, 394, 411-412
Autogenic Training 232, 276, 282, 315-316, 335, 427
autonomic nervous system (ANS) 190, 282, 315, 322-327, 331-334, 341

B

Barbiturates 46
Beer 76
Beliefs, unhelpful 90, 97, 100, 236, 429, 441
Bertrand 121-122, 218
Beta-blockers 49, 228
bilateral headache 19, 339

Biofeedback 317-344, 442
   EMG 205, 267, 319-321, 330, 431
   GSR (galvanic skin response) 339-340
   HRV (heart rate variability) 331-335
   thermal ("handwarming") 210, 342-343, 392, 338-339
   vasomotor 337-339, 342, 428
Blood vessels 24, 150-153, 178, 337-339, 425
Botox® 59-63, 89-90, 92, 197, 276, 429
Brain 18, 21-25, 39, 46-47, 57-58, 64, 80-81, 85-90, 93-95, 100-102, 106-107, 109-110, 124, 152, 155-170, 171-201, 204, 221-222, 240-241, 244-246, 254-257, 265, 267, 269-271, 273, 278-279, 281-282, 293, 298, 310-312, 320-321, 323, 340, 345-424, 432-433
Brain damage 24, 176, 279, 355
Brain injury 40, 164, 181, 189, 208, 350, 364, 366, 377-378, 404, 412, 415, 426
Brain Performance Index 378
Brain scan 51, 80, 157, 163-169, 197, 261, 298, 345-347, 375
Brainstem 24, 114, 124, 168, 174-179, 186-195, 198, 229, 245, 267, 273-274, 281, 323, 338-339, 398, 425
Breast cancer 274, 276
Breathing 137, 170, 186-187, 194, 227-229, 242, 249, 294, 316, 327-328, 330-331, 338, 427, 431
Butterbur 251-252, 427

C

Caffeine 40, 147, 242, 412
Carbon dioxide (CO_2) 137-138, 170, 228-229, 242, 338-339, 354
Case examples 262, 367, 376, 380, 385-386, 388-389, 391, 393, 402-405, 411-412
Catastrophizing 91, 112, 115, 133
Celiac disease 25, 78-79, 239-241

Index

Childhood maltreatment 105-106, 111, 158, 200-201, 240, 260, 303, 307, 309, 311, 329, 336, 439
Chirotherapy 291, 411, 428
chronic fatigue 25, 84, 123, 200, 258, 263, 324-325, 350
chronic migraine 21, 29, 31, 45, 52, 61-63, 98, 103, 116, 133, 140-141, 167, 187, 198, 208, 210, 263-264, 278, 286, 344, 352-353, 358, 385, 402, 429
chronic pain 46, 108, 115, 178, 206, 232, 258, 415, 430
Chronification 40, 46-47, 52, 63, 81, 85, 99, 105, 108, 110-111, 117, 128, 196, 210, 220, 241, 344, 358, 379, 447
Chocolate 75, 235-236, 403
Clare 83, 111-113, 116-117, 260
Cluster headache 41, 56, 282
Codeine 46
Coenzyme Q10 250, 259, 427
Coffee 37, 196, 242, 403, 427
Cognitive Behavioral Therapy (CBT) 191, 299-303, 334, 428
cognitive distortions 90-93, 97, 101, 127, 141-142, 158, 188, 207-208, 358, 378, 390, 392, 432, 439
cognitive symptoms 17, 25, 40, 190, 199, 225, 254, 350, 414
Comorbidity 21-27, 39, 42, 50, 52, 70, 78, 84, 103, 131, 152, 158, 171, 190-191, 195, 208, 211, 254, 278, 309, 334, 336, 342, 403, 411, 419, 427
Concussion 164, 189, 201, 350, 377-379
Confirmation bias 100-103, 114, 356, 390
Contingent Negative Variation (CNV) 198-199, 201
Coping-style 115, 140, 240, 306, 356, 358, 435
Copper 262, 291, 436
Cortical Spreading Depression (CSD) 180-181, 183, 191
cumulative disadvantage 84, 112-113, 208, 217, 432

D

Daisy 112-115, 117, 208, 260
Depression 17-19, 22-23, 84, 86-87, 90, 108, 116, 133, 157, 172, 201, 225, 263, 282, 294, 298, 333, 350, 368, 419
Descartes, René 156, 326
Diabetes 24, 271, 277, 343
Diarrhea 17-19, 175, 177, 190
Disability 30, 106, 199, 250
Dopamine 183, 354

E

early life stress 189, 199, 201, 240, 309, 415
EEG (Electroencephalography) 163-165, 172, 192-193, 312, 359, 370, 435
   amplifier 164, 370-372, 407
   cap 372-373
   electrode 353, 372-373, 385, 387, 406
   quantitative (QEEG) 156, 165-167, 178, 192, 371-374
   suppression 404-406
EMDR 310-311, 428
Endocrinologist 149, 275
Energy Psychology 311
Epilepsy 17, 21, 115, 134, 164, 172-174, 196, 228, 238, 242, 272, 340, 347, 352, 356, 384, 413-414
Erica 123-128, 145, 259-260, 418, 446
Estrogen 269-279, 353, 427
   dominance 274, 276-277, 279, 353-354
   conjugated equine (CEE) 275-276
Exercise (sport) 223-226, 242
explanatory style 113, 300-301

F

Family 32-35, 209, 217, 355, 380, 389, 411
Fasting 73, 76
fearful-avoidant 114, 211
Feverfew 252-253
Fibromyalgia 25, 84, 158-159, 190, 200, 294, 333-334, 351, 393, 415-419, 423, 427
Food intolerance 78, 236-238, 354
Fred 129, 147-149
freeze-response 175, 323-324, 329
functional disorders 419, 440

459

G

GABA 161
gender (migraine and ...) 29
genetic ("migraine is ...") 83, 98, 135-139, 171, 197, 270, 309, 336
George 153-154
Ginger 253, 290
Glutamate 60, 161, 180
Gluten 78-79, 239-241, 427
Goals 131-132, 187, 203, 430
God 88, 95, 128-129, 157, 442

H

Habituation 190-194, 199, 201, 423
Hair mineral analysis (HMA) 261-262, 434
Heart attack 23, 27, 223
Helplessness 95-97, 99, 133, 153, 208, 218, 329, 343, 358, 395
Henk van Haaren 67-69, 81
Herbs 123, 243, 252, 259-260
Homocysteine 258, 427
Hopelessness 97-99, 102-103, 208, 210-211, 299, 358, 395, 411, 435
Hormones 123-127, 269-279, 427
Hunger 73, 92, 189-190, 323, 421
Hunter-gatherer 94, 324, 327, 329
Hyperarousal 267
Hypervigilance 93, 106, 111, 113, 187

I

Identity 130, 220, 306, 355
interictal phase 20, 245
Irene 204-206, 209, 292, 435, 449
Iron 24, 176, 355, 427
irritable bowel syndrome (IBS) 84, 116, 157-159, 200, 229, 238-241, 324-325, 334, 419, 440

J

Jargon 108, 139
Jenny 215-216
joining the migraine revolution 443-447

K

Kevin 197, 201
Kindling 195-196
Knee-wobble disease 204

L

Larry 197, 201
Lidocaine 63, 282, 292
LoRETA (low resolution electromagnetic tomography) 166-167, 178, 192, 197, 372-374, 380,

M

Magnesium 243-248, 253, 259-260, 291, 354, 427
maladaptive schema 125, 306-307, 390, 418,
Massage 290, 293, 295, 428
Medication
    abortive 44-47, 229, 246, 253
    analgesic 47-48, 64, 106, 145, 197, 279
    anti-seizure medication 49, 134, 172, 192, 286, 413-415
    OTC 40-41, 45, 412
    preventive 49, 144-145, 287
    self- 39-41
Medication overuse 45, 52, 63, 103
    headache (MOH) 48, 64, 192, 210
Meditaping 283
Melatonin 265-266, 278, 427
metabolic syndrome 235, 241
Migraine 1-447
    menstrual 71, 271-274, 278-279, 436
Mission 131-133, 218-220, 444
Money 33, 38, 58-59, 84, 103, 106, 123, 126, 140, 209, 217-219, 292, 303, 317, 348, 430-432, 436

N

Nausea 19-20, 26, 41, 49, 89, 124, 151-152, 173, 175-177, 179, 222, 250, 257, 289-290, 418
Neck pain 17, 26-27, 40, 63, 175, 190, 222, 281, 293, 295, 324, 330, 333-334
Negativity bias 94-95, 101, 302, 304
Neglect (see Childhood maltreatment)
Neurofeedback 267, 340, 347-362
    Alpha/Theta 312-313, 428
    fMRI 298, 368, 399
    full cap 397, 402
    infralow frequency 267, 387-394

Index

infrared 267, 352-353, 355, 362-368
LoRETA 267, 368, 397-401, 428
LoRETA Z-score 400-402
low energy (LENS) 267, 403-412, 428, 430
surface Z-score 267, 396-397
symptom-based 267, 383-386
QEEG-guided 267, 375-382, 428
Z-score 267, 396-397, 400-402
Neurologist 48, 50-52, 54, 79, 84, 104, 147, 149, 158, 228, 258, 261, 265, 354-355, 375, 377, 384, 391, 393, 400, 402, 411, 435, 441
Neuron 160-163, 166, 168-170, 172, 174, 180-181, 229, 254, 286, 345-346, 359, 361, 363, 366, 407-408, 413, 425
neuronal potentials 162, 192, 388
Neuroplasticity 320-321, 345-346, 361
Neuroscience 109-110, 157-158, 210, 345-346, 359, 395
Neurotherapy 110, 157-158, 173, 303, 362, 402-403, 425-426, 428, 432-435
Neuroticism 87, 93, 111, 155, 184-185, 188, 190, 201, 225, 299, 329
Neurotransmitter 59-60, 160-163, 169-170, 183, 261, 354, 426
NSAIDs 47

O

Obstacles 90, 128-129, 135, 197, 208
Omega-3 fatty acids 254-257, 259, 331, 354
operant conditioning 46, 74, 99, 361
Opioids 46, 52, 128, 313, 418
Osmophobia 17, 19, 179
Overbreathing 170, 194, 229, 242, 249, 294, 325, 354, 427
Oxytocin 293-295, 378, 428

P

PAG (periaqueductal gray) 175-177, 183, 188, 190-191, 274
Pain killers (see medication, analgesic)
parasympathetic ANS 322, 324, 339
Partner 31-35, 145, 209, 306
PEDMIN strategy 102-103, 348
Personality 85, 87, 104, 106, 109-111, 113, 129-130, 137, 155-156, 239, 306, 313, 329, 381

PFO (patent foramen ovale) 53-59, 222, 426
Phonophobia 17, 19, 179
Photonic stimulation 205, 283
Photophobia 17, 19, 179
Physical therapy 205, 295
Placebo effect 63, 89, 171, 181-183, 191, 224, 249, 257, 356, 426
Pope, the 156, 195, 326
Postdrome 19
Pre-eclampsia 27
progressive muscle relaxation (PMR) 231-233, 316, 338
prefrontal cortex (PFC) 22-23, 88, 101, 106, 108-109, 115, 157-158, 168, 183-190, 193, 199, 204, 211, 220, 225, 240, 249, 254-255, 264-265, 267, 273-274, 298, 303, 309, 323, 348, 355, 365-367, 413, 419
Pregnancy 26-27, 56-57, 68, 70, 114, 272, 414
Priorities 148, 219, 430
Prodrome 17, 41, 56, 173
Progesterone 272-274, 276-278, 427
Progestins 275-276
psychophysiological stress-profile (PSP) 327-328
PTSD 26, 93, 106, 115, 172, 190, 200, 208, 309, 312, 333-334, 344, 349, 360, 394, 426

Q

QEEG 156, 165-167, 178, 188, 192, 197, 353, 358, 360, 371, 372-374, 375-378, 381-382, 396-397, 402, 404, 409, 435-435
Quality of life 30-31, 87, 103, 316
Quantum "bio feedback" 290

R

Reactivity 47, 78, 87, 108-109, 124, 187, 190, 208, 211, 233, 235, 260, 414, 420
Rehabilitation 206-206, 209-211, 217, 223, 324, 381, 419, 428, 435
Relaxation exercises 206-207, 231, 233, 235, 338, 342
Repetition compulsion 125
Resilience 107, 109, 154, 191, 199-200, 210, 260, 309, 343-344, 408, 415-416, 419, 423

Resources 84, 95, 209, 217-219, 389, 429, 432, 440-441, 444, 447
Riboflavin (Vitamin B2) 249, 427
Risks and side effects 43, 224, 259, 289, 356, 413-414

S

Schema therapy 127, 305-307, 428
Seizure activity 172, 177, 265, 271-272, 321, 392
Self-diagnosis 41
Sensitization 78-79, 99, 124, 190, 193-196, 198, 421
Silkenshine shampoo 150-152, 171
Sleep problems 20, 26, 93, 186, 189-190, 263-267, 290, 294, 332, 336, 351, 386, 405-406, 412
social support 84, 133, 209, 217-219, 326
social withdrawal 19
stress response 86, 185, 191, 316, 321-329, 336
Stroke 18, 24, 27, 54-55, 58, 137, 181, 190, 211, 223-224, 275-276, 320-321, 345, 351-352, 397
Suicide 22-23, 294, 299, 394, 414
Supplements 123-124, 145, 243, 247-248, 251, 257, 259-260, 262
Surgery 58, 89-90, 135, 191, 233, 275, 326, 401, 429
Swelling and inflammation 16, 21, 150, 176-178, 413, 419
sympathetic ANS 322, 327, 331, 338-339

T

Tension-type headache 23, 41, 73, 266
Testosterone 277-279, 427
Thermoimaging 168, 353, 363
tinted glasses 266, 295
Tomasso di Andrea da Pontadera 65-66, 81
Toxicity 262, 291, 354, 427
Trauma therapy 309, 312
Trembling disorder 66-68, 81
Trigger factors 65-82
Trigger points 62-63, 281-283
Triptans 33, 41, 44-45, 47-49, 51-52, 62, 192, 197-198, 287, 403, 411, 413
Twins 136, 138, 197-198, 201, 309
Tyramine 75-76

U

unhelpful beliefs 90, 97, 100, 236, 299, 258, 429, 441

V

Values 132, 148, 221, 304, 430
Victim 85, 96-97, 110, 213, 124-128, 130, 150, 208, 211, 218, 260, 355, 418, 435, 437, 439, 447
Vitamin D 258-259
Vomiting 19, 26, 89, 151-152, 173-176, 186, 228, 257, 289-290

W

Weather-sensitivity 72, 421
Work 34-35
Worrying 17, 112-113, 115, 215

X

Xenoestrogens 270-271

Y

Yubyub therapy 441-442

Z

Zinc 262, 291, 427, 436

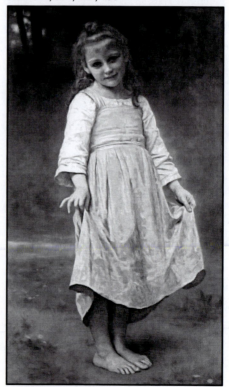

Printed by BoD in Norderstedt, Germany